Emerging and Re-emerging Infections in Travellers

Hakan Leblebicioglu • Nick Beeching
Eskild Petersen

Editors

Emerging and Re-emerging Infections in Travellers

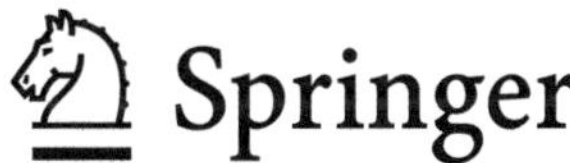
Springer

Editors
Hakan Leblebicioglu
Infectious Diseases Clinic
VM Medical Park Samsun Hospital
Samsun, Türkiye

Nick Beeching
Clinical Sciences
Liverpool School of Tropical Medicine
Liverpool, Merseyside, UK

Eskild Petersen
Faculty of Health Sciences
Aarhus University
Aarhus, Denmark

ISBN 978-3-031-49477-2   ISBN 978-3-031-49475-8   (eBook)
https://doi.org/10.1007/978-3-031-49475-8

This Springer imprint is published by the registered company Springer Nature Switzerland AG
The registered company address is: Gewerbestrasse 11, 6330 Cham, Switzerland

If disposing of this product, please recycle the paper.

Preface

Welcome to the world of emerging infections among travellers. As editors, we present a comprehensive collection of chapters, written by authors from different corners of the globe, each offering their unique insights and experiences.

In an increasingly interconnected world, the movement of people across continents has become an integral part of our lives. Travel has the potential for encountering unfamiliar pathogens and the risk of new infections not present in our home countries.

The chapters in this book cover a vast spectrum of infectious diseases, ranging from well-known infections such as dengue, influenza, and malaria, to emerging threats like Middle East Respiratory Syndrome Coronavirus (MERS-CoV) and Alkhurma Haemorrhagic Fever. Each chapter covers current knowledge, clinical manifestations, diagnostic approaches, treatment options, and prevention strategies.

The book explores the intersection between travel and infectious diseases in unique contexts such as mass gatherings, health tourism, and humanitarian aid work. It also examines the challenges posed by the emergence and spread of resistant microorganisms, as well as the crucial aspects of preparedness and response in the face of emerging infectious diseases.

As editors, we have had the privilege of collaborating with esteemed authors from diverse backgrounds, whose expertise spans continents. By bringing together this wealth of knowledge, we aim to provide a comprehensive resource for healthcare professionals, researchers, and policymakers alike.

We extend our heartfelt gratitude to all the authors who have shared their expertise and experiences, enriching this book with their invaluable insights. We would also like to express our appreciation to the publishers, who have worked tirelessly to transform this vision into a reality.

Finally, we extend our deepest gratitude to you, the readers. It is our sincere hope that *Emerging and Re-emerging Infections in Travellers* will serve as a source of inspiration, knowledge, and guidance, empowering you to navigate the uncharted territory of emerging infections and contribute to global efforts in safeguarding the health of travellers worldwide.

Samsun, Turkey	Hakan Leblebicioglu
Liverpool, UK	Nick Beeching
Aarhus, Denmark	Eskild Petersen

Contents

1 **Approach to Fever in the Returning Traveller** 1
Sofia R. Valdoleiros and Eskild Petersen

2 **Preparedness and Response for Emerging Infectious Diseases** 19
Eileen C. Farnon, Chantal B. E. M. Reusken, Bethan McDonald,
Anna Papa, and Louise Sigfrid

3 **Mass Gathering and Infectious Diseases** 41
Jaffar A. Al-Tawfiq and Ziad A. Memish

4 **Advice for Humanitarian Aid Workers** 59
Nicola Petrosillo

5 **Health Tourism and Infectious Diseases** 69
Diego Viasus and Jordi Carratalà

6 **Emergence and Spread of Resistant Microorganisms,
Related to Travel** 79
Ingeborg Fiane, Ernst Kristian Rødland, and Truls M. Leegaard

7 **Filovirus Infections in Travellers** 103
Tom E. Fletcher

8 **Crimean-Congo Haemorrhagic Fever in Travellers** 111
Resat Ozaras and Hakan Leblebicioglu

9 **Severe Fever with Thrombocytopenia Syndrome in Travellers** 125
Kato Yasuyuki

10 **Alkhurma Haemorrhagic Fever in Travellers** 131
Jaffar A. Al-Tawfiq and Ziad A. Memish

11 **Rift Valley Fever in Travellers** 143
Lucille Blumberg, Brett N. Archer, Peninah Munyua, Osama Ahmed
Hassan, David B. Wallace, and Janusz Paweska

12 **Yellow Fever in Travellers** 159
Terezinha M. P. P. Castiñeiras and Luciana G. P. Brandão

13 Viral Hepatitis in Travellers 181
J. E. Arends, Maria C. Leoni, and Andrew Ustianowski

14 Chikungunya Virus Infection in Travellers 193
Alfonso J. Rodriguez-Morales, Natalia Millan-Benavides, and
Jaime A. Cardona-Ospina

15 Dengue in Travellers 211
Huynh Trung Trieu, Angela McBride, and Sophie Yacoub

16 Zika Virus Infection in Travellers 225
Chantal B. E. M. Reusken, Barry Rockx, and Isabella Eckerle

17 West Nile Virus Infection in Travellers 259
Francesco Castelli, Corneliu Petru Popescu, and
Lina Rachele Tomasoni

18 Meningococcal Diseases in Travellers 281
Hasip Kahraman, Hüseyin Aytaç Erdem, and Oğuz Reşat Sipahi

19 Influenza in Travellers 301
Richard Pebody, Gavin Dabrera, and Joanna Ellis

**20 Middle East Respiratory Syndrome Coronavirus (MERS-CoV)
in Travellers** 311
Jaffar A. Al-Tawfiq and Ziad A. Memish

21 Multi-drug Resistant Tuberculosis in Travellers 331
Geraint Rhys Davies

22 Malaria in Travellers 343
Eskild Petersen and Martin P. Grobusch

Approach to Fever in the Returning Traveller

1

Sofia R. Valdoleiros and Eskild Petersen

Abstract

Fever is common in the ill returned traveller, with high hospitalization rates. A risk-based clinical approach to fever in the returning traveller is recommended, with initial priority given to recognizing and treating life-threatening causes of fever and identifying any infections with a high risk of transmission. Subsequently, the risk assessment should be established based on the geographic distribution of infections, risk factors for acquisition, incubation periods, and clinical findings.

Globalization and the marked increase in international travel in the last decades have increased the potential for the dissemination of infectious agents and vectors [1]. The number of travellers at a higher risk of developing infections is also growing, accompanying the rise in the immunosuppressed population (HIV infection, transplant recipients, autoimmune diseases, and other inflammatory diseases treated with immunomodulators). The likelihood of multidrug resistance is also rising and the possibility that an emerging pathogen can cause fever in the returning traveller is an additional challenge [2].

S. R. Valdoleiros
Centro Hospitalar Universitário de São João, Porto, Portugal

Faculty of Medicine, University of Porto, Porto, Portugal

ESCMID Emerging Infections Task Force, Basel, Switzerland
e-mail: sofia.valdoleiros@chsj.min-saude.pt

E. Petersen (✉)
ESCMID Emerging Infections Task Force, Basel, Switzerland

Faculty of Health Science, Institute for Clinical Medicine, University of Aarhus, Aarhus, Denmark

© The Author(s), under exclusive license to Springer Nature Switzerland AG 2024
H. Leblebicioglu et al. (eds.), *Emerging and Re-emerging Infections in Travellers*, https://doi.org/10.1007/978-3-031-49475-8_1

Fever occurs in 2–3% of European or American travellers returning to their home countries [3] and may be the only symptom of a severe or life-threatening illness [4]. In the ill returned traveller, fever is common and frequently leads to hospitalization [1, 5]. Although mortality is low (1 per 100,000) in the small proportion of patients who develop a travel-associated illness and seek medical care, the associated morbidity is significant, with high hospitalization rates [6].

Travel, especially to low-income regions, is associated with an increased risk of infections not typically seen in high-income countries, such as malaria, enteric fever, dengue, chikungunya, Zika, and schistosomiasis. As this will change the clinical approach, all febrile patients should be asked about travelling [7].

The possible causes of fever in the returning traveller are plentiful. A specific diagnosis is often difficult to establish because diagnostic tests for many diseases either perform poorly or are unavailable locally [8]. In approximately 25% or more of returned travellers, the cause for fever may not be identified [9].

For this reason, a risk-based approach is recommended, with initial priority given to recognizing and treating life-threatening causes of fever and identifying any infections that threaten public health, with a high risk of transmission [8–10]. Subsequently, the risk assessment should be established based on the knowledge of the geographic distribution of infections, risk factors for acquisition, incubation periods, and clinical findings [8–10].

1.1 Initial Evaluation

1.1.1 Does the Patient Have a Travel History?

This is the key question to be asked to all patients and especially patients with fever. A travel history opens up exposure to infections not present where the patient lives and this information is key for the healthcare professional to properly understand the situation. The evaluation is summarized in Table 1.1.

1.1.2 Is the Patient Seriously Ill?

As for all emergency admissions, it should be assessed if the patient is seriously ill. Glasgow Coma Scale, blood pressure, pulse, temperature, respiratory rate, and peripheral oxygen saturation are essential parameters in the initial evaluation, in order to evaluate whether the patient may be a candidate for intensive care.

1.1.3 Medical Emergencies and Life-threatening Diseases

Malaria is the most common life-threatening tropical disease associated with fever in returned travellers [9]. As so, fever in a traveller returning from a malaria-endemic country must be evaluated immediately.

Table 1.1 Initial evaluation of the febrile returned traveller

Medical emergencies	Hemodynamic instability (monitor blood pressure) Respiratory distress (respiratory rate and peripheral oxygen saturation) Haemorrhagic manifestations (petechiae, ecchymosis, conjunctiva) Neurologic manifestations such as altered mental status (Glasgow Coma Scale), neck stiffness, or focal deficits
Isolation measures	Implement transmission-based precautions based on the clinical presentation and likely pathogens
Localizing symptoms	Associated symptoms Date of illness onset and temporal relation to the trip Previous received healthcare (such as medications or hospitalizations)
Host factors	Age and sex Comorbidities and chronic diseases, including immunosuppressive conditions Pregnancy Immunization status, including pretravel vaccines Routine medications Over-the-counter medications Recent antimicrobials Herbal, complementary, and alternative medicines
Pretravel advice	Adherence to effective insect measures, such as repellent and bed nets Adherence to malaria chemoprophylaxis
Travel history[a]	Destination, itinerary and visited areas Travel purpose (tourism, visiting friends or relatives, business, research, education, missionary/volunteer work, providing medical care or receiving medical care) Duration of travel and date of return from travel Type of environment Type of accommodation Recreational activities (safari, hiking, ocean exposure, freshwater exposure, swimming pools and hot tubs, rafting/boating and other adventure activities) Exposures (type of eaten foods, source of drinking water, animal or insect bites, stings, or scratches, sexual activities, tattoos or piercings received while travelling)

[a] Should go back at least a year, but may go back several years (for instance if TB, HIV or schistosomiasis are suspected)

Other life-threatening diseases include avian (H5N1) influenza, Middle East respiratory syndrome coronavirus (MERS-CoV), viral haemorrhagic fevers (yellow fever, severe dengue, Ebola, Lassa, Marburg, and Crimean-Congo haemorrhagic fevers), Japanese encephalitis, Rift Valley fever, rabies, anthrax, enteric fever, leptospirosis, relapsing fever, melioidosis, Oroya fever, scrub typhus, rickettsioses, plague, and East African sleeping sickness [8].

1.1.4 Isolation

In the initial evaluation of the febrile returning traveller, risk assessment for highly transmissible pathogens is a critical first step. If viral haemorrhagic fevers such as

Ebola, Marburg, Lassa, and Crimean-Congo are considered (according to the patient's travel itinerary and symptoms) or infections with airborne transmission, for instance pulmonary tuberculosis, isolation should be implemented to prevent nosocomial outbreaks [8]. Infections with a risk of airborne transmission are shown in Table 1.2.

Transmission-based precautions must be applied based on the clinical presentation and likely pathogens [11]. Certain clinical syndromes carry a sufficiently high risk to warrant their use empirically while awaiting confirmatory tests (Table 1.3).

Table 1.2 Type of precautions recommended for selected infections

Disease	Type of isolation precaution[a]
Colonization or infection with multidrug-resistant microorganisms (e.g. methicillin-resistant *Staphylococcus aureus*, carbapenem-resistant *Enterobacteriaceae*)	Contact
COVID-19, MERS-CoV, and SARS	Airborne + Contact
Diphtheria	
Cutaneous	Contact
Pharyngeal	Droplet
Ebola, Marburg, Lassa, Crimean-Congo, and Chapare haemorrhagic fevers	Airborne + Contact
Influenza	Droplet
Measles	Airborne
Meningococcal infections	Droplet
Mpox	Airborne + Contact
Pneumonic plague	Droplet
Poliomyelitis	Contact
Tuberculosis	
Pulmonary or laryngeal	Airborne
Extrapulmonary, draining lesion	Airborne + Contact

Contact precautions: A single-patient room is preferred. Healthcare personnel wear a gown and gloves for all interactions that may involve contact with the patient or potentially contaminated areas in the patient's environment

Droplet precautions: A single-patient room is preferred, but special air handling and ventilation are not required. Healthcare personnel wear a surgical face mask (a respirator, for instance N95, is not necessary) for close contact with the patient. If the patient is transported outside of the room, a mask should be worn and respiratory hygiene/cough etiquette followed

Airborne precautions: The preferred placement of the patient is in an airborne infection isolation room, a single-patient room that is equipped with special air handling and ventilation capacity. Healthcare personnel wear a respirator (for instance N95 or equivalent). Whenever possible, non-immune healthcare worker (HCWs) should not care for patients with vaccine-preventable airborne diseases (e.g. measles, chickenpox, and smallpox)

COVID-19 Coronavirus disease 2019, *MERS-CoV* Middle East respiratory syndrome coronavirus, *SARS* Severe acute respiratory syndrome

[a] Standard precautions should always be applied

Table 1.3 Clinical syndromes warranting empiric transmission-based precautions

Clinical syndrome in addition to fever	Potential pathogens	Type of isolation precaution[a]
Acute diarrhoea with a likely infectious cause	Enteric pathogens	Contact if incontinent or diapered patient
Cough and weight loss	*M. tuberculosis*	Airborne
Cough/fever/pulmonary infiltrate in any lung location in a patient with a history of recent travel to countries with active outbreaks of SARS	SARS-CoV-1	Airborne + Contact
Cough/fever/pulmonary infiltrate in any lung location in a patient with a history of recent travel to countries with active outbreaks of MERS-CoV	MERS-CoV	Airborne + Contact
Meningitis	*N. meningitidis* *M. tuberculosis*	Droplet if *N. meningitidis* is a possibility Airborne if *M. tuberculosis* is a possibility, in the presence of pulmonary infiltrate
Rash, macular, papular, vesicular or pustular	Mpox	Airborne + Contact if Mpox is a possibility
Rash, maculopapular with cough and coryza	Measles	Airborne + Contact if measles is a possibility
Rash, petechial/ecchymotic	*N. meningitidis* Viral haemorrhagic fevers (Ebola, Lassa, Marburg viruses)	Droplet if *N. meningitidis* is a possibility Airborne + Contact if viral haemorrhagic fever is a possibility

Contact precautions: A single-patient room is preferred. Healthcare personnel wear a gown and gloves for all interactions that may involve contact with the patient or potentially contaminated areas in the patient's environment

Droplet precautions: A single-patient room is preferred, but special air handling and ventilation are not required. Healthcare personnel wear a surgical face mask (a respirator is not necessary) for close contact with the patient. If the patient is transported outside of the room, a mask should be worn and respiratory hygiene/cough etiquette followed

Airborne precautions: The preferred placement of the patient is in an airborne infection isolation room, a single-patient room that is equipped with special air handling and ventilation capacity. Healthcare personnel wear a respirator, for instance N95 or equivalent. Whenever possible, nonimmune HCWs should not care for patients with vaccine-preventable airborne diseases (e.g. measles, chickenpox, and smallpox)

[a] Standard precautions should always be applied

If implemented when the patient arrives at the healthcare facility, these measures reduce transmission opportunities [11].

Public health officials should be alerted as per local guidelines, considering the possibility that the traveller may be infected with a pathogen of public health importance at the origin or destination and the possibility that the traveller may have been contagious.

1.1.5 Presenting Symptoms and Physical Examination

Fever should be characterized by measured temperature, pattern (sustained, intermittent, biphasic, or relapsing), and response to antipyretics. Associated symptoms, such as nausea, vomiting, diarrhoea, rash, respiratory symptoms, genitourinary symptoms, localized pain, and neurologic manifestations, should be thoroughly explored.

A complete physical examination that includes vital signs, neurologic examination, haemorrhagic manifestations, rash or other skin lesions, jaundice, retinal or conjunctival changes, organomegaly, lymphadenopathy, and genital lesions should be conducted.

1.1.6 Host Factors

Baseline history should include comorbidities (including immunosuppression factors, such as diabetes mellitus, HIV infection and CD4+ T cell count, transplantation, malignancy, and asplenia) and medications (especially immunosuppressive therapy), as these can affect the patient's immune response to preventive vaccines and infection or predispose the individual to specific diseases. The patient's immunization status should be documented. Drug and toxin history, including antimicrobials, should be noted.

1.1.7 Pretravel Advice

The patient should be inquired about receiving pretravel advice, immunizations, adherence to recommendations, and malaria chemoprophylaxis, including compliance and duration.

1.1.8 Travel History

The travel purpose (tourism, visiting friends or relatives, business, research, education, missionary/volunteer work, providing or receiving medical care) should be addressed, as it is associated with different risks. For example, missionaries and healthcare personnel are at higher risk for contracting diseases that require prolonged or closer exposure, like tuberculosis, whereas the adventure traveller that goes to remote destinations engages in high-risk activities and is at higher risk for vector-transmitted diseases [10]. People visiting friends or relatives are a particular category of travellers, as they are less likely to seek pretravel advice and take prophylactic measures, but typically stay for more extended periods, possibly in rural environments, and have more exposure to the local population and contaminated food and water.

The travel history should be thoroughly explored and include the itinerary and visited areas, type of environment and accommodation, activities and exposures (such as eating and drinking places, recreational activities, and unprotected sexual intercourses), and the travel duration.

1.2 Differential Diagnosis

In a traveller, the probability of common diseases with a global distribution (such as respiratory tract infections or urinary tract infections) to be the cause of fever is about as high as more exotic illnesses [7, 10]. Noninfectious, travel-related diseases should also be considered (for example, deep venous thrombosis of the lower extremities in air travellers on long flights) [10].

Three main factors should be used to narrow the differential diagnosis: (1) clinical findings, (2) locations of exposure, and (3) the incubation period.

1.2.1 Clinical Findings

In association with fever, certain signs, symptoms, or laboratory findings can suggest specific infections (Table 1.4) [9].

Table 1.4 Clinical syndrome or findings and infectious diseases to consider

Clinical syndrome or findings	Infections to consider
Fever and rash	Dengue Zika Chikungunya Rickettsial infections Acute schistosomiasis Enteric fever Meningococcemia Acute HIV infection Measles Varicella Mpox
Fever and haemorrhage	Viral haemorrhagic fevers (such as dengue, yellow fever, Ebola, Lassa, Marburg, and Crimean-Congo haemorrhagic fevers) Meningococcemia Leptospirosis Rickettsial infections
Fever and diarrhoea	Traveller's diarrhoea (Enterotoxigenic *E. coli*, norovirus, *Giardia, Cryptosporidium, Campylobacter, Shigella*, nontyphoidal *Salmonella*) Intestinal amebiasis Cholera (persistent, voluminous diarrhoea)

(continued)

Table 1.4 (continued)

Clinical syndrome or findings	Infections to consider
Fever and abdominal pain (without diarrhoea)	Enteric fever Amebic or pyogenic liver abscess Non-travel-related causes (appendicitis, urinary tract infection, cholecystitis, cholangitis, pancreatitis)
Fever and arthralgia or myalgia (sometimes persistent)	Chikungunya Dengue Zika Ross River virus Muscular sarcocystosis Trichinellosis
Fever and eosinophilia	Acute schistosomiasis Drug hypersensitivity reaction Fascioliasis Filariasis Sarcocystosis Trichinellosis Angiostrongyliasis Other parasitic infections (Helminths)
Fever and respiratory symptoms/pulmonary infiltrates	Influenza and other common bacterial and viral pathogens Legionellosis Tuberculosis Acute schistosomiasis Q fever Leptospirosis COVID-19, MERS-CoV, and SARS-CoV-2 Acute histoplasmosis Coccidioidomycosis Psittacosis Melioidosis Pneumonic plague (rare)
Fever and altered mental status/ central nervous system involvement	Cerebral malaria Arboviral encephalitides (for example, Japanese encephalitis, West Nile virus) Meningococcal meningitis Pneumococcal meningitis Rabies African trypanosomiasis Scrub typhus Angiostrongyliasis Tick-borne encephalitis (TBE)
Flaccid paralysis of recent onset	Poliomyelitis
Fever and jaundice	Acute viral hepatitis (A, B, C, E) Yellow fever, severe dengue and other viral haemorrhagic fevers Severe malaria Leptospirosis Liver flukes Acute cholangitis (non-travel related)

Table 1.4 (continued)

Clinical syndrome or findings	Infections to consider
Mononucleosis syndrome	Epstein-Barr virus infection Cytomegalovirus infection Acute toxoplasmosis Acute HIV infection
Fever persisting >2 weeks	Malaria Enteric fever Epstein-Barr virus infection Cytomegalovirus infection Toxoplasmosis Acute HIV infection Acute schistosomiasis Brucellosis Tuberculosis Q fever Visceral leishmaniasis Abscess Noninfectious causes

COVID-19 Coronavirus disease 2019, *MERS* Middle East respiratory syndrome coronavirus, *SARS* Severe acute respiratory syndrome

1.2.2 Locations of Exposure

In the febrile returning traveller, the destination is one of the strongest diagnostic predictors for tropical diseases [12], since specific diseases are limited to or are more prevalent in certain locations, even within the same country [10]. Hence, the geographic area of travel determines the relative likelihood of major causes of fever [7, 9, 13] (Table 1.5). As previously discussed, specific activities may constitute additional risk factors, and preparation before travel (such as vaccinations and malaria prophylaxis) reduces the probability of some infections.

After travelling to sub-Saharan Africa and other tropical areas, malaria is the most common cause of acute undifferentiated fever [9]. Dengue is the most common cause of febrile illness after travelling to Latin America or Asia [9]. Other arboviral infections are causes of fever in travellers, such as chikungunya and Zika viruses. Viral haemorrhagic fevers other than dengue and yellow fever (such as Ebola, Lassa, Marburg, and Crimean-Congo haemorrhagic fevers) are essential to identify but rare in travellers. Some bacterial infections, like leptospirosis, meningococcemia, and rickettsial infections, can also cause fever and haemorrhage and should be considered in order to institute prompt treatment. Especially among travellers hospitalized abroad, infection or colonization with drug-resistant pathogens is possible. Special attention should also be taken to current outbreaks in the traveller's destination.

Table 1.5 Common causes of fever by geographic area

Geographic area	Common diseases	Other rare infections
North Africa, Europe, Mediterranean Middle East	Brucellosis MERS-CoV Q fever Toscana (sandfly fever) West Nile fever	Visceral leishmaniasis
Africa, Sub-Saharan	Acute schistosomiasis Dengue HIV infection Malaria (primarily *P. falciparum*) Rickettsiae (main cause of fever in southern Africa)	African trypanosomiasis Amebic liver abscess Brucellosis Chikungunya Dengue Zika Enteric fever Meningococcal meningitis Other arboviruses (e.g. Rift Valley fever, West Nile fever) Viral haemorrhagic fever (Lassa, Ebola, Marburg, Crimean-Congo haemorrhagic fever, yellow fever) Visceral leishmaniasis
America, Latin Caribbean	Chikungunya Dengue Enteric fever Malaria (primarily *P. vivax*) Zika	Bartonellosis Brucellosis Chagas disease Coccidioidomycosis Hantavirus Histoplasmosis Leishmaniasis Leptospirosis Paracoccidioidomycosis Yellow fever
America, North	–	Babesiosis Coccidioidomycosis Ehrlichiosis Histoplasmosis Lyme disease Rocky Mountain Spotted fever West Nile fever
Asia, South and Central	Dengue Enteric fever Malaria (primarily non-*falciparum*)	Chikungunya Crimean-Congo haemorrhagic fever Japanese encephalitis Other arboviruses (Nipah virus, Kyasanur Forest disease) Q fever Rickettsiae Sandfly fever Scrub typhus Visceral and cutaneous leishmaniasis

Table 1.5 (continued)

Geographic area	Common diseases	Other rare infections
Asia, Southeast	Chikungunya Dengue Enteric fever Malaria (primarily non-*falciparum*) Zika (emerging)	Hantavirus Japanese encephalitis Leptospirosis Melioidosis Other arboviruses (Nipah virus) Paragonimiasis Scrub typhus Talaromycosis
Australia	–	Barmah Forest virus infection Dengue Melioidosis Murray Valley encephalitis Q fever Rickettsiae Ross River fever
Europe, Eastern Scandinavia	Lyme disease	Hantavirus Tick-borne encephalitis Tularemia

1.2.3   Incubation Period

Since each infection has a characteristic incubation period (although the range is extensive in some diseases), the onset of symptoms and its relation to the trip should be determined, in order to establish the likely incubation period. The incubation period will allow the clinician to narrow the differential diagnosis (Table 1.6).

Although most common travel-related infections have a short incubation period and the majority of ill travellers will seek medical care within one month of return from their destination [9], it should be noted that some infections can manifest months or even years after initial infection.

Table 1.6 Travel-associated infections by incubation period

Disease	Usual incubation period (range)
Incubation period ≤14 days	
Anthrax[a]	1–7 days (can be >2 weeks)
Bartonellosis[a]	1–3 weeks
Brucellosis[a]	2–4 weeks (5 days to 5 months)
Chagas disease (acute), vector-borne exposure	1–2 weeks
Chapare haemorrhagic fever (CHHF)[a]	4–21 days
Chikungunya	2–4 days (1–14 days)
Coccidioidomycosis[a]	1–3 weeks
COVID-19	4–5 days (1–14 days)
Crimean-Congo haemorrhagic fever	1–13 days (1–3 days after a tick bite; 3–7 days following contact with blood and body fluids)
Dengue	4–8 days (3–14 days)
Diphtheria	2–5 days (1–10 days)
Ebola virus disease[a]	6–12 days (2–21 days)
Enteric fever (typhoid and paratyphoid fevers)[a]	7–18 days (6–45 days)
Hantavirus infection[a]	Haemorrhagic fever with renal syndrome (HFRS): 2–4 weeks (few days to 2 months) Hantavirus pulmonary syndrome (HPS): 2 weeks (few days to 2 weeks)
Histoplasmosis (acute)[a]	10–14 days (3–25 days)
HIV infection (acute)[a]	10–28 days (10 days to 6 weeks)
Influenza	2 days (1–4 days)
Japanese encephalitis[a]	5–15 days
Lassa fever[a]	1–3 weeks
Legionellosis	5–6 days (2–12 days)
Leptospirosis[a]	7–12 days (2–26 days)
Lyme disease[a]	7–12 days for erythema migrans; longer for other manifestations
Malaria, *P. falciparum*[a]	6–30 days (98% onset within 3 months of travel)
Malaria, *P. vivax*[a]	8 days to months (almost half have onset >30 days after completion of travel)
Marburg fever	5–10 days
Measles[a]	10–14 days (8–21 days)
Melioidosis[a]	2 days to 3 weeks (days to months)
Meningococcal infections	3–4 days (2–10 days)
Mpox[a]	5–13 days (4–21 days)
Oropouche virus disease	4–8 days (3–12 days)
Plague	2–7 days for bubonic (1–14 days)
Poliomyelitis	4–10 days
Psittacosis[a]	7–14 days (4–28 days)
Q fever[a]	18–21 days (4–39 days)
Rabies[a]	1–2 months (4 days to years)
Relapsing fever[a]	7–8 days (2–18 days)
Rickettsial infections[a]	6–7 days (3–18 days)

Table 1.6 (continued)

Disease	Usual incubation period (range)
Scrub typhus (*Orientia* spp)[a]	8–12 days (3–21 days)
Tick-borne encephalitis[a]	8 days (4–28 days)
Toxoplasmosis[a]	1–3 weeks (5–23 days)
Trichinosis[a]	10–20 days (few days to >2 months)
Trypanosomiasis, African[a]	1–3 weeks Rhodesiense: <3 weeks Gambiense: weeks to months
Tularemia	3–5 days (1–14 days)
West Nile virus encephalitis	2–14 days
Yellow fever	1–6 days (3–14 days)
Zika virus infection	5–6 days (3–14 days)
Incubation period 14 days to 6 weeks	
Amebic liver abscess[b]	Weeks to months
Chagas disease (acute), transfusion- and transplant-associated[b]	Weeks to 4 months
Chapare haemorrhagic fever (CHHF)	4–21 days
Ebola virus disease	6–12 days (2–21 days)
Enteric fever (typhoid and paratyphoid fevers)[b]	7–18 days (6–45 days)
Hantavirus infection[b]	Haemorrhagic fever with renal syndrome (HFRS): 2–4 weeks (few days to 2 months) Hantavirus pulmonary syndrome (HPS): 2 weeks (few days to 2 weeks)
Hepatitis A[b]	28–30 days (15–50 days)
Hepatitis C[b]	6–9 weeks (2 weeks to 6 months)
Hepatitis E[b]	26–42 days (2–9 weeks)
Histoplasmosis (acute)	10–14 days (3–25 days)
HIV infection (acute)	10–28 days (10 days to 6 weeks)
Japanese encephalitis	5–15 days
Lassa fever	1–3 weeks
Leishmaniasis, visceral[b]	2–10 months (10 days to years)
Leptospirosis	7–12 days (2–26 days)
Lyme disease	7–12 days for erythema migrans; longer for other manifestations
Malaria[b]	Weeks to months
Measles[a]	10–14 days (8–21 days)
Melioidosis[b]	2 days to 3 weeks (days to months)
Mpox[a]	5–13 days (4–21 days)
Psittacosis	7–14 days (4–28 days)
Q fever	18–21 days (4–39 days)
Rabies[b]	1–2 months (4 days to years)
Relapsing fever	7–8 days (2–18 days)
Rickettsial infections	6–7 days (3–18 days)
Schistosomiasis (acute)[b]	14–84 days
Scrub typhus (*Orientia* spp)	8–12 days (3–21 days)

(continued)

Table 1.6 (continued)

Disease	Usual incubation period (range)
Tick-borne encephalitis	8 days (4–28 days)
Toxoplasmosis	1–3 weeks (5–23 days)
Trichinosis[b]	10–20 days (few days to >2 months)
Trypanosomiasis, African	1–3 weeks Rhodesiense: <3 weeks Gambiense: weeks to months
Trypanosomiasis, African[b]	1–3 weeks Rhodesiense: <3 weeks Gambiense: weeks to months
Tuberculosis[b]	Months to years (4 weeks to decades)
Incubation period >6 weeks	
Amebic liver abscess	Weeks to months
Chagas disease (acute), transfusion- and transplant-associated	Weeks to 4 months
Enteric fever (typhoid and paratyphoid fevers)	7–18 days (6–45 days)
Fascioliasis	6–12 weeks
Hantavirus infection	Haemorrhagic fever with renal syndrome (HFRS): 2–4 weeks (few days to 2 months) Hantavirus pulmonary syndrome (HPS): 2 weeks (few days to 2 weeks)
Hepatitis A	28–30 days (15–50 days)
Hepatitis B	90 days (60–150 days)
Hepatitis C	6–9 weeks (2 weeks to 6 months)
Hepatitis E	26–42 days (2–9 weeks)
HIV infection	10 days to years before symptoms appear
Leishmaniasis, visceral	2–10 months (10 days to years)
Malaria	Weeks to months
Melioidosis	2 days to 3 weeks (days to months)
Rabies	1–2 months (4 days to years)
Schistosomiasis (acute)	14–84 days
Trichinosis	10–20 days (few days to >2 months)
Trypanosomiasis, African	1–3 weeks Rhodesiense: <3 weeks Gambiense: weeks to months
Tuberculosis	Months to years (4 weeks to decades)

[a] Incubation period may exceed 14 days
[b] Incubation period may exceed 6 weeks

1.3 Investigation

1.3.1 First-Tier Laboratory Tests

Initial laboratory tests to be performed in all patients include a complete blood cell count (including white blood cell count, thrombocytes, and haemoglobin) with differential (to analyse for leukocytosis, leukopenia, anaemia, thrombocytopenia, and eosinophilia), liver enzyme and function tests, renal function tests, electrolytes, glycemia, pH, and bicarbonate. In the severely ill patient, lactate should be evaluated.

Urine and blood cultures should also be conducted and urine for white blood cells.

Because the most common life-threatening tropical disease associated with fever in returned travellers is malaria [9], it should always be excluded in people who have visited endemic areas in recent months. A rapid diagnostic test for dengue should also be done if relevant.

1.3.2 Second-Tier Laboratory Tests

Other laboratory tests may be warranted depending on the previous risk assessment (Table 1.7).

Table 1.7 Laboratory evaluation for fever in the returning traveller

First-tier laboratory tests	Complete blood count with differential (white blood cells, haemoglobin, haematocrit, and platelets)
	Liver enzyme and function tests
	Renal function tests
	Electrolytes
	Glycaemia
	pH and bicarbonate
	Lactate (if severely ill)
	Urinalysis (white blood cells, protein, nitrate)
	Rapid diagnostic test and blood smears for malaria (if travel to endemic area)
	Rapid diagnostic tests for dengue (if relevant)
	Blood cultures
Second-tier laboratory tests (to consider according to risk assessment)	Urine culture
	Stool culture and/or examination for blood, faecal leukocytes, ova, and parasites
	Serologic tests depending on exposure
	Serum PCR for dengue virus, Zika virus, Chikungunya, and yellow fever (if relevant)
	Examination of cerebrospinal fluid plus PCR and culture
	Urinary antigens for *S. pneumoniae* and *Legionella*
	PCR for SARS-CoV-2, SARS-CoV-1, MERS-CoV, influenza, and other respiratory virus
	Sputum culture
	Chest radiograph
	Abdominal ultrasonography
	Other imaging studies
	Blood smears for *Babesia*, *Borrelia*, filaria
	Bone marrow aspirate/biopsy
	Biopsy of skin lesion, lymph nodes, other masses

1.4 Conclusion

Because a history of travel will change the clinical approach to a febrile patient, all patients presenting with fever should be inquired about travelling. However, common illnesses with a worldwide distribution (such as respiratory and urinary tract infections) are as likely to be the most common source of fever in travellers as in non-travellers.

The febrile returning traveller poses a diagnostic challenge for the clinician. A risk-based approach is advisable, with initial priority given to recognizing life-threatening causes of fever and infections that may represent public health threats. The need for admission to an intensive care unit should be immediately assessed if the patient is severely ill; the need for isolation to prevent nosocomial transmission should also be evaluated at admission.

A detailed history is essential for risk assessment. Differential diagnosis should be conducted according to the geographic distribution of infections, risk factors for acquisition, incubation periods, and clinical findings. Malaria is the most common cause of fever in the international traveller and should always be excluded if the patient travelled to endemic areas.

Declaration of Conflict of Interest We declare that we have no conflicts of interest.

References

1. Grobusch MP, Weld L, Goorhuis A, Hamer DH, Schunk M, Jordan S, et al. Travel-related infections presenting in Europe: a 20-year analysis of EuroTravNet surveillance data. Lancet Reg Health Eur. 2020;1:100001.
2. Hagmann SHF, Angelo KM, Huits R, Plewes K, Eperon G, Grobusch MP, et al. Epidemiological and clinical characteristics of international travelers with enteric fever and antibiotic resistance profiles of their isolates: a GeoSentinel analysis. Antimicrob Agents Chemother. 2020;64(11):e01084–20.
3. Boggild K, Freedman D. Infections in returning travelers. In: Bennett J, Dolin R, Blaser M, editors. Mandell, Douglas, and Bennett's principles and practice of infectious diseases, 9th ed. Elsevier; 2020.
4. Wilson ME, Freedman DO. Etiology of travel-related fever. Curr Opin Infect Dis. 2007;20:449–53.
5. Wilson ME, Weld LH, Boggild A, Keystone JS, Kain KC, von Sonnenburg F, et al. Fever in returned travelers: results from the GeoSentinel surveillance network. Clin Infect Dis. 2007;44:1560–8.
6. Kotlyar S, Rice BT. Fever in the returning traveler. Emerg Med Clin North Am. 2013;31:927–44.
7. Petersen E, Chen LH, Schlagenhauf-Lawlor P. Infectious diseases: a geographic guide. London: Wiley; 2017.
8. Thwaites GE, Day NP. Approach to fever in the returning traveler. N Engl J Med. 2017;376:548–60.
9. Wilson ME. Chapter 11—Posttravel evaluation. In: CDC Yellow Book, Centers for Disease Control and Prevention. 2019.
10. Speil C, Mushtaq A, Adamski A, Khardori N. Fever of unknown origin in the returning traveler. Infect Dis Clin North Am. 2007;21:1091–113, x.

11. Siegel JD, Rhinehart E, Jackson M, Chiarello L; the Healthcare Infection Control Practices Advisory Committee. 2007 guideline for isolation precautions: preventing transmission of infectious agents in healthcare settings. https://www.cdc.gov/infectioncontrol/guidelines/isolation/index.html.
12. Bottieau E, Clerinx J, Van den Enden E, Van Esbroeck M, Colebunders R, Van Gompel A, et al. Fever after a stay in the tropics: diagnostic predictors of the leading tropical conditions. Medicine (Baltimore). 2007;86:18–25.
13. Johnston V, Stockley JM, Dockrell D, Warrell D, Bailey R, Pasvol G, et al. Fever in returned travellers presenting in the United Kingdom: recommendations for investigation and initial management. J Infect. 2009;59:1–18.

Preparedness and Response for Emerging Infectious Diseases

Eileen C. Farnon, Chantal B. E. M. Reusken, Bethan McDonald, Anna Papa, and Louise Sigfrid

Abstract

Emerging and re-emerging infectious diseases cause a risk both to populations in which these diseases occur and to travellers. This chapter reviews the mechanisms of clinical, laboratory, and public health outbreak preparedness and response, global health security and the International Health Regulations (2005). New efforts to improve multi-disciplinary research responses during epidemics to advance knowledge into effective interventions are described, as well as challenges to effective outbreak detection and response and actions needed.

E. C. Farnon
Center for Global Health, Institut Pasteur, Paris, France
e-mail: efarnon@taskforce.org

C. B. E. M. Reusken
Centre for Infectious Disease Control, National Institute for Public Health and the Environment (RIVM), Bilthoven, The Netherlands
e-mail: chantal.reusken@rivm.nl

B. McDonald
Centre for Tropical Medicine and Global Health, University of Oxford, Oxford, UK
e-mail: bethan.mcdonald@phc.ox.ac.uk

A. Papa
Department of Microbiology, Aristotle University of Thessaloniki, Thessaloniki, Greece
e-mail: annap@auth.gr

L. Sigfrid (✉)
Policy and Practice Research Group, Pandemic Sciences Institute, University of Oxford, Oxford, UK
e-mail: louise.sigfrid@ndm.ox.ac.uk

H. Leblebicioglu et al. (eds.), *Emerging and Re-emerging Infections in Travellers*, https://doi.org/10.1007/978-3-031-49475-8_2

2.1 Background

Emerging and re-emerging infectious diseases pose a risk to travellers, as well as to residents of countries who may be exposed to infections imported by returning travellers. These infectious diseases may be newly emerging or re-emerging diseases which had previously been controlled or absent in the traveller's home country. In either circumstance, imported infectious diseases may be poorly recognized by clinicians and public health systems, and delays in diagnosis, treatment, and control may lead to local transmission. This may in turn result in an outbreak or epidemic, and even in the imported disease becoming endemic, as in the cases of the introduction of chikungunya virus (CHIKV) and Zika virus (ZIKV) in the Americas where both viruses are now firmly established [1, 2].

As international travel and trade have increased, countries and their endemic infections have become much more interconnected. Today an infection can spread rapidly across the globe via air travel, as was seen during the SARS outbreak in 2002–2003, and to a greater extent during the COVID-19 pandemic. The emergence of CHIKV in the Indian Ocean region in 2005, followed by an expansion to the Western Hemisphere in 2013, again took the public health community by surprise [3]. This was followed by the introduction of ZIKV, thought to be introduced by travellers, which resulted in hundreds of thousands of infections in the Western Hemisphere [4]. Both emerging infectious diseases caused large outbreaks when introduced into areas with naïve populations. ZIKV was associated with congenital complications, such as microcephaly, spontaneous abortion, and neurologic complications, such as Guillain-Barre syndrome, that had not previously been identified in the limited number of cases detected during previous outbreaks [5]. The mpox outbreak in traditionally non-endemic regions in 2022, further emphasized the risk of introduction of travel-imported cases into new regions. It also emphasized the need for investment into clinical trials to identify effective treatments and prophylaxis for infectious diseases affecting populations in any region.

Vaccine-preventable diseases like measles have also caused large outbreaks in countries which previously had limited numbers of cases, to the point of threatening their elimination status. This has been due largely to increasing vaccine hesitancy among populations in these countries, the importation of cases from endemic countries [6, 7] and in some instances, the breakdown of public health systems due to war and conflict. Another concern that requires intensified focus is the emergence of antimicrobial resistance (AMR), which threatens the effective prevention and treatment of infectious diseases [8].

Finally, diseases of high consequence due to their morbidity, mortality or lack of approved effective vaccines or therapeutics, have resulted in the importation of cases by travellers into other countries, sometimes resulting in local transmission. During the 2014–2016 Ebola virus disease (EVD) outbreak in West Africa, a combination of factors, including delayed identification of cases, lack of access to timely diagnostics and resources to implement effective infection prevention and control (IPC), weak governmental and healthcare systems, and distrust between authorities and populations fuelled the spread of the disease. Thousands of people experienced EVD, including a large proportion of healthcare workers. Border screening and monitoring of returned travellers may have mitigated the transmission to other countries [9]. The outbreak highlighted the need to integrate social sciences, health promotion and community engagement in outbreak preparedness and response, ensuring that efforts are targeted and adapted to the context of each outbreak, including the local culture and politics.

In this increasingly interconnected world, there is a need to strengthen preparedness across disciplines to improve our capacity to identify and respond to emerging infectious disease outbreaks. The COVID-19 pandemic highlighted how a new infection could rapidly spread across the globe, overwhelming healthcare and public health systems, and causing widespread disruption to societies. It illustrates the need for early detection to inform rapid and appropriate control measures. The pandemic also highlighted the need to strengthen global preparedness and capacity to develop new diagnostics, vaccines and medical countermeasures and ensure equitable access globally.

2.2 Clinical Preparedness and Response

What can clinicians do to be prepared for newly emerging and re-emerging infectious diseases? Prevention remains the mainstay of travel medicine. Immunization for pathogens known to be endemic in patients' travel destinations, as well as for routine infectious diseases, and prevention through behavioural measures to prevent food-borne, vector-borne, zoonotic, and sexually transmitted diseases remain important and cost-effective means to reduce the threat of infectious diseases among travellers [10]. Frontline clinicians should keep abreast of current outbreaks worldwide to inform the differential diagnosis of returned travellers to ensure timely identification of imported cases. Moreover, clinicians are advised to refer patients to travel and tropical medicine clinics for pre-travel consultation and post-travel evaluation for ill returned travellers when needed [2, 11]. There are many expert sources for clinicians and patients for pre-travel advice, including national and international websites that provide up-to-date information on current outbreaks globally (Box 2.1).

Box 2.1 Travel Risk Assessments
For information about travel risks consult with:
- travel or tropical medicine clinic
- local or national public health agency
- up-to-date national or international certified websites, e.g.:
  - Centers for Disease Control and Prevention (CDC)[a]
  - National Travel Health Network and Centre (NaTHNaC)[b]
  - Pro-Med International Society for Infectious Diseases[c]
  - The World Health Organization (WHO)[d]

[a] www.promedmail.org/
[b] https://travelhealthpro.org.uk/about
[c] https://wwwnc.cdc.gov/travel
[d] https://www.who.int/ith/en/

Clinicians should ask patients with syndromes suggesting infectious aetiologies about recent travel, activities, ill contacts, animal exposures and previous vaccinations and prophylactic medications in addition to their symptoms. Based on this information, clinicians should formulate a differential diagnosis, and order appropriate testing and infection control precautions. Treating clinicians should additionally notify and consult with their public health authorities if the differential diagnosis includes high-hazard or unknown pathogens, so that the appropriate response may be implemented, even before microbiologic confirmation is obtained. For high-hazard pathogens, testing may be required in reference laboratories with special collection and shipping requirements. Early notification of cases of possible imported infectious diseases to public health authorities improves the likelihood of timely detection, treatment, and public health response, by triggering appropriate actions locally, nationally, and internationally when needed [12] (Box 2.2). For emerging infectious disease outbreaks where information changes rapidly and imported diseases for which local knowledge on management may be limited, clinicians are advised to consult current clinical guidelines to guide differential diagnosis and treatment or consult with specialist travel clinics. For example, the World Health Organization (WHO) developed 'living' guidelines in response to the COVID-19 pandemic in which newly available evidence is rapidly assessed and incorporated.

For unusual infections, there may be special infection prevention control (IPC) precautions to be aware of when evaluating and treating patients to reduce risk of healthcare-associated transmission. The evidence for the risk of transmission from different body fluids and even the mode of transmission may be limited at the early stages of outbreaks of emerging infectious diseases. Therefore, standard and transmission-based precautions based on the best available evidence should always be implemented, in consultation with public health authorities when needed. When initially evaluating patients and collecting and shipping diagnostic specimens, clinicians should seek advice on appropriate isolation precautions, personal protective equipment needed, sample collection and shipping requirements. Communicating with primary care clinics, care homes, hospitals, laboratory, and health authorities as appropriate is critical in these instances to avoid accidental exposures. Failing to adhere to isolation and IPC measures, may lead to unnecessary risks to staff, with risks of lengthy quarantine of staff members and risks to vulnerable patients.

Diseases transmitted person-to-person require contact tracing to ensure follow-up and management of exposed persons according to their level of risk. The responsibility for contact tracing may vary among countries. In many, a national public health institute or a local health authority is responsible for following up contacts and implementing necessary public health measures, whereas in others this may be the responsibility of the treating clinician, or a combination. Clinicians should contact their hospital infection control department and health authorities for guidance when needed.

> **Box 2.2 Clinical Management of Suspected Infectious Diseases in Returning Travellers**
> - Use IPC precautions (standard and transmission-based as indicated)
> - Promptly examine the patient
> - Ask about travel and vaccination history to help guide differential diagnostics
> - Take samples for diagnostics
> - If suspicion of an infection that is part of mandatory reporting or an emerging infection that may pose a risk of transmission, rapidly:
>   - Inform your local microbiologist
>   - Inform the relevant local authority/public health institute
> - Ensure samples are referred to the appropriate reference laboratory and public health authorities are alerted as needed
> - Consult up-to-date clinical management guidelines to inform evidence-based care
> - Inform and provide advice to the patient and any accompanying contacts
> - Inform your healthcare colleagues and IPC team
> - Treat the patient according to best available evidence guidelines
>
> **Notify relevant local authorities promptly; do not wait for diagnosis to be confirmed.**
>
> Abbreviations: *IPC* Infection prevention and control

2.3 Laboratory Preparedness and Response

A timely and accurate diagnosis of cases is one of the main pillars for clinical and public health response to an infectious disease emergence [13]. As such, laboratory systems are recognized as one of the core capacities of the International Health Regulations (IHR, 2005) [14]. An adequate national laboratory response requires inter-epidemic preparedness activities focused on building capacity and identifying and overcoming logistical barriers to sample collection, shipping, testing, interpretation, and reporting of results, to ensure capability to respond to outbreaks [13]. In addition to national laboratory systems strengthening, international sharing of samples and knowledge is required to facilitate efficient confirmatory testing and response, as well as development of diagnostic tests and medical countermeasures.

Rapid diagnostic tests are available for several emerging infectious diseases, including COVID-19, dengue and malaria. Although not as accurate as the molecular methods, they are quick and easy-to-use and are of great help as they can be done by the patients themselves or at the point of care. The COVID-19 pandemic showed that they are an essential part of a comprehensive response strategy [15].

Building lab capacity requires compliance of diagnostic laboratories with accreditation schemes (e.g. ISO 15189), participation in training and external quality assessment (EQA) through proficiency testing and establishment of platforms for data sharing (e.g. sequence data, test validation data). National and international prioritization exercises [16] can provide focus to these inter-epidemic activities, while international laboratory preparedness networks can offer support in addressing these issues. Examples of such networks include the WHO Laboratory task force for high threat pathogens, the laboratory part of SHARP (Strengthened International Health Regulations and Preparedness) in the EU, and the European Centre for Disease Prevention and Control (ECDC) funded European expert laboratory network for emerging viral diseases (EVD-LabNet) [17–19]. EVD-LabNet supports preparedness and response in expert laboratories to strengthen diagnostic testing, surveillance and clinical and public health outbreak response (Box 2.3).

Box 2.3 EVD-LabNet[a] Laboratory Network for Emerging Viral Diseases
EVD-LabNet provides access to:

(a) essential background information on target viruses;
(b) reference diagnostics within the network;
(c) state-of-the-art European diagnostic portfolio and diagnostic capacity and capability;
(d) training courses and workshops based on needs within the network;
(e) EQA through proficiency panels and assistance with corrective actions based on panel outcomes;
(f) yearly meetings to strengthen the coherence of the network and to provide a platform for knowledge exchange.

Abbreviations: *EQA* External quality assessment
[a] https://www.evd-labnet.eu/

Laboratories should be informed when receiving clinical samples from travellers and collaborate with clinicians for the selection of the most appropriate sample types and testing methods (molecular and/or serological), as well as for the interpretation of the results taking into account patients' signs and symptoms, date of illness onset, immunocompromising conditions, vaccination and travel history including possible exposures (Table 2.1).

In cases when a high-risk pathogen is suspected, laboratories must be informed promptly to apply enhanced precaution measures (e.g. work in biosafety level 3 or 4 facilities) [20]. National reference laboratories must be prepared for diagnostics for "exotic" pathogens and be aware of the current global epidemiology which is changing over time [21]. Since the diagnosis is challenging, and several pathogens are included in the differential diagnosis, a syndromic approach is usually applied [22]. As an example, diagnostics for dengue virus, ZIKV, and CHIKV should be

Table 2.1 Questions to inform diagnostic triage[a]

What are the risk factors?	• Recent travel history? Activities undertaken? Risk contacts? • Previous vaccinations? • Seasonality and ongoing outbreaks? • Immunosuppression?
What is the time-point during the course of infection when specimens should be collected?	• When was the illness onset? • What are the kinetics of pathogen shedding and antibody responses in persons with different disease states (asymptomatic, mild, moderate, severe, acute, convalescent)? • How are infection kinetics influenced by host factors (e.g. pregnancy, immunosuppression, co-morbidities)?
What is the type of specimens adequate for the suspected pathogen and required for the available diagnostic tests?	• What is the concentration of the pathogen in various body compartments, fluids and secreta during the progression of the disease? • How are pathogen loads influenced by host factors (e.g. pregnancy, immunosuppression, co-morbidities)?
What are the available in-house and/or commercial laboratory tests (including rapid tests) to confirm or rule out a diagnosis?	• What is the limit of detection of the various diagnostic methods used for the different specimens and related to stage of illness? • Specificity?

[a] Adapted from Reusken CB, Ieven M, Sigfrid L, et al. Clin Microbiol Infect. 2018;24(3):221–228

applied in a traveller with a rash coming back from endemic areas (however, not forgetting other causes of febrile rash illness, like varicella or measles virus which may be more common in countries with outbreaks of vaccine-preventable diseases). The use of multiplex molecular and serological methods is very helpful, while the recent technology of next generation sequencing is promising as an all-in-one diagnostic test [23]. Since it is difficult for every laboratory to have in place all diagnostic methods for every pathogen, collaboration with other laboratories is needed. Therefore, networking among laboratories and defining a process to send samples to regional or national reference laboratories is very important for knowledge and reagents exchange and support in case confirmatory testing is needed.

2.4   Public Health Preparedness and Response

Systems of public health preparedness vary among different countries but operate on the same basic principles. At the local level, health authorities collect data on cases and clusters of diseases of public health importance as part of routine disease surveillance systems. These data are reported electronically or manually by clinical laboratories, hospitals and primary care clinics, and by individual clinicians. Clinicians and microbiologists are required to report diseases of public health significance to their national public health institutes or relevant local authorities. These indicator (disease)-based surveillance data are verified by the public health agency, which may contact infection preventionists and clinicians for additional information or request additional testing to classify a case according to its case definition for the notifiable disease [24]. A case definition is a set of standard criteria for classifying the likelihood of a person having a particular disease for public health surveillance and outbreak response purposes. Case definitions developed for nationally notifiable diseases or during outbreaks of novel disease syndromes ensure comparability by applying the same objective criteria to classify all cases as suspected/possible, probable, or confirmed, allowing for description of case characteristics and investigation of the source of the outbreak and potential risk factors for disease. The line listing of cases (including the "who, what, where, when" from the case reports) and their classifications is de-identified and shared with regional and national institutes on a regular basis. In some cases, national data are shared at an international level, as in the case of The European Surveillance System (TESSy) run by the European Centre for Disease Control [25]. All countries globally are also required to report all diseases and events of international concern to WHO as part of the IHR [26].

Public health surveillance data are used to identify outbreaks of notifiable diseases or syndromes when cases exceed a defined threshold, and inform the need for national, regional, or global control measures. In addition to tracking diseases over time, these data are used to inform targeted allocation of resources and to assess the impact of public health interventions like vaccination programmes.

The early warning functions of surveillance are fundamental for national, regional and global health security. Recent outbreaks such as the mpox and Sudan Ebola virus outbreaks in 2022 demonstrate the importance of effective national surveillance and response systems. The IHR, 2005 underscore the commitment to the goal of global security and oblige all WHO Member States to establish and implement effective surveillance and response systems to detect, assess, report, and respond to public health events of national and international importance [27]. They additionally require 196 countries, including the 194 WHO Member States, to report public health events that may constitute a public health emergency of international concern (PHEIC) to WHO.

In addition, public health agencies at the national and international level often conduct event-based surveillance (EBS) to detect outbreaks quickly, for unusual cases or clusters, which may represent newly introduced diseases of unknown aetiology or imported diseases which are not under routine public health surveillance and may pose a public health threat [28]. EBS collects and evaluates reports, stories, rumours, and other information about health events that could be a serious risk to public health. It compiles information from different sources, including media, social media, and internet use to identify potential outbreak signals, which are then verified by the public health agency [29]. Finally, syndromic surveillance systems may be used by public health agencies to enable early detection of outbreaks before the causative agent is identified, e.g. syndromes of undifferentiated fever or encephalitis, or track a disease of public health importance like polio using the broad syndrome of acute flaccid paralysis surveillance in order to capture all possible cases. These different types of surveillance complement each other: EBS and syndromic surveillance have the potential to identify outbreaks early, whereas traditional indicator-based surveillance does not capture suspected cases until the case-patients

The four international agencies, the Food and Agriculture Organization of the United Nations (FAO), the World Organisation for Animal Health (OIE), the UN Environment Programme (UNEP) and the World Health Organization (WHO) signed an agreement in 2022 to strengthen cooperation to sustainably balance and optimize the health of humans, animals, plants and the environment.

The Quadripartite memorandum of understanding provides a legal and formal framework for the four organizations to tackle the challenges at the human, animal, plant and ecosystem interface using a more integrated and coordinated approach. This framework will also contribute to reinforce national and regional health systems and services.

These organisations work in close collaboration to combat health risks at the human-animal-ecosystems interface, in the context of the One Health approach, particularly endemic and epidemic zoonoses and antimicrobial resistance.

These health threats pose risks to public health, animal health and global health security.

Prevention, detection, assessment, and response to pathogens transmitted through contact between humans, animals, food, water, and contaminated environments cannot effectively be addressed by one health sector alone. Thus, continuous communication and collaboration among all sectors responsible for health are required.

* https://www.who.int/news/item/29-04-2022-quadripartite-memorandum-of-understanding-(mou)-signed-for-a-new-era-of-one-health-collaboration

Fig. 2.1 The quadripartite collaboration for One Health*. (https://www.who.int/news/item/29-04-2022-quadripartite-memorandum-of-understanding-(mou)-signed-for-a-new-era-of-one-health-collaboration)

seek medical attention. All systems need verification to ensure that the cases meet a specific case definition and are most credible when supported by laboratory confirmation. With the recognition that >60% of infectious diseases are zoonotic [30], i.e. transmitted from animals to humans, and the impact of the environment on health, there is increased recognition of the importance of an integrated One Health approach to disease prevention, surveillance, and control (Fig. 2.1). For example, West Nile virus (WNV) might be detected in birds, mosquitoes, or horses before it is detected in human populations. A signal from either surveillance system can initiate prevention and control measures to prevent further transmission.

The goal of surveillance systems with respect to epidemics is to identify outbreaks early; to characterize the cases and the geographic and temporal evolution of the outbreak. During an outbreak, active surveillance may also be implemented using active case-finding (door-to-door, triage and screening at healthcare facilities, border screening, etc.) and contact tracing to identify all possible cases in an outbreak area. Surveillance data collected during outbreaks, as well as applied epidemiological studies on the affected populations, can be analysed on an ongoing basis to inform control measures. Characterizing the affected populations, their location, and identifying potential risk factors for hospitalization, complications and death can facilitate the implementation of appropriate public health interventions and the measurement of their impact. For example, during the 2009 pH1N1 outbreak, groups thought to be at risk of severe complications and death included those at the extremes of age and pregnant women, and both medical and "non-pharmaceutical" interventions, such as school closures could be targeted at these populations with the aim to achieve the greatest impact. Epidemiologic studies conducted during outbreaks can be limited given their preliminary nature and often small sample sizes, and this should be taken into consideration when interpreting their results to inform appropriate outbreak control measures in different contexts. In the case of pH1N1, later meta-analyses found pregnancy to be a risk factor for hospitalization but not for other severe outcomes or mortality [31, 32].

2.4.1 The Role of Clinicians, Microbiologists and Communities in Public Health Surveillance and Response

It is often the astute clinician or microbiologist who first identifies cases of unusual, travel-associated epidemic- and pandemic-prone diseases. Clinicians have a responsibility to implement measures including appropriate infection control, while simultaneously alerting public health authorities and obtaining testing at the appropriate reference laboratory, in a coordinated effort to identify and contain the disease. This is how travel- or laboratory-associated cases of viral haemorrhagic fever (VHF) have been identified in non-endemic countries in Europe and the United States [33, 34]. During the 2014–2016 West African Ebola outbreak, screening processes using syndromic case definitions were implemented for travellers returning from outbreak-affected areas to facilitate rapid identification and isolation of potential case-patients to reduce the risk of further transmission. These screening systems depended heavily on the participation of the medical community to identify patients with risk of exposure, initiate isolation and testing and alert public health authorities [35].

2.4.2 Outbreak Response

In the event an outbreak is detected, the relevant local or regional public health authority will generally lead and coordinate the response to control and contain the outbreak. If the outbreak crosses local or regional jurisdictions, is of national concern, or is beyond their capacity to respond, the response may be coordinated at national level. Likewise, responses to outbreaks crossing national borders are often coordinated by WHO. The response will be coordinated in collaboration with a range of organizations as needed. Organizations that may be involved depending on the nature and scale of the outbreak includes local and/or national public health authority, primary care, hospitals, laboratories, epidemiologists, environmental, agriculture and wildlife health agencies, police or other security agency and communication leads. Ensuring harmonized, effective, and proactive communication using standardized, clear messages is important to build trust, reduce risk of misinformation, as well as unnecessary fear and worry. Clear messaging guides people to the correct services depending on risk of exposure, and ensures cases are directed to the appropriate level of care, while reducing the risk of services being overwhelmed by the worried well, thereby avoiding unnecessary strain on health services and the outbreak response. The steps in an outbreak investigation are outlined in Figs. 2.2 and 2.3.

The WHO Emergency Medical Teams (EMT) Initiative assists organizations and member states build capacity and strengthen health systems by coordinating the deployment of "quality assured" medical teams during emergencies. The EMT Initiative places a strong focus on helping every country develop its own teams which can deploy where needed on shortest notice [36]. The Global Health Cluster

- Verify information - establish the existence of an outbreak
- Verify the diagnosis
- Develop a working case definition
- Systematically find cases and record information
- Perform descriptive epidemiology
- Develop hypotheses
- Evaluate hypotheses epidemiologically
- Compare with laboratory and/or environmental studies
- Implement multi-agency control measures
- Continuously communicate findings to all stakeholders
- Declare outbreak over
- Prepare outbreak report and incorporate lessons learnt

Fig. 2.2 Epidemiologic steps of an outbreak investigation. When a country requires international support in controlling an outbreak, the response may be supported or coordinated by WHO, an agency of the United Nations. WHO can provide different types of support if requested, in collaboration with the affected country's Ministry of Health along with partner organizations and UN agencies and regional public health agencies as required (Fig. 2.3)

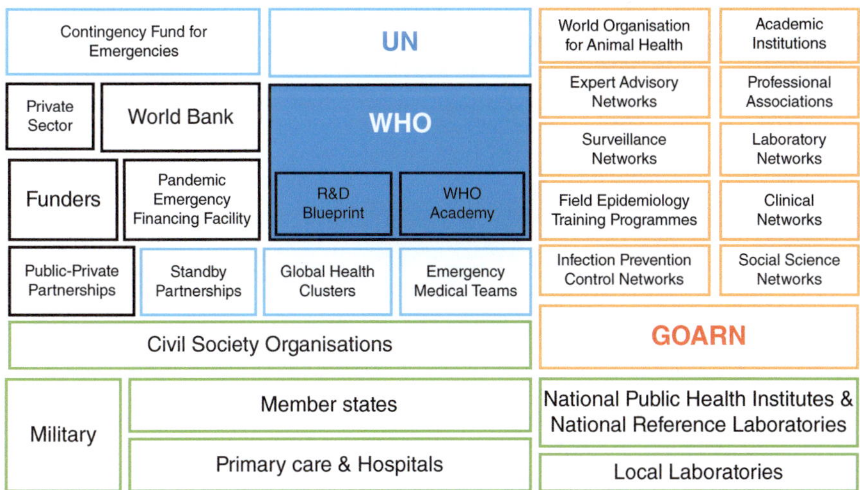

Fig. 2.3 Global outbreak preparedness and response infrastructure. Abbreviations: *WHO* World Health Organization, *UN* United Nations, *GOARN* Global Outbreak Alert and Response Network, *R&D* Research & Development

is a platform for organizations to work in partnership to ensure collective action results in timelier, more effective, and predictable responses to humanitarian emergencies, with WHO as the Cluster Lead Agency for Health [37]. Clusters are groups of humanitarian organizations, both UN and non-UN, in each of the main sectors of humanitarian action (e.g. water, health, and logistics) with clear responsibilities for coordination [38]. Standby partners are non-UN organizations which provide a mechanism for rapidly deploying extra highly skilled specialist personnel if required to support the emergency work of WHO and the Health Cluster [39].

Responding to epidemics does not just require manpower but also sustained and flexible funding. The WHO Contingency Fund for Emergencies, using donations from member states, provides WHO with resources to respond immediately to disease outbreaks and humanitarian crises with health consequences. The ability to respond quickly—in as little as 24 h—before other funding is mobilized can assist in early mitigation of health emergencies, saving lives and resources [40]. Many other funding organizations and initiatives, including donations by the public to non-governmental organizations, are vital for outbreak preparedness and response. Security forces from the UN or other agencies are rarely used and only when deemed necessary, e.g. in conflict situations to provide safety and protection to affected populations and responders.

The Global Outbreak Alert and Response Network (GOARN), overseen by WHO and the GOARN Steering Committee, is comprised of >200 partner organizations which respond to outbreaks. GOARN coordinates their efforts and supports individuals from these organizations to respond when needed to provide their expertise to responses (Fig. 2.4). GOARN can deploy epidemiologists, laboratory staff, infection prevention and control experts, clinicians, communication specialists, and other experts and support staff to assist with outbreak investigation and response [41]. GOARN teams are only deployed when a country's own capacity is exceeded and a request for assistance from the country is made to WHO.

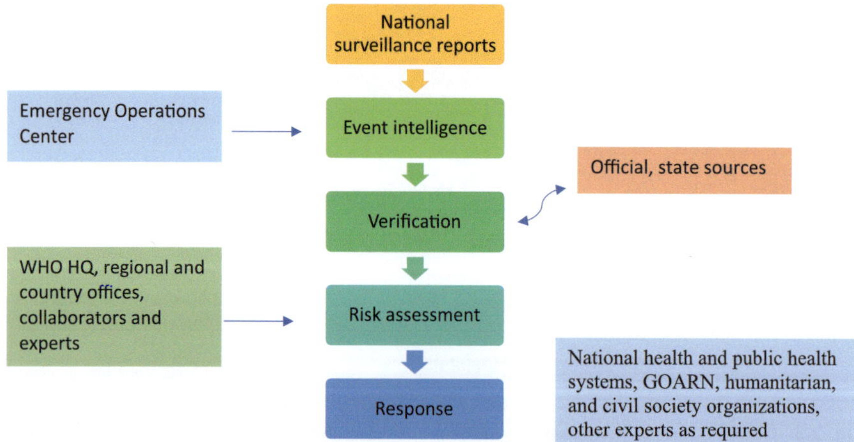

Fig. 2.4 WHO system of Global Outbreak Alert and Response Network (GOARN) operations. Abbreviations: *WHO* World Health Organization, *HQ* Headquarters, *GOARN* Global Outbreak Alert and Response Network

2.5 Global Health Security and the International Health Regulations (IHR)

With trade and travel expanding on a global level, the opportunity for greater disease spread also increases. The public health and economic impact due to infectious diseases can cause great harm to humans and severely damage a country's economy. The IHR 2005 is an agreement between 196 countries, including the 194 WHO Member States to work together for global health security. It is an agreement to prevent, protect against, control, and respond to the international spread of disease, and to reduce the risk of disease spread at international airports, ports, and ground crossings, while avoiding unnecessary interference with international traffic and trade.

Member states are guided, and committed to build their capacities to detect, assess and report public health events. Under the IHR (2005), all 196 participating countries are required to have the ability to detect, assess, report, and respond to public health events [26] (Box 2.4). The IHR require countries to designate a National IHR Focal Point for communications with WHO, to establish and maintain core capacities for surveillance and response, including at designated points of entry. The IHR also introduce important safeguards to protect the rights of travellers in relation to the treatment of personal data, informed consent and non-discrimination in the application of health measures under the regulations.

Box 2.4 IHR (2005) Requirements

IHR (2005) requires that all countries have the ability to do the following:

- **Detect:** Make sure surveillance systems and laboratories can detect potential threats
- **Assess:** Work together with other countries to make decisions in public health emergencies
- **Report:** Report specific diseases, plus any potential international public health emergencies, through participation in a network of National Focal Points
- **Respond:** Respond to public health events

IHR includes specific measures countries can take at ports, airports and ground crossings to limit the spread of health risks to neighbouring countries, and to prevent unwarranted travel and trade restrictions.

Abbreviations: *IHR* International Health Regulations

Under the IHR, all states are required to notify WHO of all events that are assessed as possibly constituting a public health emergency of international concern (PHEIC) within 24 hours. A PHEIC is defined as an extraordinary event that poses a risk to the public health of more than one state because of the international spread of the disease, thereby potentially requiring a coordinated international response. The assessment by states to whether an event within their territories is notifiable to WHO, is determined by following the algorithm in Annex 2 of the IHR, 2005 in which two of the four following criteria are met [42].

1. Is the public health impact of the event serious?
2. Is the event unusual or unexpected?
3. Is there a significant risk of international spread?
4. Is there a significant risk of international travel or trade restrictions?

Cases of some diseases always require reporting under the IHR, while others become notifiable when they represent an unusual risk or situation. Those that are always notifiable include smallpox; poliomyelitis due to wild-type poliovirus, human influenza caused by a new subtype, severe acute respiratory syndrome (SARS). Other potentially notifiable events include outbreaks of cholera, pneumonic plague, yellow fever, viral haemorrhagic fevers, West Nile fever, or other biological, radiological, or chemical events that meet reporting criteria using the algorithm [43].

The decision to declare a PHEIC is taken by the WHO Director General. When a PHEIC is declared, WHO coordinates an immediate international response. Given that many countries do not yet have the capacity to meet all the IHR requirements, WHO and partner organizations are working with countries to improve their capacity to detect, assess, report, and respond to public health threats and thereby improve Global Health Security (GHS). Launched in 2014, the Global Health Security Agenda (GHSA) is a partnership among countries, international organizations, and non-governmental organizations to improve countries' capacity to prevent, detect and respond to infectious disease threats by measuring and improving IHR core capacities with a standardized approach using the process below [44]. Being adequately prepared to manage these infectious disease outbreaks is a challenge for many countries. IHR (2005) Monitoring and Evaluation Framework (MEF) provides a roadmap for assessing a country's health security capacity, enabling them to identify areas for improvement [45].

It includes a four-step process:

1. States Parties Self-Assessment Annual Reporting (SPAR)
2. Joint External Evaluations (JEE)
3. After Action Reviews (AAR)
4. Simulation Exercises (SimEx)

During the COVID-19 pandemic, Intra-Action Review (IAR) was added to the MEF process as a temporary, voluntary process for countries to conduct an interim evaluation and improvement of their response. In the future, this process may be used for other long-term public health events [43]. As of 2024, seven PHEICs have been declared by the IHR Emergency Committee (Fig. 2.5). An unintended negative consequence of a PHEIC can occur when countries implement travel and trade restrictions. This can hinder the public health response and humanitarian relief by

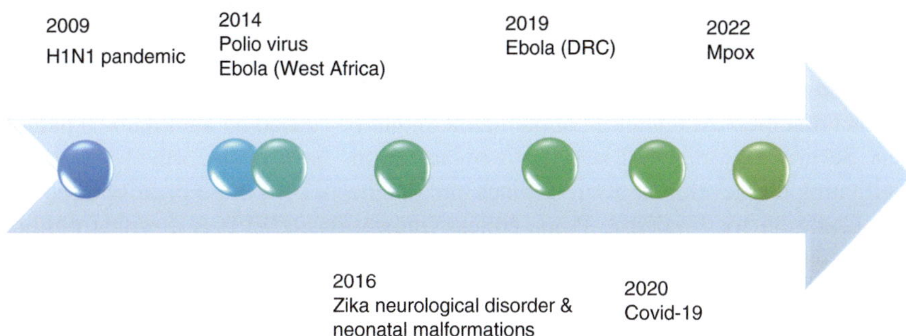

Fig. 2.5 Public health emergencies of international concern declarations. Abbreviations: *DRC* Democratic Republic of Congo

closing borders and ceasing flights in and out of affected countries. Moreover, these restrictions have serious implications for affected countries' economies and response and recovery resources.

Despite the IHR it is estimated that only a third of countries globally have sufficient **capacity to assess, detect, and respond to public health emergencies** [43]. In light of the impact of the COVID-19 pandemic, WHO's 194 Member States established a process to draft and negotiate a new convention, agreement, or other international instrument on pandemic preparedness and response. This was driven by the need to ensure communities, governments, and all sectors of society—within countries and globally—are better prepared and protected, to prevent and respond to future pandemics. The great loss of human life, disruption to households and societies and impact on development are among the factors cited by governments to support the need for lasting action to prevent a repeat of such crises. At the heart of the proposed accord is the need to ensure equity in both access to the tools needed to prevent pandemics (including technologies like vaccines, personal protective equipment, information, and expertise) and access to healthcare for all people [46].

2.6 Clinical Research During Epidemics

In addition to increasing global health security and improving IHR capacity through improvement in public health infrastructure, increased emphasis has been placed on clinical research and development (R&D) to combat infectious disease threats. Many emerging infectious diseases are rare or neglected tropical diseases for which few if any therapeutics and vaccines exist. Clinical and epidemiologic observational studies can provide important information to characterize new and emerging infectious diseases and identify risk factors for severe disease to inform early identification of cases and public health management. Furthermore, clinical trials conducted during outbreaks can identify optimal supportive care and treatment strategies, to inform clinical management to improve individual and epidemic outcomes.

The WHO R&D blueprint, launched in 2016, provides a list of priority diseases for prioritizing therapeutics and vaccine research and development [16]. The list is reviewed on a regular basis and in 2018 'disease X' was added to the list to highlight the fact that the next epidemic or pandemic might be caused by an unknown pathogen. Several major global non-profit organizations have been formed which are facilitating the development of vaccines and diagnostics for these priority diseases. The Coalition for Epidemic Preparedness Innovations (CEPI) is a global public-private partnership launched in 2017 to accelerate development of vaccines and other biologic countermeasures against epidemic and pandemic threats so they can be accessible to all in need during outbreaks [47]. The Foundation for Innovative New Diagnostics (FIND), seeks to ensure equitable access to reliable diagnosis around the world, with a focus on diseases affecting developing countries; pandemic threats is one of its core programme areas [48]. The Global Research Collaboration for Infectious Disease Preparedness (GLOPID-R) is an international network of major research funders created in 2013 to coordinate funding for a timely, effective and equitable research response during outbreaks, in addition to promoting preparedness and readiness to respond [49].

Efforts to engage clinicians in conducting clinical studies during outbreaks has increased through the development of clinical trials consortia established to conduct important necessary clinical research studies during outbreaks. For rare diseases, epidemics often present the only opportunity to conduct research to learn more about the disease and test diagnostic methods, clinical management strategies, including medical countermeasures such as therapeutics, vaccines, as well as behavioural and community-based control measures. One example is the clinical trial of four Ebola therapeutics during the 2018–2019 Ebola virus disease outbreak in the Democratic Republic of Congo (DRC) [50]. To strengthen capacity and capability for research responses to epidemics and pandemics, consortia such as the African coaLition for Epidemic Research, Response and Training (ALERRT) network have been funded to provide training and support for multiple disciplines to conduct multi-site clinical studies led by regional researchers during outbreaks [51]. The PREPARE partnership was formed to strengthen preparedness to emerging and re-emerging infectious diseases across Europe, by setting up syndromic studies of infectious diseases that are open and ready to recruit patients at the start of an outbreak. Further, by providing training and strengthening clinical and laboratory networks across Europe [52]. The Australian Partnership for Preparedness Research on Infectious Disease Emergencies (APPRISE) is a similar research consortium for Australia. Advancing Clinical Evidence in Infectious Diseases (Advance-ID) is a network of >30 hospitals across Asia which conducts collaborative infectious disease clinical research to strengthen research capacity and improve evidence for the optimal prescribing of antibiotics for antimicrobial-resistant infections [53].

There is an increased recognition for the need to sustain networks and consortia beyond traditional short-term project funding, to sustain capability to respond. The European Clinical Research Alliance on Infectious Diseases (ECRAID) is an example of a European clinical research network for infectious diseases, building on the PREPARE partnership, sustained via public and private funding. These consortia aim to strengthen preparedness to be ready to respond to new and emerging outbreaks, by improving research capacity and preparedness for outbreak response, advancing knowledge, and generating evidence to inform new diagnostic tests and optimal therapies. This approach will not only advance clinical research on emerging and neglected infectious diseases but can also facilitate integration of trials into clinical practices and result in greater awareness among clinicians, resulting in faster implementation of effective research, clinical and public health responses. Healthcare sites and staff interested in taking part in research can join regional networks to stay updated on activities and opportunities to participate in studies.

Experience from previous epidemics indicates that the clinical research response is often delayed and fragmented, failing to enroll sufficient patients to generate actionable evidence [54]. This was evident during the H1N1 pandemic in 2009, when the opportunity to conduct clinical trials on medical countermeasures was missed [55]. In contrast, during the Ebola outbreak in West Africa (2013–2016), substantive clinical research was undertaken. However, the rapid launch of several clinical trials led to the unintended consequence of multiple trials competing for enrolment of patients [56]. Improvements in rapid research responses were seen in some regions during the COVID-19 pandemic. Diagnostic tests were developed within a week; effective therapeutics (dexamethasone) identified within 138 days and effective vaccines in just over 300 days after the WHO declared a PHEIC. However, the pandemic also highlighted many challenges, including political ones, as well as the proliferation of uncoordinated and often underpowered trials which were competing for patients, and many failed to meet their aims, wasting valuable resources [57]. There were few trials based in lower resourced settings [58] and inequity in access to trial outputs such as vaccines. In the face of a global threat, most efforts were national or regional, with little international cooperation [59, 60]. In the wake of the pandemic, there have been many calls to action, including calls for better coordination of clinical trials [61–63]. Sustaining clinical research networks globally and integrating research into healthcare would help facilitate timely research responses to generate new evidence to inform clinical and public health management to improve patient and epidemic outcomes. However, more work is needed to coordinate our responses, and improve global collaboration.

2.7   Challenges and Actions Needed

Clinicians and microbiologists play a key role in the early identification, notification and response to new and emerging infectious diseases imported by travel. They alert public health authorities of potential public health threats and contribute to the clinical response. Effective coordination and communication, in addition to expertise and a well-trained workforce is key for effective public health response. Domestically, national Ministries of Health depend on local and regional clinicians, labs, and health departments for effective responses. Internationally, GOARN has contributed to the improved organization and coordination of responses among the many different organizations which respond to large outbreaks, such as the 2014–2016 Ebola outbreak in West Africa and later outbreaks in the Democratic Republic of Congo and Uganda.

However, effective coordination on the ground is still largely dependent on political will, for national governments and the global community to fund these responses and for the affected countries to lead within their own infrastructure and effect evidence-based recommendations. When strong leadership and trust is absent, proposed control measures may not be adopted, and those that are may be limited in their effectiveness. This situation is exacerbated in areas experiencing violent conflict, which can directly challenge the response and result in widespread mistrust of governmental authorities and international assistance among the affected populations. An effective response requires it to be tailored to the context of the outbreak. Trust is critical for effective community engagement; likewise, international agencies need to trust local communities and organizations to guide them on how to best operate in the local context.

The promise of clinical trials has never been more exciting than now, given new mechanisms and willingness to collaborate among multiple scientific disciplines and partners, both public and private, to combat the threat of epidemic- and pandemic-prone emerging and re-emerging infectious diseases. However, given the short window of time during which a trial must start enrolment before an outbreak ends, rigorous preparation of all the logistics is essential so that barriers such as ethical and regulatory approvals are addressed, and clinicians and laboratory staff are engaged and trained in advance. Doing this effectively entails strengthening of research capacity at local level and engaging with appropriate ethical and regulatory authorities ahead of outbreaks in countries likely to experience them [64]. Research should be integrated into clinical care during outbreaks wherever possible, as it is the foundation of evidence-based care.

Finally, the great challenge of emerging infections remains the unknown, whether it be new diseases for which the mode of transmission is unknown, and for which no known treatments or vaccines exist; to the unknown aspect of where known diseases like yellow fever may emerge next due to increased global travel and trade [65]. Strengthening country and global preparedness and developing a well-trained workforce and partners who are accustomed to collaborating with one another is essential to quickly detect, assess, report, and respond to travel-associated cases of infectious diseases and outbreaks in a timely and coordinated manner, to prevent further transmission and improve outcomes. This is the essence of global health security, and the efforts to build country IHR capacity must continue to build and maintain this security. The best efforts may not prevent new infectious diseases from occurring but will greatly mitigate the morbidity and mortality from outbreaks.Declaration of InterestWe declare no conflict of interest.

References

1. Powers AM. Risks to the Americas associated with the continued expansion of chikungunya virus. J Gen Virol. 2015;96(Pt 1):1–5. https://doi.org/10.1099/vir.0.070136-0.
2. Faria NR, Quick J, Claro IM, et al. Establishment and cryptic transmission of Zika virus in Brazil and the Americas. Nature. 2017;546(7658):406–10. https://doi.org/10.1038/nature22401.
3. Zeller H, Van Bortel W, Sudre B. Chikungunya: its history in Africa and Asia and its spread to new regions in 2013-2014. J Infect Dis. 2016;214(Suppl 5):S436–40.

4. Gubler DJ, Vasilakis N, Musso D. History and emergence of Zika virus. J Infect Dis. 2017;216(Suppl 10):S860–7. https://doi.org/10.1093/infdis/jix451.

5. Musso D, Gubler DJ. Zika Virus. Clin Microbiol Rev. 2016;29(3):487–524. https://doi.org/10.1128/CMR.00072-15.

6. Phadke VK, Bednarczyk RA, Salmon DA, Omer SB. Association between vaccine refusal and vaccine-preventable diseases in the United States: a review of measles and pertussis. JAMA. 2016;315(11):1149–58. https://doi.org/10.1001/jama.2016.1353.

7. O'Connor P, Jankovic D, Muscat M, et al. Measles and rubella elimination in the WHO region for Europe: progress and challenges. Clin Microbiol Infect. 2017;23(8):504–10. https://doi.org/10.1016/j.cmi.2017.01.003.

8. WHO. Antimicrobial resistance. https://www.who.int/news-room/fact-sheets/detail/antimicrobial-resistance. Accessed 13 Jan 2023.

9. Cohen NJ, Brown CM, Alvarado-Ramy F, et al. Travel and border health measures to prevent the international spread of Ebola. MMWR Suppl. 2016;65(Suppl 3):57–67. https://doi.org/10.15585/mmwr.su6503a9.

10. Schlagenhauf P, Weld L, Goorhuis A, et al. Travel-associated infection presenting in Europe (2008-12): an analysis of EuroTravNet longitudinal, surveillance data, and evaluation of the effect of the pre-travel consultation. Lancet Infect Dis. 2015;15(1):55–64. https://doi.org/10.1016/S1473-3099(14)71000-X.

11. Eclerle I, Briciu VT, Egönül Ö, et al. Emerging souvenirs-clinical presentation of the returning traveller with imported arbovirus infections in Europe. Clin Microbiol Infect. 2018;24(3):240–5. https://doi.org/10.1016/j.cmi.2018.01.007.

12. Findlater A, Bogoch II. Human mobility and the global spread of infectious diseases: a focus on air travel. Trends Parasitol. 2018;34:772–83. https://doi.org/10.1016/j.pt.2018.07.004.

13. Reusken CB, Ieven M, Sigfrid L, et al. Laboratory preparedness and response with a focus on arboviruses in Europe. Clin Microbiol Infect. 2018;24(3):221–8. https://doi.org/10.1016/j.cmi.2017.12.010.

14. WHO. Annex 1. International health regulations (2005), 3rd ed. Geneva: WHO Press; 2005.

15. WHO. Use of SARS-CoV-2 antigen-detection rapid diagnostic tests for COVID-19 self-testing. https://www.who.int/publications/i/item/WHO-2019-nCoV-Ag-RDTs-Self_testing-2022.1. Accessed 13 Jan 2023.

16. WHO. R&D blueprint; list of priority diseases. https://www.who.int/activities/prioritizing-diseases-for-research-and-development-in-emergency-contexts. Accessed 13 Jan 2023.

17. WHO. Laboratory task force for high threat pathogens. https://www.who.int/europe/initiatives/better-labs-for-better-health/laboratory-task-force-for-high-threat-pathogens. Accessed 15 Jan 2023.

18. SHARP. Workshop on laboratory preparedness and responsiveness held online. https://sharpja.eu/about-us/work-packages/laboratory-preparedness-and-responsiveness-wp7/#WP7. Accessed 15 Jan 2023.

19. EVD-LabNet. https://www.ecdc.europa.eu/en/about-us/partnerships-and-networks/disease-and-laboratory-networks/evd-labnet. Accessed 13 Jan 2023.

20. Bartolini B, Cruber CE, Koopmans M, et al. Laboratory management of Crimean-Congo haemorrhagic fever virus infections: perspectives from two European networks. Euro Surveill. 2019;24(5):1800093. https://doi.org/10.2807/1560-7917.

21. Cleton N, Koopmans M, Reimerink J, et al. Come fly with me: review of clinically important arboviruses for global travellers. J Clin Virol. 2012;55(3):191–203. https://doi.org/10.1016/j.jcv.2012.07.004.

22. Papa A, Kotrotsiou T, Papadopoulou E, et al. Challenges in laboratory diagnosis of acute viral central nervous system infections in the era of emerging infectious diseases: the syndromic approach. Expert Rev Anti Infect Ther. 2016;14(9):829–36.

23. Jerome H, Taylor C, Sreenu VB, et al. Metagenomic next-generation sequencing aids the diagnosis of viral infections in febrile returning travellers. J Infect. 2019;79(4):383–8. S0163-4453(19)3024207. https://doi.org/10.1016/j.jinf.2019.08.003.

24. Lesson 1: introduction to epidemiology. In: Principles of epidemiology in public health practice, 3rd ed. https://www.cdc.gov/csels/dsepd/ss1978/lesson1/section5.html. Accessed 13 Jan 2023.
25. ECDC. Tools: surveillance atlas for infectious diseases. https://www.ecdc.europa.eu/en/data-tools. Accessed 13 Jan 2023.
26. WHO. Strengthening health security by implementing the International Health Regulations. 2005. https://www.who.int/ihr/about/en/. Accessed 1 Aug 2019.
27. World Health Organization. Communicable disease surveillance and response systems: guide to monitoring and evaluating. World Health Organization. 2006. https://apps.who.int/iris/handle/10665/69331.
28. O'Shea J. Digital disease detection: a systematic review of event-based internet biosurveillance systems. Int J Med Inform. 2017;101:15–22. https://doi.org/10.1016/j.ijmedinf.2017.01.019.
29. CDC. Global Health Protection and Security: event based surveillance. https://www.cdc.gov/globalhealth/healthprotection/gddopscenter/how.html. Accessed 13 Jan 2023.
30. Taylor LH, Latham SM, Woolhouse ME. Risk factors for human disease emergence. Philos Trans R Soc Lond Ser B Biol Sci. 2001;356(1411):983–9. https://doi.org/10.1098/rstb.2001.0888.
31. Mertz D, Geraci J, Winkup J. Pregnancy as a risk factor for severe outcomes from influenza virus infection: a systematic review and meta-analysis of observational studies. Vaccine. 2017;35(4):521–8. https://doi.org/10.1016/j.vaccine.2016.12.012.
32. Mertz D, Kim TH, Johnstone J, et al. Populations at risk for severe or complicated influenza illness: systematic review and meta-analysis. BMJ. 2013;347:f5061. https://doi.org/10.1136/bmj.f5061.
33. Timen A, Koopmans M, Vossen AC, et al. Response to imported case of Marburg hemorrhagic fever, the Netherlands. Emerg Infect Dis. 2009;15(8):1171–5. https://doi.org/10.3201/eid1508.090015.
34. CDC. Imported case of Marburg hemorrhagic fever—Colorado, 2008. MMWR. 2009;58(49):1377–81.
35. Van Beneden CA, Pietz H, Kirkcaldy RD, et al. Early identification and prevention of the spread of Ebola—United States. MMWR Suppl. 2016;65(Suppl 3):75–84.
36. WHO. Emergency medical teams. https://www.who.int/emergencies/partners/emergency-medical-teams. Accessed 13 Jan 2023.
37. WHO. Health cluster. https://healthcluster.who.int/. Accessed 13 Jan 2023.
38. WHO. Humanitarian health action: questions and answers about WHO's role in humanitarian health action. https://www.who.int/news-room/questions-and-answers/item/emergencies-humanitarian-health-action.
39. WHO. Standby partners. https://www.who.int/emergencies/partners/standby-partners. Accessed 13 Jan 2023.
40. WHO. Contingency Fund for Emergencies (CFE). https://www.who.int/emergencies/funding/contingency-fund-for-emergencies. Accessed 13 Jan 2023.
41. GOARN. Global outbreak alert and response network. https://goarn.who.int/. Accessed 13 Jan 2023.
42. WHO. Annex 2. International health regulations (2005)—3rd ed. Geneva: WHO Press; 2005.
43. CDC. International health regulations. https://www.cdc.gov/globalhealth/healthprotection/ghs/ihr/index.html. Accessed 3 Jan 2023.
44. CDC. The global health security agenda. https://www.cdc.gov/globalhealth/security/ghsa-genda.htm. Accessed 13 Jan 2023.
45. WHO. IHR monitoring and evaluation framework. https://extranet.who.int/sph/ihr-monitoring-evaluation. Accessed 13 Jan 2023.
46. WHO events. https://www.who.int/news-room/events/detail/2022/04/12/default-calendar/public-hearings-regarding-a-new-international-instrument-on-pandemic-preparedness-and-response. Accessed 3 Jan 2023.
47. CEPI. Creating a world in which epidemics are no longer a threat to humanity. https://cepi.net/about/whyweexist/. Accessed 13 Jan 2023.

48. FIND. https://www.finddx.org/. Accessed 13 Jan 2023.
49. GLOPID-R. Our work. https://www.glopid-r.org/our-work/. Accessed 13 Jan 2023.
50. WHO. Democratic Republic of the Congo begins first-ever multi-drug Ebola trial. https://www.who.int/news-room/detail/26-11-2018-democratic-republic-of-the-congo-begins-first-ever-multi-drug-ebola-trial. Accessed 13 Jan 2023.
51. ALERRT. ALERRT: The African coaLition for Epidemic Research, Response and Training. https://www.alerrt.global/. Accessed 13 Jan 2023.
52. PREPARE. PREPARE: Platform for European Preparedness Against (Re-)emerging Epidemics https://www.prepare-europe.eu/. Accessed 13 Jan 2023.
53. ADVANcing Clinical Evidence in Infectious Diseases (ADVANCE-ID). https://sph.nus.edu.sg/2022/11/advancing-clinical-evidence-in-infectious-diseases-advance-id/. Accessed 3 Jan 2022.
54. Gobat N, Amuasi J, Yazdanpanah Y, Sigfid L, Davies H, Byrne J-P, et al. Advancing preparedness for clinical research during infectious disease epidemics. Eur Respir Soc. 2019;5:00227.
55. Lurie N, Manolio T, Patterson AP, Collins F, Frieden T. Research as a part of public health emergency response. Mass Med Soc. 2013;368:1251–5.
56. Rojek AM, Horby PW. Offering patients more: how the West Africa Ebola outbreak can shape innovation in therapeutic research for emerging and epidemic infections. Philos Trans R Soc B Biol Sci. 2017;372(1721):20160294.
57. National Academies of Sciences, Engineering, and Medicine. Integrating clinical research into epidemic response: the Ebola experience. 2017.
58. McLean AR, Rashan S, Tran L, Arena L, Lawal A, Maguire BJ, et al. The fragmented COVID-19 therapeutics research landscape: a living systematic review of clinical trial registrations evaluating priority pharmacological interventions. Wellcome Open Res. 2022;7(24):24.
59. Angus DC. Optimizing the trade-off between learning and doing in a pandemic. JAMA. 2020;323(19):1895–6.
60. Park JJ, Mogg R, Smith GE, Nakimuli-Mpungu E, Jehan F, Rayner CR, et al. How COVID-19 has fundamentally changed clinical research in global health. Lancet Glob Health. 2021;9(5):e711–20.
61. UK Government. Pandemic preparedness partnership report to the G7. 100 days mission to respond to future pandemic threats. 2021. https://www.gov.uk/government/publications/100-days-mission-to-respond-to-future-pandemic-threats. Accessed 15 Jan 2023.
62. UK Government Department of Health and Social Care. G7 therapeutics and vaccines clinical trials charter. 2021. https://www.gov.uk/government/publications/g7-health-ministers-meeting-june-2021-communique/g7-therapeutics-and-vaccines-clinical-trials-charter. Accessed 15 Jan 2023.
63. WHO. WHA resolution 75.8. Strengthening clinical trials to provide high-quality evidence on health interventions and to improve research quality and coordination. 2022.
64. Saxena A, Horby P, Amuasi J, et al. Ethics preparedness: facilitating ethics review during outbreaks—recommendations from an expert panel. BMC Med Ethics. 2019;20(1):29. https://doi.org/10.1186/s12910-019-0366-x.
65. Brent SE, Watts A, Cetron M, et al. International travel between global urban centres vulnerable to yellow fever transmission. Bull World Health Organ. 2018;96(5):343–354B. https://doi.org/10.2471/BLT.17.205658.

Mass Gathering and Infectious Diseases

3

Jaffar A. Al-Tawfiq and Ziad A. Memish

Abstract

In the recent years, there had been an increased travel and increased gathering of people for various activities such as religious, sports, rites, musical, and other reasons. Thus, there is a need to develop a new discipline for mass gathering medicine. There are multiple definitions for mass gatherings (MGs). One definition states that MG is as an event attended by more than 1000 individuals, and another definition requires the attendance of 25,000 people. The World Health Organization (WHO) defines MG as any event that will gather enough people to strain the public health planning and response capacities of the host community, city, or country. MG requires careful planning and surveillance. One of the most widely used surveillance strategies for monitoring communicable diseases dur-

J. A. Al-Tawfiq
Specialty Internal Medicine, Johns Hopkins Aramco Healthcare, Dhahran, Saudi Arabia

Quality and Patient Safety Department, Johns Hopkins Aramco Healthcare,
Dhahran, Saudi Arabia

Departemnt of Medicine, Indiana University School of Medicine, Indianapolis, IN, USA

Department of Medicine, Johns Hopkins University School of Medicine,
Baltimore, MD, USA
e-mail: jaffar.tawfiq@jhah.com

Z. A. Memish (✉)
College of Medicine, Alfaisal University, Riyadh, Saudi Arabia

King Saud Medical City, Riyadh, Saudi Arabia

Hubert Department of Global Health, Rollins School of Public Health, Emory University,
Atlanta, GA, USA

© The Author(s), under exclusive license to Springer Nature
Switzerland AG 2024
H. Leblebicioglu et al. (eds.), *Emerging and Re-emerging Infections in
Travellers*, https://doi.org/10.1007/978-3-031-49475-8_3

ing MG is syndromic surveillance. This strategy has been shown to be effective in early recognition, leading to rapid intervention and prevention of large outbreaks related to the spread of infectious diseases.

3.1 Introduction

In the recent years, there had been an increased travel and increased gathering of people for various activities such as religious, sports, rites, musical and other reasons. Thus, there is a need to develop a new discipline for mass gathering medicine. This new discipline of medicine was highlighted at the World Health Assembly of Ministers of Health in Geneva in May 2014 [1]. This discipline deals with identifying the risk of health hazards associated with mass gathering, developing strategies to mitigate this risk, and activities to promote safe mass gathering events. This chapter review main features, planning strategies, and prevention of infections at mass gatherings (MGs).

3.2 Definition

There are multiple definitions for mass gatherings (MGs). One definition states that mass gathering is as an event attended by more than 1000 individuals, and another definition requires the attendance of 25,000 people [2–4]. Mass gathering can be defined as the occurrence of a preplanned public events taking place for a limited period of time and attended by >25,000 people [2]. One paper refers to mass gathering as any gathering of a large numbers of people attending a focused meeting at a specific site for a finite time [5]. The World Health Organization (WHO) definition of MG is the following "as a planned or spontaneous event that gathers substantial numbers of attendees who might strain the health planning and response capacities of the host community, city, or country" [6]. Mass gatherings can be classified as spontaneous events such as large funerals and rites [4]. These events have the potential to strain public planning and response resources of the community, city or nation hosting the event [7]. These strains arise from the preparations and planning for security, transportation, housing, providing safe food and water supply and waste management and preventing the potential for communicable diseases spread.

3.3 Brief Description of Major Mass Gathering Events

There are two major types of MGs. The first is spontaneous mass gatherings such as the Pope's funeral. The second type is planned mass gatherings. These planned mass gatherings may take place at different locations (the Olympics and World Cup) or take place at the same location, such as the Hajj pilgrimage in Saudi Arabia, and Arbaeen in Iraq [8–17], and the Hindu Kumbh Mela, religious pilgrimage festival

[18–23]. The annual Hajj pilgrimage takes place in Makkah, Kingdom of Saudi Arabia, and attracts millions of pilgrims from more than 180 countries. Hajj is one of the five obligatory pillars of Islam. However, it is an obligatory duty once in a Muslim's lifetime only if he/she is able and capable of performing Hajj [15, 24]. The Hajj starts with visiting Makkah followed by specified rituals as shown in Fig. 3.1. The Hajj spans an obligatory 5 days in the twelfth month of the Islamic calendar, 8th–12th Dhu'l Hijjah [15]. Pilgrims wear simple garments (white for male pilgrims), and their activities include a series of rituals and rites together as an expression of unity, equality, and solidarity irrespective of nationality, ethnic origin, sex, and social class. Pilgrims fulfil each of the required rituals by visiting and doing prayers in a particular order at several of the holy sites in Makkah, commencing at the Ka'aba in the grand mosque. Although most pilgrims walk during the Hajj, some may use buses or trains. Disabled or elderly individuals are pushed along in wheelchairs or carried on shoulders. During the Hajj, pilgrims participate in religious activities in the holy cities of Makkah and Medina and their pilgrimage mandates sleeping in Mina where they stay in tents. Pilgrims then move to Mount Arafat devoting their time to prayer from sunrise to dusk, while staying in tents. Leaving to Muzdalifah after sunset, pilgrims gather pebbles for the Jamarat ceremony to throw at three stone pillars (symbolic of the devil) and then move on to Makkah [10] (Fig. 3.1).

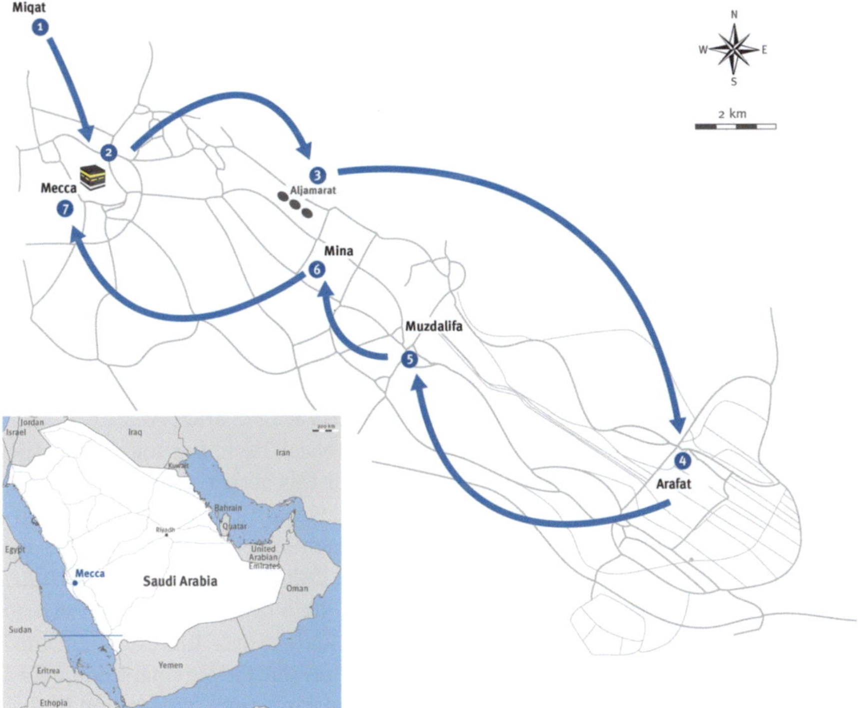

Fig. 3.1 The different stages of the Hajj

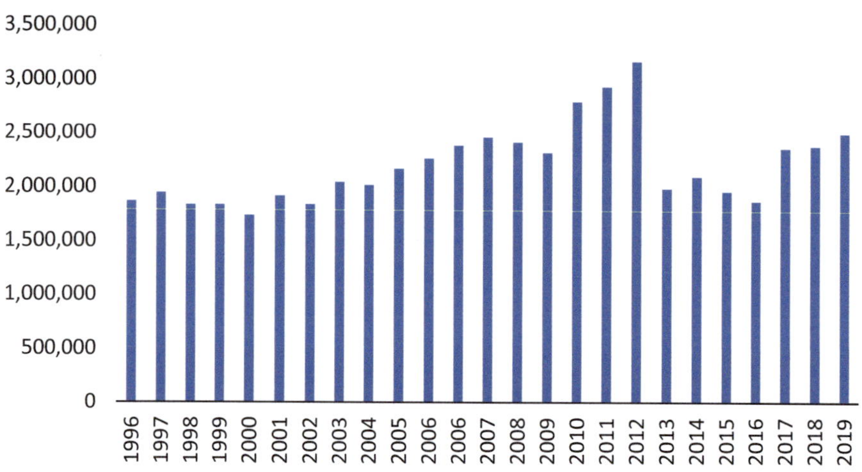

Fig. 3.2 Annual number of Hajj pilgrimage (1996–2019)

On the other hand, the Umrah is a mini-pilgrimage which can be carried out at any time of the year. However, the month of Ramadan, when Muslims perform obligatory fasting, is the busiest period for Umrah. The number of Hajj pilgrims in 2019 was 2,500,000 foreign visitors from over 180 countries, with 500,000 domestic Hajj pilgrims. The annual number of Hajj pilgrims is shown in Fig. 3.2. In contrast Umrah attracts more than six million pilgrims each year [25]. Over the last few decades there has been a significant increase in the number of external and internal pilgrims for both Hajj and Umrah. The number of Hajj pilgrims in 1920 was 58,584 and increased to 3,161,573 in 2012 [10]. Pilgrims enter Saudi Arabia through 15 ports of entry, and 94% enter through Jeddah and Medina airports, and 5% enter through 11 land ports, and 1% enter through 2 seaports [10].

Other religious mass gathering events outside of Kingdom of Saudi Arabia (KSA) include Kumbh Mela in India, Grand Magal in Senegal and Arbaeen in Iraq [26]. The Kumbh Mela is the Hindu religious pilgrimage and is considered one of the largest mass gathering [18–23]. Kumbh Mela attracts 120 million pilgrims or more for up to 2 months. This gathering takes place at one of the following rivers: the Ganga (Ganges) River (Haridwar district), Godavari River (Nasik district), Kshipra River (Ujjain district), and Sangam River (Prayag district, Allahabad) [1].

The grand magal mass gathering is an annual festival of the indigenous Senegalese Muslim brotherhood, the Mourides [27]. Each year this activity brings millions of individuals gathering in the holy city of Touba, Senegal [27]. The Arbaeen mass gathering in Iraq is an annual ceremony that commemorates the 40th day after the anniversary of Imam Hussein's martyrdom [16, 26, 28]. It is estimated that the total number of visitors was 19–22 million and most of them take part in an 80 km road walk from the city of Najaf to the city of Karbala [29]. However, this event remained relatively neglected by global public health authorities due the regional Middle East focus and frequent interruptions to attendance of pilgrims from outside Iraq [26].

3.4   Evaluating the Risk During Mass Gathering

One of the surveillance strategies used during MG events is syndromic surveillance for communicable diseases leading to early recognition, prompt application of preventative strategies, and halting outbreak development [10, 30, 31]. Such a strategy has a limited importance in countries with strong clinical and laboratory notification systems [32]. In addition, it is important to plan for the need to use postexposure prophylaxes and ensure the availability of vaccines, immunoglobulins, and antibiotics [33]. It is important to note that a preplanned mass gathering is a moving target and needs constant preparedness [7]. It needs to be highlighted that not all MG events have the same risks for developing infectious diseases outbreaks. For example, during sport events the occurrence of infectious diseases are extremely low as was seen during the Olympic Games in Atlanta in 1996 and in Sydney in 2000 where infectious diseases accounted for 1% of healthcare visits [34]. Public health emergency operations centre and emergency operations centres are critical infrastructure to deliver public health functions and to mount adequate response during emergencies [35].

3.5   Risk of Respiratory Illness

Respiratory infections, both upper and lower, due to viruses and bacteria are fairly common during MG events. The spread of respiratory infections during the annual Hajj has been studied extensively over the years and rates as high as 40–80% have been reported (depending on the diagnostic tests used) and hence is of a great concern for Hajj planners and the global public health community. The potential of dissemination of known viruses among pilgrims and newly emerging viruses with the potential spread to other countries is of great concern [11, 36, 37]. There are multiple contributing factors for the occurrence of such events and include close proximity between pilgrims, crowded accommodation, and congregation [9, 10].

There are multiple studies that systematically investigated the occurrence of respiratory infections among pilgrims performing the Hajj in Saudi Arabia [38–60]. Some of these studies were conducted prior to departure to KSA, some were done in KSA and the others were done on returning pilgrims to their home countries. The majority of reported cases were due to rhinovirus, influenza A and coronavirus 229E [61]. The average percentage of patients with specified viruses among pilgrims from different studies utilizing PCR for the detection of respiratory viruses is shown in Fig. 3.3. Outbreak of influenza was also described in the World Youth Day in Sydney, Australia, in July 2008 [44, 45, 62, 63]. During the outbreak, the following strains were identified: oseltamivir-resistant influenza A (H1N1) viruses, oseltamivir-sensitive influenza A (H1N1) viruses, influenza A (H3N2) viruses, and strains from both influenza B lineages (B/Florida/4/2006-like and B/Malaysia/2506/2004-like) [45].

In addition to common viruses, bacterial pathogens play a significant role in respiratory infections during MG events with *S. pneumoniae* and *Hemophilus*

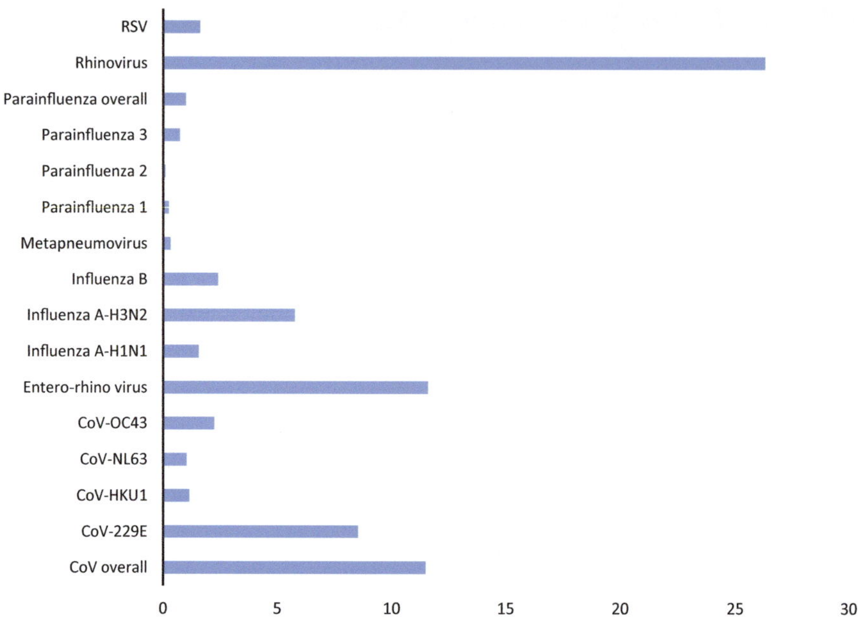

Fig. 3.3 The average percentage of patients with specified viruses among pilgrims from different studies

influenzae infections being commonly isolated among infected pilgrims [11, 12, 37, 64, 65]. The data on *S. pneumoniae* is limited and one study showed an overall carriage rate of *S. pneumoniae* in the pre- and post-Hajj of 4.4% and 7.5%, respectively [65]. The coverage of 23-valent pneumococcal polysaccharide vaccine (PPV23) and of the 7-valent pneumococcal conjugate vaccine (PCV7), PCV10, and PCV13 were 54.8%, 17.4%, 20%, and 39.1%, respectively [65].

3.6 Outbreaks of Meningococcal Disease

Meningococcal disease outbreaks have been linked to MG events over the years [8, 66–69]. The first reported meningococcal outbreak caused by *Neisseria meningitidis* serogroup A was reported in 1987 Hajj season [70–72], followed by another outbreak of meningococcal disease serogroup W135 in the year 2000 [67, 73, 74]. One of the major contributing factors was the increased prevalence of asymptomatic *N. meningitidis* carriage [8, 70]. Following the initial outbreak in 1987, mandatory vaccination for all Hajj pilgrims with bivalent AC meningococcal polysaccharide vaccine was implemented, in addition to annual vaccination campaigns for all the residents living in the Hajj areas. The vaccine recommendation was expanded to quadrivalent (A, C, Y, W135) after the 2000–2001 meningococcal outbreak due to W135 serotypes. In addition, mandatory oral ciprofloxacin prophylaxis for all pilgrims from sub-Saharan African meningitis belt, Indian subcontinent countries and all local pilgrims on completion of Hajj and prior to returning to their homes were adopted by the authorities of the Saudi Arabia [30, 64, 70, 75, 76]. Subsequent studies showed that 2.5% of pilgrims were positive for *N. meningitidis* on arrival and only 0.15% of them remained positive after the Hajj [77]. There were four studies showing no increase in the carriage rate of *N. meningitidis* after the Hajj [78–81] and one study showed a rate of 0.6% among non-paired cohort [42]. It was then decided to stop ciprofloxacin prophylaxis for the Indian subcontinent and local pilgrims on completion of Hajj.

Although, the majority of the literature on mass gathering and *N. meningitidis* comes from the Hajj pilgrimage, there are few studies of the transmission of *N. meningitidis* during other mass gathering. In one study, the carrier rate of *N. meningitidis* was 8% among 1020 Swedish teenagers who participated in the Jamboree during the 23rd World Scout Jamboree in 2015 [82]. During that event there was six cases of meningococcal disease due to *N. meningitidis* [19, 82, 83]. There were four cases of meningococcal disease among rugby match spectators in United Kingdom [84].

3.7 Middle East Respiratory Syndrome Coronavirus (MERS-CoV) During Mass Gatherings

Middle East Respiratory Syndrome Coronavirus (MERS-CoV) emerged in 2012 in KSA and this virus was of a major concern regarding the possibility of the development of pandemic. In fact, the 2012 Hajj season was only few weeks from the description of the first MERS-CoV case. Multiple studies were conducted by health authorities in KSA to determine the possibility of MERS-CoV spread from the Hajj and no transmission of MERS-CoV was documented during the Hajj seasons [42, 54, 55, 81, 85–98]. However, very infrequently MERS-CoV cases were reported among pilgrims performing Umrah with history of contact with camels in Makkah [99, 100].

3.8 Risk of Severe Acute Respiratory Syndrome Coronavirus 2 (SARS-CoV-2) During Mass Gatherings

Since the emergence of the SARS-CoV-2 in late 2019 and its pandemic effect in 2020, there had been concerns about inadequacies of all global public health systems and the global preparedness [101]. The World Health Organization (WHO) published interim guidelines for the planning for mass gatherings at the time of the current COVID-19 pandemic [102] and recommendations to deal with such events [103, 104]. However, due to the global lockdown measures and travel restrictions had to lead to either delay or cancellation of mass gathering events [105] such as the 2020 Olympic Games from 2020 to 2021 [106]. The 2020 Hajj was a symbolic one restricted to a limited number of local Saudi pilgrims observing strict infection control measures including hand hygiene and social distancing performing religious rites [101]. However, with the ease of restrictions globally the 2021 and 2022 Hajj pilgrims were escalated with appropriate preventive measures including the requirements of COVID-19 vaccination [107]. One study during the escalation of the Hajj pilgrimage in 2021 showed that non-mandatory pre- and post-Hajj PCR test was positive in 41 (0.07%) of 58,428 pilgrims [108].

3.9 Measles Outbreaks During Mass Gatherings

Although, there are no outbreaks of measles during the Hajj pilgrimage. Measles outbreaks were reported in other MGs [109] and one such outbreak occurred among the international youth sporting event in the United States of America and resulted in multiple cases in eight states [110], measles among attendees of a church gathering in the 2010 Taizé festival in France [111, 112]. Another outbreak was described among attendees of a Church meeting in Indiana, USA, in 2005 [111]. In 1991, 26 cases of measles were linked to the International Special Olympics Games in the Minneapolis-St. Paul metropolitan [113]. In 2007, there were 7 epidemiologically linked cases of measles to international youth sporting event in Pennsylvania, Michigan, and Texas [114].

3.10 Risk of Diarrhoeal Disease

One of the earliest mass gathering-associated disease was the 1817–1824 Asia cholera pandemic [115] and was associated with Kumbh Mela. Many studies showed increased bacterial load in the river water associated with the act of defecation and urination at the time of mass gathering [19, 83, 116]. The 2013 Kumbh Mela was associated with an incidence of 5% of diarrhoeal diseases [115, 117]. In 2005, a large outbreak of cholera occurred in the Senegal and there were 27,000 cases and the outbreak was thought to be linked to the 2005 Grand Magal de Touba mass gathering [118].

In the Hajj pilgrimage, a study of 117 pilgrims showed that the acquisition of enteropathogenic *Escherichia coli* (EPEC), enteroaggregative *E. coli* (EAEC), and Shiga-like toxin-producing *E. coli* were 29.9%, 10.2%, and 6.5% pilgrims, respectively [119]. There are multiple studies addressing the occurrence of diarrhoeal disease among pilgrims [120–126]. Hajj-diarrhoeal disease is usually associated with one bacterial agent such as *Salmonella* spp., Shigella/enteroinvasive *Escherichia coli* and enterotoxigenic *E. coli* [1]. In the Riga Cup 2015 junior ice-hockey competition, there was a total of 214 salmonellosis cases in seven countries [127].

3.11 Risk of Spread of Antimicrobial Resistance

One of the concern with globalization is the possibility the spread of antimicrobial resistant (AMR) bacteria during mass gatherings [9, 10, 17, 30, 64, 93, 128, 129]. In the 2015 Kumbh Mela mass gathering, there was a significant increase in *blaNDM-1* gene carrying bacteria in the bank of the Ganges [115]. In addition, a novel antibiotic-resistant *Corynebacterium godavarianum* was isolated from the Godavari River [83].

There are few studies addressing the prevalence of multi-drug resistant organisms (MDRO) among attendees of mass gatherings. One study showed that the prevalence of the bla_{CTX-M} gene in rectal samples was 10% and 33% in the pre-Hajj and post-Hajj [130]. In the same study, there was an increase in the number of pilgrims harbouring ceftriaxone and ticarcillin-clavulanic acid resistant *E. coli* [130]. The rate of acquisition of *A. baumannii* with bla_{OXA-72} and *E. coli* with bla_{NDM-5} in a French cohort travelling to the 2014 Hajj [131]. During the 2014–2015 Hajj, the bla_{CTX-M} gene in *E. coli* isolates was reported among 47% of pilgrims attending hospitals for urinary tract infections [132]. Imipenem-resistant bacteria were also reported during the 2014–2015 Hajj in *A. baumannii*, *E. coli*, *K. pneumoniae*, and *P. aeruginosa* [131, 133, 134].

Salmonella enterica which were resistant to ceftriaxone, gentamycin and colistin were isolated from two pilgrims [135]. Screening for the *mcr-1* plasmid-mediated colistin resistance gene was conducted in 2013 and 2014, and showed a prevalence of 1–2% before-Hajj and 9% after-Hajj and *E. coli* and *K. pneumoniae* were isolated from pilgrims carrying the *mcr-1* genes [136].

3.12 Travel Advice for Those Attending Mass Gatherings

Each year the Saudi Ministry of Health publishes the Hajj requirements for each Hajj season and such previous recommendations were published [9, 30]. There are mandatory vaccines such as meningococcal and poliomyelitis vaccines and other recommended vaccines such as influenza vaccine. Vaccination is an effective method for the reduction of the risk of respiratory tract infection [1, 11, 40, 41].

It is important that attendees of mass gathering adhere to personal hygiene, cough etiquette and hand hygiene to prevent respiratory tract infections [11, 30]. Compliance with hand hygiene was 77.4%, use of disposable handkerchiefs was 89.8%, and use of face masks was 79.6% in one study [124]. Although, other practices such as social distancing and contact avoidance were associated reduced risk of respiratory illness, these practices are difficult to implement in mass gathering events [11].

To avoid diarrhoeal disease, it is important to observe factors leading to inadequate standards of food hygiene, shortage of water, the presence of asymptomatic carriers of pathogenic agents, and poorly stored food [64]. It is important also to have a thorough inspections of the quality of drinking water, inspection of water treatment plants, examinations of water supply sources and tanks as being done during the Hajj pilgrimage [137]. A detailed inspection of food preparation workers at various sites should be a priority for public health authority [10]. It is advisable that attendees of mass gathering also look into ways for prevention, oral rehydration strategies, antimotility agents, and emergency antibiotic use for travellers' diarrhoea.

Box Key Websites for Travellers and Healthcare Workers
1. Saudi Hajj: https://www.saudiembassy.net/hajj
2. ECDC Risk assessment. https://ecdc.europa.eu/sites/portal/files/documents/risks-diseases-hajj-saudi-arabia-rapid-risk-assessment-24-august-2018.pdf
3. CDC and Hajj: https://wwwnc.cdc.gov/travel/yellowbook/2018/select-destinations/saudi-arabia-hajj-umrah-pilgrimage

Acknowledgments None.

Declarations of Conflict of Interest None.

References

1. Memish ZA, Zumla A, McCloskey B, Heymann D, Al Rabeeah AA, Barbeschi M, et al. Mass gatherings medicine: international cooperation and progress. Lancet. 2014;383:2030–2. https://doi.org/10.1016/S0140-6736(14)60225-7.
2. Arbon P, Bridgewater FH, Smith C. Mass gathering medicine: a predictive model for patient presentation and transport rates. Prehosp Disaster Med. 2001;16:150–8.
3. Michael JA, Barbera JA. Mass gathering medical care: a twenty-five year review. Prehosp Disaster Med. 1997;12:305–12.
4. Al-Tawfiq JA, Memish ZA. Mass gathering medicine: a leisure or necessity? Int J Clin Pract. 2012;66:530–2. https://doi.org/10.1111/j.1742-1241.2012.02923.x.
5. Memish ZA, Stephens GM, Steffen R, Ahmed QA. Emergence of medicine for mass gatherings: lessons from the Hajj. Lancet Infect Dis. 2012;12:56–65. https://doi.org/10.1016/S1473-3099(11)70337-1.
6. WHO. What is WHO's role in mass gatherings? WHO. 2016. https://www.who.int/features/qa/mass-gatherings/en/. Accessed 19 June 2019.
7. Elachola H, Gozzer E, Zhuo J, Sow S, Kattan R, Mimesh SA, et al. Mass gatherings: a one-stop opportunity to complement global disease surveillance. J Health Specialties. 2016;4:178. https://doi.org/10.4103/2468-6360.186487.
8. Al-Tawfiq JA, Clark TA, Memish ZA. Meningococcal disease: the organism, clinical presentation, and worldwide epidemiology. J Travel Med. 2010;17:3–8. https://doi.org/10.1111/j.1708-8305.2010.00448.x.
9. Al-Tawfiq JA, Gautret P, Memish ZA. Expected immunizations and health protection for Hajj and Umrah 2018—an overview. Travel Med Infect Dis. 2017;19:2–7. https://doi.org/10.1016/j.tmaid.2017.10.005.
10. Memish ZA, Zumla A, Alhakeem RF, Assiri A, Turkestani A, Al Harby KD, et al. Hajj: infectious disease surveillance and control. Lancet. 2014;383:2073–82. https://doi.org/10.1016/S0140-6736(14)60381-0.
11. Al-Tawfiq JAJA, Zumla A, Memish ZAZA. Respiratory tract infections during the annual Hajj: potential risks and mitigation strategies. Curr Opin Pulm Med. 2013;19:192–7. https://doi.org/10.1097/MCP.0b013e32835f1ae8.
12. Al-Tawfiq JA, Gautret P, Benkouiten S, Memish ZA. Mass gatherings and the spread of respiratory infections. Lessons from the Hajj. Ann Am Thorac Soc. 2016;13:759–65. https://doi.org/10.1513/AnnalsATS.201511-772FR.

13. Zumla A, Mwaba P, Bates M, Al-Tawfiq JA, Maeurer M, Memish ZA. The Hajj pilgrimage and surveillance for Middle East respiratory syndrome coronavirus in pilgrims from African countries. Trop Med Int Health. 2014;19:838–40. https://doi.org/10.1111/tmi.12318.

14. Gautret P, Benkouiten S, Al-Tawfiq JA, Memish ZA. The spectrum of respiratory pathogens among returning Hajj pilgrims: myths and reality. Int J Infect Dis. 2016;47:83–5. https://doi.org/10.1016/j.ijid.2016.01.013.

15. Memish ZA, Al-Tawfiq JA, Al-Rabeeah AA. Hajj: preparations underway. Lancet Glob Heal. 2013;1(6):e331. https://doi.org/10.1016/S2214-109X(13)70079-2.

16. Karampourian A, Ghomian Z, Khorasani-Zavareh D. Exploring challenges of health system preparedness for communicable diseases in Arbaeen mass gathering: a qualitative study. F1000Res. 2018;7:1448. https://doi.org/10.12688/f1000research.15290.1.

17. Gautret P. Influenza risk at Muslim pilgrimages in Iraq and Saudi Arabia. Travel Med Infect Dis. 2018;21:1–2. https://doi.org/10.1016/j.tmaid.2017.10.016.

18. Barnett I, Khanna T, Onnela J-P. Social and spatial clustering of people at humanity's largest gathering. PLoS One. 2016;11:e0156794. https://doi.org/10.1371/journal.pone.0156794.

19. Jani K, Dhotre D, Bandal J, Shouche Y, Suryavanshi M, Rale V, et al. World's largest mass bathing event influences the bacterial communities of Godavari, a Holy River of India. Microb Ecol. 2018;76:706–18. https://doi.org/10.1007/s00248-018-1169-1.

20. Greenough PG. The Kumbh Mela stampede: disaster preparedness must bridge jurisdictions. BMJ. 2013;346:f3254. https://doi.org/10.1136/bmj.f3254.

21. Sridhar S, Gautret P, Brouqui P. A comprehensive review of the Kumbh Mela: identifying risks for spread of infectious diseases. Clin Microbiol Infect. 2015;21:128–33. https://doi.org/10.1016/j.cmi.2014.11.021.

22. Baranwal A, Anand A, Singh R, Deka M, Paul A, Borgohain S, et al. Managing the Earth's biggest mass gathering event and WASH conditions: Maha Kumbh Mela (India). PLoS Curr. 2015;7. https://doi.org/10.1371/currents.dis.e8b3053f40e774e7e3fdbe1bb50a130d.

23. Cariappa MP, Singh BP, Mahen A, Bansal AS. Kumbh Mela 2013: healthcare for the millions. Med J Armed Forces India. 2015;71:278–81. https://doi.org/10.1016/j.mjafi.2014.08.001.

24. Gatrad AR, Sheikh A. Hajj: journey of a lifetime. BMJ. 2005;330:133–7. https://doi.org/10.1136/bmj.330.7483.133.

25. Benkouiten S, Al-Tawfiq JA, Memish ZA, Albarrak A, Gautret P. Clinical respiratory infections and pneumonia during the Hajj pilgrimage: a systematic review. Travel Med Infect Dis. 2019;28:15–26. https://doi.org/10.1016/j.tmaid.2018.12.002.

26. Shafi S, Azhar E, Al-Abri S, Sharma A, Merali N, Al-Tawfiq JA, et al. Infectious diseases threats at the Arba'een—a neglected but one of the largest annually recurring mass gathering religious events. Int J Infect Dis. 2022;123:210–1. https://doi.org/10.1016/J.IJID.2022.09.010.

27. Sokhna C, Mboup BM, Sow PG, Camara G, Dieng M, Sylla M, et al. Communicable and non-communicable disease risks at the Grand Magal of Touba: the largest mass gathering in Senegal. Travel Med Infect Dis. 2017;19:56–60. https://doi.org/10.1016/j.tmaid.2017.08.005.

28. Al-Lami F, Al-Fatlawi A, Bloland P, Nawwar A, Jetheer A, Hantoosh H, et al. Pattern of morbidity and mortality in Karbala hospitals during Ashura mass gathering at Karbala, Iraq, 2010. East Mediterr Health J. 2013;19 Suppl 2:S13–8.

29. Taher A, Abo-ghniem TN, Albujeer ANN, Almahafdha A, Khoshnevisan M-H. Oral hygiene and mass gathering of Iraqi and nonIraqi visitors in Arbaeen; a random sample survey for 3500 visitor. Res Rev J Dent Sci. 2017;5:92–5.

30. Al-Tawfiq JA, Memish ZA. Mass gathering medicine: 2014 Hajj and Umra preparation as a leading example. Int J Infect Dis. 2014;27:26–31. https://doi.org/10.1016/j.ijid.2014.07.001.

31. Centers for Disease Control and Prevention (CDC). Surveillance for early detection of disease outbreaks at an outdoor mass gathering-Virginia, 2005. MMWR Morb Mortal Wkly Rep. 2006;55:71–4.

32. Khan K, Freifeld CC, Wang J, Mekaru SR, Kossowsky D, Sonricker AL, et al. Preparing for infectious disease threats at mass gatherings: the case of the Vancouver 2010 Olympic winter games. CMAJ. 2010;182:579–83. https://doi.org/10.1503/cmaj.100093.

33. Weiss BP, Mascola L, Fannin SL. Public health at the 1984 summer Olympics: the Los Angeles County experience. Am J Public Health. 1988;78:686–8. https://doi.org/10.2105/AJPH.78.6.686.
34. Al-Tawfiq JA, Memish ZA. Mass gatherings and infectious diseases. Prevention, detection, and control. Infect Dis Clin North Am. 2012;26:725–37. https://doi.org/10.1016/j.idc.2012.05.005.
35. Elachola H, Al-Tawfiq JA, Turkestani A, Memish ZA. Public health emergency operations center—a critical component of mass gatherings management infrastructure. J Infect Dev Ctries. 2016;10:785–90. https://doi.org/10.3855/jidc.8332.
36. Abubakar I, Gautret P, Brunette GW, Blumberg L, Johnson D, Poumerol G, et al. Global perspectives for prevention of infectious diseases associated with mass gatherings. Lancet Infect Dis. 2012;12:66–74. https://doi.org/10.1016/S1473-3099(11)70246-8.
37. Gautret P, Benkouiten S, Al-Tawfiq JA, Memish ZA. Hajj-associated viral respiratory infections: a systematic review. Travel Med Infect Dis. 2016;14:92–109. https://doi.org/10.1016/j.tmaid.2015.12.008.
38. Alherabi AZ. Impact of pH1N1 influenza A infections on the otolaryngology, head and neck clinic during Hajj, 2009. Saudi Med J. 2011;32:933–8.
39. Kraaij-Dirkzwager M, Timen A, Dirksen K, Gelinck L, Leyten E, Groeneveld P, et al. Middle East respiratory syndrome coronavirus (MERS-CoV) infections in two returning travellers in the Netherlands, May 2014. Euro Surveill. 2014;19:20817.
40. Haworth E, Barasheed O, Memish ZA, Rashid H, Booy R. Prevention of influenza at Hajj: applications for mass gatherings. J R Soc Med. 2013;106:215–23. https://doi.org/10.1258/jrsm.2012.120170.
41. Razavi SM, Salamati P. Prevention of influenza at Hajj: applications for mass gatherings. J R Soc Med. 2013;106:386. https://doi.org/10.1177/0141076813504327.
42. Memish ZA, Assiri A, Turkestani A, Yezli S, Al Masri M, Charrel R, et al. Mass gathering and globalization of respiratory pathogens during the 2013 Hajj. Clin Microbiol Infect. 2015;21(571):e1–8. https://doi.org/10.1016/j.cmi.2015.02.008.
43. Gundlapalli AV, Rubin MA, Samore MH, Lopansri B, Lahey T, McGuire HL, et al. Influenza, Winter Olympiad, 2002. Emerg Infect Dis. 2006;12:144–6. https://doi.org/10.3201/eid1201.050645.
44. van Hal SJ, Foo H, Blyth CC, McPhie K, Armstrong P, Sintchenko V, et al. Influenza outbreak during Sydney World Youth Day 2008: the utility of laboratory testing and case definitions on mass gathering outbreak containment. PLoS One. 2009;4:e6620. https://doi.org/10.1371/journal.pone.0006620.
45. Blyth CC, Foo H, van Hal SJ, Hurt AC, Barr IG, McPhie K, et al. Influenza outbreaks during world youth day 2008 mass gathering. Emerg Infect Dis. 2010;16:809–15. https://doi.org/10.3201/eid1605.091136.
46. Gautret P, Parola P, Brouqui P. Relative risk for influenza like illness in French Hajj pilgrims compared to non-Hajj attending controls during the 2009 influenza pandemic. Travel Med Infect Dis. 2013;11:95–7. https://doi.org/10.1016/j.tmaid.2013.03.003.
47. Ziyaeyan M, Alborzi A, Jamalidoust M, Moeini M, Pouladfar GR, Pourabbas B, et al. Pandemic 2009 influenza A (H1N1) infection among 2009 Hajj pilgrims from southern Iran: a real-time RT-PCR-based study. Influenza Other Respir Viruses. 2012;6:e80–4. https://doi.org/10.1111/j.1750-2659.2012.00381.x.
48. Lim HC, Cutter J, Lim WK, Ee A, Wong YC, Tay BK. The influenza A (H1N1-2009) experience at the inaugural Asian Youth Games Singapore 2009: mass gathering during a developing pandemic. Br J Sports Med. 2010;44:528–32. https://doi.org/10.1136/bjsm.2009.069831.
49. Botelho-Nevers E, Gautret P, Benarous L, Charrel R, Felkai P, Parola P. Travel-related influenza A/H1N1 infection at a rock festival in Hungary: one virus may hide another one. J Travel Med. 2010;17:197–8. https://doi.org/10.1111/j.1708-8305.2010.00410.x.
50. Mandourah Y, Al-Radi A, Ocheltree AH, Ocheltree SR, Fowler RA. Clinical and temporal patterns of severe pneumonia causing critical illness during Hajj. BMC Infect Dis. 2012;12:117. https://doi.org/10.1186/1471-2334-12-117.

51. Shi P, Keskinocak P, Swann JL, Lee BY. The impact of mass gatherings and holiday traveling on the course of an influenza pandemic: a computational model. BMC Public Health. 2010;10:778. https://doi.org/10.1186/1471-2458-10-778.
52. Ishola DA, Phin N. Could influenza transmission be reduced by restricting mass gatherings? Towards an evidence-based policy framework. J Epidemiol Glob Health. 2011;1:33–60. https://doi.org/10.1016/j.jegh.2011.06.004.
53. Yavarian J, Shafiei Jandaghi NZ, Naseri M, Hemmati P, Dadras M, Gouya MM, et al. Influenza virus but not MERS coronavirus circulation in Iran, 2013–2016: comparison between pilgrims and general population. Travel Med Infect Dis. 2017;21:51. https://doi.org/10.1016/j.tmaid.2017.10.007.
54. Kandeel A, Deming M, Elkreem EA, El-Refay S, Afifi S, Abukela M, et al. Pandemic (H1N1) 2009 and Hajj pilgrims who received predeparture vaccination, Egypt. Emerg Infect Dis. 2011;17:1266–8. https://doi.org/10.3201/eid1707.101484.
55. Rashid H, Shafi S, Haworth E, El Bashir H, Memish ZA, Sudhanva M, et al. Viral respiratory infections at the Hajj: comparison between UK and Saudi pilgrims. Clin Microbiol Infect. 2008;14:569–74. https://doi.org/10.1111/j.1469-0691.2008.01987.x.
56. Rashid H, Shafi S, Booy R, El Bashir H, Ali K, Zambon M, et al. Influenza and respiratory syncytial virus infections in British Hajj pilgrims. Emerg Health Threats J. 2008;1:e2. https://doi.org/10.3134/ehtj.08.002.
57. El-Sheikh SM, El-Assouli SM, Mohammed KA, Albar M. Bacteria and viruses that cause respiratory tract infections during the pilgrimage (Haj) season in Makkah, Saudi Arabia. Trop Med Int Health. 1998;3:205–9.
58. Memish ZA, Assiri AM, Hussain R, Alomar I, Stephens G. Detection of respiratory viruses among pilgrims in Saudi Arabia during the time of a declared influenza A(H1N1) pandemic. J Travel Med. 2012;19:15–21. https://doi.org/10.1111/j.1708-8305.2011.00575.x.
59. Khan K, Memish ZA, Chabbra A, Liauw J, Hu W, Janes DA, et al. Global public health implications of a mass gathering in Mecca, Saudi Arabia during the midst of an influenza pandemic. J Travel Med. 2010;17:75–81. https://doi.org/10.1111/j.1708-8305.2010.00397.x.
60. Ashshi A, Azhar E, Johargy A, Asghar A, Momenah A, Turkestani A, et al. Demographic distribution and transmission potential of influenza A and 2009 pandemic influenza A H1N1 in pilgrims. J Infect Dev Ctries. 2014;8:1169–75.
61. Al-Tawfiq JA, Benkouiten S, Memish ZA. A systematic review of emerging respiratory viruses at the Hajj and possible coinfection with Streptococcus pneumoniae. Travel Med Infect Dis. 2018;23:6–13. https://doi.org/10.1016/j.tmaid.2018.04.007.
62. Foo H, Blyth CC, van Hal S, McPhie K, Ratnamohan M, Fennell M, et al. Laboratory test performance in young adults during influenza outbreaks at World Youth Day 2008. J Clin Virol. 2009;46:384–6. https://doi.org/10.1016/j.jcv.2009.09.019.
63. Fizzell J, Armstrong PK. Blessings in disguise: public health emergency preparedness for World Youth Day 2008. Med J Aust. 2008;189:633–6.
64. Al-Tawfiq JA, Memish ZA. The Hajj: updated health hazards and current recommendations for 2012. Euro Surveill. 2012;17:20295.
65. Memish ZA, Al-Tawfiq JA, Almasri M, Akkad N, Yezli S, Turkestani A, et al. A cohort study of the impact and acquisition of nasopharyngeal carriage of Streptococcus pneumoniae during the Hajj. Travel Med Infect Dis. 2016;14:242–7. https://doi.org/10.1016/j.tmaid.2016.05.001.
66. Lucidarme J, Scott KJ, Ure R, Smith A, Lindsay D, Stenmark B, et al. An international invasive meningococcal disease outbreak due to a novel and rapidly expanding serogroup W strain, Scotland and Sweden, July to August 2015. Euro Surveill. 2016;21:30395. https://doi.org/10.2807/1560-7917.ES.2016.21.45.30395.
67. Wilder-Smith A, Goh KT, Barkham T, Paton NI. Hajj-associated outbreak strain of Neisseria meningitidis serogroup W135: estimates of the attack rate in a defined population and the risk of invasive disease developing in carriers. Clin Infect Dis. 2003;36:679–83. https://doi.org/10.1086/367858.

68. Aguilera J-F, Perrocheau A, Meffre C, Hahné S, W135 Working Group. Outbreak of serogroup W135 meningococcal disease after the Hajj pilgrimage, Europe, 2000. Emerg Infect Dis. 2002;8:761–7. https://doi.org/10.3201/eid0805.010422.
69. Dull PM, Abdelwahab J, Sacchi CT, Becker M, Noble CA, Barnett GA, et al. *Neisseria meningitidis* serogroup W-135 carriage among US travelers to the 2001 Hajj. J Infect Dis. 2005;191:33–9. https://doi.org/10.1086/425927.
70. al-Gahtani YM, el Bushra HE, al-Qarawi SM, al-Zubaidi AA, Fontaine RE. Epidemiological investigation of an outbreak of meningococcal meningitis in Makkah (Mecca), Saudi Arabia, 1992. Epidemiol Infect. 1995;115:399–409.
71. Moore PS, Reeves MW, Schwartz B, Gellin BG, Broome CV. Intercontinental spread of an epidemic group A Neisseria meningitidis strain. Lancet. 1989;2:260–3.
72. Novelli VM, Lewis RG, Dawood ST. Epidemic group A meningococcal disease in Haj pilgrims. Lancet. 1987;2:863.
73. Lingappa JR, Al-Rabeah AM, Hajjeh R, Mustafa T, Fatani A, Al-Bassam T, et al. Serogroup W-135 meningococcal disease during the Hajj, 2000. Emerg Infect Dis. 2003;9:665–71. https://doi.org/10.3201/eid0906.020565.
74. Taha M-K, Giorgini D, Ducos-Galand M, Alonso J-M. Continuing diversification of Neisseria meningitidis W135 as a primary cause of meningococcal disease after emergence of the serogroup in 2000. J Clin Microbiol. 2004;42:4158–63. https://doi.org/10.1128/JCM.42.9.4158-4163.2004.
75. Memish ZA. Meningococcal disease and travel. Clin Infect Dis. 2002;34:84–90. https://doi.org/10.1086/323403.
76. Shibl A, Tufenkeji H, Khalil M, Memish Z, Meningococcal Leadership Forum (MLF) Expert Group. Consensus recommendation for meningococcal disease prevention for Hajj and Umra pilgrimage/travel medicine. East Mediterr Health J. 2013;19:389–92.
77. Memish ZA, Al-Tawfiq JA, Almasri M, Azhar EI, Yasir M, Al-Saeed MS, et al. Neisseria meningitidis nasopharyngeal carriage during the Hajj: a cohort study evaluating the need for ciprofloxacin prophylaxis. Vaccine. 2017;35:2473–8. https://doi.org/10.1016/j.vaccine.2017.03.027.
78. Alborzi A, Oskoee S, Pourabbas B, Alborzi S, Astaneh B, Gooya MM, et al. Meningococcal carrier rate before and after hajj pilgrimage: effect of single dose ciprofloxacin on carriage. East Mediterr Health J. 2008;14:277–82.
79. Wilder-Smith A, Barkham TMS, Chew SK, Paton NI. Absence of Neisseria meningitidis W-135 electrophoretic type 37 during the Hajj, 2002. Emerg Infect Dis. 2003;9:734–7. https://doi.org/10.3201/eid0906.020725.
80. Wilder-Smith A, Barkham TMS, Earnest A, Paton NI. Acquisition of W135 meningococcal carriage in Hajj pilgrims and transmission to household contacts: prospective study. BMJ. 2002;325:365–6.
81. Benkouiten S, Charrel R, Belhouchat K, Drali T, Nougairede A, Salez N, et al. Respiratory viruses and bacteria among pilgrims during the 2013 Hajj. Emerg Infect Dis. 2014;20:1821–7. https://doi.org/10.3201/eid2011.140600.
82. Jacobsson S, Stenmark B, Hedberg ST, Mölling P, Fredlund H. Neisseria meningitidis carriage in Swedish teenagers associated with the serogroup W outbreak at the World Scout Jamboree, Japan 2015. APMIS. 2018;126:337–41. https://doi.org/10.1111/apm.12819.
83. Jani K, Khare K, Senik S, Karodi P, Vemuluri VR, Bandal J, et al. Corynebacterium godavarianum sp. nov., isolated from the Godavari river, India. Int J Syst Evol Microbiol. 2018;68:241–7. https://doi.org/10.1099/ijsem.0.002491.
84. Orr H, Kaczmarski E, Sarangi J, Pankhania B, Stuart J, Outbreak Investigation Team. Cluster of meningococcal disease in rugby match spectators. Commun Dis Public Health. 2001;4:316–8.
85. Refaey S, Amin MM, Roguski K, Azziz-Baumgartner E, Uyeki TM, Labib M, et al. Cross-sectional survey and surveillance for influenza viruses and MERS-CoV among Egyptian pil-

grims returning from Hajj during 2012-2015. Influenza Other Respir Viruses. 2017;11:57–60. https://doi.org/10.1111/irv.12429.

86. Atabani SF, Wilson S, Overton-Lewis C, Workman J, Kidd IM, Petersen E, et al. Active screening and surveillance in the United Kingdom for Middle East respiratory syndrome coronavirus in returning travellers and pilgrims from the Middle East: a prospective descriptive study for the period 2013–2015. Int J Infect Dis. 2016;47:10–4. https://doi.org/10.1016/j.ijid.2016.04.016.

87. ProMed. Novel coronavirus—Eastern Mediterranean (03): Saudi comment, 2013. http://promedmail.org/post/20130326.1603038.

88. Aberle JH, Popow-Kraupp T, Kreidl P, Laferl H, Heinz FX, Aberle SW. Influenza A and B viruses but not MERS-CoV in Hajj pilgrims, Austria, 2014. Emerg Infect Dis. 2015;21:726–7. https://doi.org/10.3201/eid2104.141745.

89. Griffiths K, Charrel R, Lagier J-C, Nougairede A, Simon F, Parola P, et al. Infections in symptomatic travelers returning from the Arabian peninsula to France: a retrospective cross-sectional study. Travel Med Infect Dis. 2016;14:414–6. https://doi.org/10.1016/j.tmaid.2016.05.002.

90. Ma X, Liu F, Liu L, Zhang L, Lu M, Abudukadeer A, et al. No MERS-CoV but positive influenza viruses in returning Hajj pilgrims, China, 2013–2015. BMC Infect Dis. 2017;17:715. https://doi.org/10.1186/s12879-017-2791-0.

91. Al-Abdallat MM, Rha B, Alqasrawi S, Payne DC, Iblan I, Binder AM, et al. Acute respiratory infections among returning Hajj pilgrims—Jordan, 2014. J Clin Virol. 2017;89:34–7. https://doi.org/10.1016/j.jcv.2017.01.010.

92. Koul PA, Mir H, Saha S, Chadha MS, Potdar V, Widdowson M-A, et al. Influenza not MERS CoV among returning Hajj and Umrah pilgrims with respiratory illness, Kashmir, north India, 2014–15. Travel Med Infect Dis. 2017;15:45–7. https://doi.org/10.1016/j.tmaid.2016.12.002.

93. Al-Tawfiq JA, Smallwood CAH, Arbuthnott KG, Malik MSK, Barbeschi M, Memish ZA. Emerging respiratory and novel coronavirus 2012 infections and mass gatherings. East Mediterr Health J. 2013;19:48–54. https://doi.org/10.26719/2013.19.supp1.s48.

94. Gautret P, Charrel R, Belhouchat K, Drali T, Benkouiten S, Nougairede A, et al. Lack of nasal carriage of novel corona virus (HCoV-EMC) in French Hajj pilgrims returning from the Hajj 2012, despite a high rate of respiratory symptoms. Clin Microbiol Infect. 2013;19:E315–7. https://doi.org/10.1111/1469-0691.12174.

95. Barasheed O, Rashid H, Alfelali M, Tashani M, Azeem M, Bokhary H, et al. Viral respiratory infections among Hajj pilgrims in 2013. Virol Sin. 2014;29:364–71. https://doi.org/10.1007/s12250-014-3507-x.

96. Baharoon S, Al-Jahdali H, Al Hashmi J, Memish ZA, Ahmed QA. Severe sepsis and septic shock at the Hajj: etiologies and outcomes. Travel Med Infect Dis. 2009;7:247–52. https://doi.org/10.1016/j.tmaid.2008.09.002.

97. Memish ZA, Assiri A, Almasri M, Alhakeem RF, Turkestani A, Al Rabeeah AA, et al. Prevalence of MERS-CoV nasal carriage and compliance with the Saudi health recommendations among pilgrims attending the 2013 Hajj. J Infect Dis. 2014;210:1067–72. https://doi.org/10.1093/infdis/jiu150.

98. Annan A, Owusu M, Marfo KS, Larbi R, Sarpong FN, Adu-Sarkodie Y, et al. High prevalence of common respiratory viruses and no evidence of Middle East respiratory syndrome coronavirus in Hajj pilgrims returning to Ghana, 2013. Trop Med Int Health. 2015;20:807–12. https://doi.org/10.1111/tmi.12482.

99. Sridhar S, Brouqui P, Parola P, Gautret P. Imported cases of Middle East respiratory syndrome: an update. Travel Med Infect Dis. 2015;13:106–9. https://doi.org/10.1016/j.tmaid.2014.11.006.

100. Al-Tawfiq JA, Zumla A, Memish ZA. Travel implications of emerging coronaviruses: SARS and MERS-CoV. Travel Med Infect Dis. 2014;12:422–8. https://doi.org/10.1016/j.tmaid.2014.06.007.

101. Al-Tawfiq JA, El-Kafrawy SA, McCloskey B, Azhar EI. COVID-19 and other respiratory tract infections at mass gathering religious and sporting events. Curr Opin Pulm Med. 2022;28:192–8. https://doi.org/10.1097/MCP.0000000000000859.

102. World Health Organization. Key planning recommendations for mass gatherings in the context of the current COVID-19 outbreak 2020. https://www.who.int/publications/i/item/10665-332235. Accessed 2 Oct 2021.

103. Adami PE, Cianca J, McCloskey B, Derman W, Steinacker JM, O'Connor F, et al. Infectious diseases outbreak management tool for endurance mass participation sporting events: an international effort to counteract the COVID-19 spread in the endurance sport setting. Br J Sports Med. 2021;55:181–2. https://doi.org/10.1136/bjsports-2020-103091.

104. Morimura N, Mizobata Y, Sugita M, Takeda S, Kiyozumi T, Shoko T, et al. Medicine at mass gatherings: current progress of preparedness of emergency medical services and disaster medical response during 2020 Tokyo Olympic and Paralympic Games from the perspective of the Academic Consortium (AC2020). Acute Med Surg. 2021;8:e626. https://doi.org/10.1002/ams2.626.

105. Revollo B, Blanco I, Soler P, Toro J, Izquierdo-Useros N, Puig J, et al. Same-day SARS-CoV-2 antigen test screening in an indoor mass-gathering live music event: a randomised controlled trial. Lancet Infect Dis. 2021;21:1365–72. https://doi.org/10.1016/s1473-3099(21)00268-1.

106. Hoang VT, Al-Tawfiq JA, Gautret P. The Tokyo Olympic Games and the risk of COVID-19. Curr Trop Med Reports. 2020;7:126–32. https://doi.org/10.1007/s40475-020-00217-y.

107. Al-Tawfiq JA, Kattan RF, Memish ZA. Escalating the 2022 Hajj during the third year of the COVID-19 pandemic. J Travel Med. 2022;29:taac059. https://doi.org/10.1093/jtm/taac059.

108. Alahmari AA, Khan AA, Alamri FA, Almuzaini YS, Alradini FA, Almohamadi E, et al. Hajj 2021: Role of mitigation measures for health security. J Infect Public Health. 2022, 15:1350. https://doi.org/10.1016/J.JIPH.2022.09.006.

109. Gautret P, Steffen R. Communicable diseases as health risks at mass gatherings other than Hajj: what is the evidence? Int J Infect Dis. 2016;47:46–52. https://doi.org/10.1016/j.ijid.2016.03.007.

110. Chen T-H, Kutty P, Lowe LE, Hunt EA, Blostein J, Espinoza R, et al. Measles outbreak associated with an International Youth Sporting Event in the United States, 2007. Pediatr Infect Dis J. 2010;29:794–800. https://doi.org/10.1097/INF.0b013e3181dbaacf.

111. Parker AA, Staggs W, Dayan GH, Ortega-Sánchez IR, Rota PA, Lowe L, et al. Implications of a 2005 measles outbreak in Indiana for sustained elimination of measles in the United States. N Engl J Med. 2006;355:447–55. https://doi.org/10.1056/NEJMoa060775.

112. Pfaff G, Lohr D, Santibanez S, Mankertz A, van Treeck U, Schonberger K, et al. Spotlight on measles 2010: measles outbreak among travellers returning from a mass gathering, Germany, September to October 2010. Euro Surveill. 2010;15:19750.

113. Ehresmann KR, Hedberg CW, Grimm MB, Norton CA, Macdonald KL, Osterholm MT. An outbreak of measles at an International Sporting Event with airborne transmission in a Domed Stadium. J Infect Dis. 1995;171:679–83. https://doi.org/10.1093/infdis/171.3.679.

114. Centers for Disease Control and Prevention (CDC). Multistate measles outbreak associated with an International Youth Sporting Event—Pennsylvania, Michigan, and Texas, August–September 2007. MMWR Morb Mortal Wkly Rep. 2008;57:169–73.

115. Memish ZA, Steffen R, White P, Dar O, Azhar EI, Sharma A, et al. Mass gatherings medicine: public health issues arising from mass gathering religious and sporting events. Lancet. 2019;393:2073–84. https://doi.org/10.1016/S0140-6736(19)30501-X.

116. Jani K, Ghattargi V, Pawar S, Inamdar M, Shouche Y, Sharma A. Anthropogenic activities induce depletion in microbial communities at urban sites of the river Ganges. Curr Microbiol. 2018;75:79–83. https://doi.org/10.1007/s00284-017-1352-5.

117. David S, Roy N. Public health perspectives from the biggest human mass gathering on earth: Kumbh Mela, India. Int J Infect Dis. 2016;47:42–5. https://doi.org/10.1016/j.ijid.2016.01.010.

118. Finger F, Genolet T, Mari L, de Magny GC, Manga NM, Rinaldo A, et al. Mobile phone data highlights the role of mass gatherings in the spreading of cholera outbreaks. Proc Natl Acad Sci U S A. 2016;113:6421–6. https://doi.org/10.1073/pnas.1522305113.

119. Sow D, Dogue F, Edouard S, Drali T, Prades S, Battery E, et al. Acquisition of enteric pathogens by pilgrims during the 2016 Hajj pilgrimage: a prospective cohort study. Travel Med Infect Dis. 2018;25:26–30. https://doi.org/10.1016/j.tmaid.2018.05.017.

120. Al-Jasser FS, Kabbash IA, Almazroa MA, Memish ZA. Patterns of diseases and preventive measures among domestic hajjis from central, Saudi Arabia. Saudi Med J. 2012;33:879–86.

121. Meysamie A, Ardakani HZ, Razavi SM, Doroodi T. Comparison of mortality and morbidity rates among Iranian pilgrims in Hajj 2004 and 2005. Saudi Med J. 2006;27:1049–53.

122. Razavi SM, Sabouri-Kashani A, Ziaee-Ardakani H, Tabatabaei A, Karbakhsh M, Sadeghipour H, et al. Trend of diseases among Iranian pilgrims during five consecutive years based on a syndromic surveillance system in Hajj. Med J Islam Repub Iran. 2013;27:179–85.

123. Gautret P, Soula G, Delmont J, Parola P, Brouqui P. Common health hazards in French pilgrims during the Hajj of 2007: a prospective cohort study. J Travel Med. 2009;16:377–81. https://doi.org/10.1111/j.1708-8305.2009.00358.x.

124. Gautret P, Vu Hai V, Sani S, Doutchi M, Parola P, Brouqui P. Protective measures against acute respiratory symptoms in French pilgrims participating in the Hajj of 2009. J Travel Med. 2011;18:53–5. https://doi.org/10.1111/j.1708-8305.2010.00480.x.

125. Valerio L, Arranz Y, Hurtado B, Roure S, Reina MD, Martínez-Cuevas O, et al. [Epidemiology and risk factors associated with religious pilgrimage to Saudi Arabia. Results of a prospective cohort 2008-2009]. Gac Sanit. 2012;26:251–255. https://doi.org/10.1016/j.gaceta.2011.09.011.

126. Saeed KMI, Mofleh J, Rasooly MH, Aman MI. Occurrence of acute respiratory infection, diarrhea and jaundice among Afghan pilgrims, 2010. J Epidemiol Glob Health. 2012;2:215–20. https://doi.org/10.1016/j.jegh.2012.11.003.

127. Pesola A, Pärn T, Huusko S, Perevoščikovs J, Ollgren J, Salmenlinna S, et al. Multinational outbreak of Salmonella enteritidis infection during an international youth ice hockey competition in Riga, Latvia, preliminary report, March and April 2015. Euro Surveill. 2015;20:21133. https://doi.org/10.2807/1560-7917.ES2015.20.20.21133.

128. Leangapichart T, Rolain JM, Memish ZA, Al-Tawfiq JA, Gautret P. Emergence of drug resistant bacteria at the Hajj: a systematic review. Travel Med Infect Dis. 2017;18:3–17. https://doi.org/10.1016/j.tmaid.2017.06.008.

129. Patel D. The Hajj and Umrah: health protection matters. Travel Med Infect Dis. 2017;19:1. https://doi.org/10.1016/j.tmaid.2017.10.013.

130. Leangapichart T, Dia NM, Olaitan AO, Gautret P, Brouqui P, Rolain J-M. Acquisition of extended-spectrum β-lactamases by Escherichia coli and Klebsiella pneumoniae in gut microbiota of pilgrims during the Hajj pilgrimage of 2013. Antimicrob Agents Chemother. 2016;60:3222–6. https://doi.org/10.1128/AAC.02396-15.

131. Leangapichart T, Gautret P, Griffiths K, Belhouchat K, Memish Z, Raoult D, et al. Acquisition of a high diversity of bacteria during the Hajj pilgrimage, including Acinetobacter baumannii with blaOXA-72 and Escherichia coli with blaNDM-5 carbapenemase genes. Antimicrob Agents Chemother. 2016;60:5942–8. https://doi.org/10.1128/AAC.00669-16.

132. Alyamani EJ, Khiyami AM, Booq RY, Majrashi MA, Bahwerth FS, Rechkina E. The occurrence of ESBL-producing Escherichia coli carrying aminoglycoside resistance genes in urinary tract infections in Saudi Arabia. Ann Clin Microbiol Antimicrob. 2017;16:1. https://doi.org/10.1186/s12941-016-0177-6.

133. Marglani OA, Alherabi AZ, Herzallah IR, Saati FA, Tantawy EA, Alandejani TA, et al. Acute rhinosinusitis during Hajj season 2014: prevalence of bacterial infection and patterns of antimicrobial susceptibility. Travel Med Infect Dis. 2016;14:583–7. https://doi.org/10.1016/j.tmaid.2016.11.004.

134. Haseeb A, Faidah HS, Bakhsh AR, Al Malki WH, Elrggal ME, Saleem F, et al. Antimicrobial resistance among pilgrims: a retrospective study from two hospitals in Makkah, Saudi Arabia. Int J Infect Dis. 2016;47:92–4. https://doi.org/10.1016/j.ijid.2016.06.006.

135. Olaitan AO, Dia NM, Gautret P, Benkouiten S, Belhouchat K, Drali T, et al. Acquisition of extended-spectrum cephalosporin- and colistin-resistant Salmonella enterica subsp. enterica

serotype Newport by pilgrims during Hajj. Int J Antimicrob Agents. 2015;45:600–4. https://doi.org/10.1016/j.ijantimicag.2015.01.010.

136. Leangapichart T, Gautret P, Brouqui P, Mimish Z, Raoult D, Rolain J-M. Acquisition of mcr-1 plasmid-mediated colistin resistance in Escherichia coli and Klebsiella pneumoniae during Hajj 2013 and 2014. Antimicrob Agents Chemother. 2016;60:6998. https://doi.org/10.1128/AAC.01486-16.

137. Gautret P, Benkouiten S, Sridhar S, Al-Tawfiq JA, Memish ZA. Diarrhea at the Hajj and Umrah. Travel Med Infect Dis. 2015;13:159–66. https://doi.org/10.1016/j.tmaid.2015.02.005.

Advice for Humanitarian Aid Workers

Nicola Petrosillo

Abstract

Humanitarian aid workers are a valuable asset in developing countries; they deliver much-needed help to those in need and are often essential to ensure basic health levels. However, geographical areas where they are deployed often present high concentrations of potentially infectious human vectors (patients, healthcare workers, households of infected individuals, etc.…) and healthcare facilities where proper protection is often inadequate. These factors should be well addressed and mitigated before deployment. The institution that organizes the deployment should assist the aid workers in their own personal decision-making process by ensuring that their decision is fully considered and informed. Moreover, the organization should have a minimum set of operational standards in place to ensure the health and security of aid workers. Information on all possible risks, training, vaccination, and medical prophylaxis should be ensured. On-site training, availability of personal protective equipments in case of direct care of infected individuals, a pre-return in-country screening and assistance in case of injuries or blood/body fluid exposures should be provided. Finally, after deployment, aid workers should be advised to seek medical care and to inform their physicians of the recent travel and work, if they sustained injuries or infectious exposures or become ill after returning.

N. Petrosillo (✉)
Fondazione Policlinico Universitario Campus Bio-Medico, Rome, Italy
e-mail: nicola.petrosillo@inmi.it

H. Leblebicioglu et al. (eds.), *Emerging and Re-emerging Infections in Travellers*, https://doi.org/10.1007/978-3-031-49475-8_4

4.1   Background

At the beginning of the Ebola virus disease epidemic in Western Africa in 2013, World Health Organization (WHO) declared that there was a need for several thousand healthcare workers to contain the epidemic, because the "single most important" problem causing difficulties in a rapid management of the situation was "not having enough people on the ground" [1]. In few weeks and months later a surge of healthcare workers, including physicians, nurses, and people supporting humanitarian aid, including logistics, administrative, informatics, statisticians, etc.… were voluntarily deployed at West Africa to provide clinical care and to support disease control efforts. In some cases all this occurred at considerable personal risk for the humanitarian aid workers. Since the start of this outbreak, 881 confirmed Ebola virus disease (EVD) cases among healthcare workers have been reported in the three most affected countries (i.e. Guinea, Liberia, and Sierra Leone), including 513 (58.2%) deaths [2]. Outside of these three countries, infected healthcare workers have been reported from Mali (two), Nigeria (11), Spain (one, infected in Spain while caring for an evacuated EVD patient), UK (three, infected in Sierra Leone), USA (nine cases, including one death; two of the cases were infected in the US), and Italy (two, infected in Sierra Leone). Therefore, during the 2013–2015 EVD epidemic in West Africa, another ethical and clinical problem occurred, i.e. the management of healthcare workers, deployed in Africa for the epidemic, who acquired EVD during the care of infected patients. As of 24 June 2015, 65 individuals were evacuated or repatriated worldwide from the EVD-affected countries. Of these, 38 individuals have been evacuated or repatriated to Europe.

More recently in 2018, in the Democratic Republic of Congo another Ebola virus disease outbreak was occured. This latest EVD outbreak in the Democratic Republic of the Congo accounted for 3665 EVD cases with a total of 2387 deaths (overall case fatality rate 65.1%), and now is declared over, with no new cases reported for 42 days after the burial of the last and only confirmed case on 16 August 2022 [3]. On 20 September 2020, another EVD outbreak occurred in Uganda. As of 22 November 2022, there had been 141 confirmed cases of Ebola virus disease (EVD), including 55 deaths (case fatality rate: 39%). Among these, at least 19 healthcare workers were infected, of whom 7 died [4].

The occurrence of EVD in deployed health workers highlighted the need for organizations participating in the EVD response to carefully carry out their responsibility to ensure a safe work and stay of deployed volunteers. An evaluation of the ability of each aid organization to give protection to volunteers under all the complex environmental situations during the EVD outbreak was sometimes lacking, or partial or confusing.

In circumstances as that of an epidemic of highly transmissible infections, like Ebola or Marburg, health workers have a double obligation, i.e. to provide the best medical care to improve patient survival, but also to provide symptom relief and palliation when required. In the context of patients with EVD, clinical care must be strengthened whilst minimizing the risk of onwards transmission to others, including humanitarian health workers.

The specific risks and situations experienced by aid workers include those related to their safety and security, i.e. exposure to the disaster or conflict environment and difficulties in sanitation facilities and living accommodations, that lead to high levels of insecurity, and those related to mental health, i.e. stressful environments and working long hours often under adverse or extreme conditions [5].

Between 2016 and 2018, a questionnaire was presented to the International Committee of the Red Cross workers. Participants to the survey were queried about their experience abroad including security incidents (the primary objective), health, and malaria prevention. Security incidents were reported by 12% (95/796) of them; 78 out of the 95 incidents (83%) were related to armed threats and attacks. Accidents or injuries occurred for 7.5% (60/796), mostly sporting activities and road accidents. Fifteen percent of participants (119/795) reported to engage in risky behaviours, including driving too fast or inebriated, and unsafe sex. Compliance to malaria prophylaxis was low 43% (113/263). Over 40% found the mission more stressful than expected, and a third of participants reported worsened health on their return [6].

To face the health risk among humanitarian aid workers travelling in areas with high rates of communicable diseases, several national and international agencies developed recommendations [5, 7–9].

Humanitarian aid traveller must first address their personal health and welfare before, during, and after travel. Knowledge of preparation for all the usual elements associated with travel to the area are the milestones for minimizing any health risk during their stay, including risks due to precipitated events (wars, natural disasters, etc.), overworking in extreme conditions, limited availability of food, water, accommodation and travel, stress and ethical issues faced during their job.

4.2 Pre-travel Advice and Considerations

First of all, the institution that organizes the deployment should assist the individuals in their own personal decision-making process by ensuring that their decision is fully considered and informed.

Three points are crucial in the final decision of travelling as humanitarian aid worker [10]:

1. Knowledge, skills and experiences should be assessed in the volunteer, not only regarding her/his clinical role, but also in her/his personal capacities for facing difficult conditions including stress, unfamiliar environments, and basic living conditions. Trainees should not be deployed because they lack supervision in such contexts, often cannot practice independently, and can have insurance limitations. As a consequence, if trainees are deployed standard of care in medical humanitarian aid could be inferior to that provided in developed countries, and unpreparedness can affect their own health and well-being.
2. Physical and mental health status should be full assessed before deployment, including vaccinations, prophylactic medications and a full travel health assessment by a travel medicine specialist.

3. The risks associated with deployment should be well known, understood and accepted by the humanitarian aid worker. This does not mean that the volunteer should feel alone and abandoned during the deployment. Capabilities and medical contingency plans of the home organization in terms of responsibility for individual's health, safety and security, including medical assistance and evacuation, should be well known and understood by the humanitarian aid worker. All this should be part of the individual's assessment as a component of her/his final decision to be deployed.

In a systematic literature review performed to assess the information available on pre-deployment interventions and recommendations such as vaccinations and other health preserving measures in volunteers and professionals deploying abroad in humanitarian relief missions [11]. Costa et al. reported that training and preparation pre-deployment is mostly regarded as very important in all the articles reviewed, but not all organizations provide pre-deployment information and sometimes the aid workers felt lost in the country after arrival. In the reviewed literature, 30–85% of humanitarian aid workers felt adequately prepared and medical pre-deployment check-up was performed in 42–100% of cases. Moreover, pre-deployment vaccinations did not fully cover all the aid workers (range of coverage from 50 to 83%). With regard to prophylaxis only 60% aid workers took malaria chemoprophylaxis as recommended and 85% used a mosquito net; 6% had unprotected sex intercourse. Eventhough aid workers had a better understanding in travel risks and way of transmission than other travellers, the most important finding of the review was the fact that humanitarian aid workers felt insufficiently prepared. Moreover, the organizations had non-standardized practices for the screening for appropriateness, and presented strong differences in the educational practice and field preparation [12]. The pre-deployment process is therefore different among organizations, and those organizations with great resources likely give a better training that, by definition, is costly and time-consuming.

In the systematic review by Costa [12], psychological support was needed by most of the humanitarian aid workers due to the traumatic events witnessed. Of note, in a longitudinal study among expatriate humanitarian aid workers in a representative sample of 19 non-governmental organizations Lopes Cardozo et al. [13] commonly evidenced psychological distress, depression, anxiety, and burnout. Two hundred twelve, 169, and 154 humanitarian aid workers participated at pre-deployment, post-deployment, and within 3–6 months after deployment assessments, respectively. Anxiety and depression symptoms were reported by less than 4% and 10.4% of participants, respectively, before deployment compared to 11.8% and 19.5% at post-deployment ($p = 0.0027$ and $p = 0.0117$, respectively). Depression still remained in 20.1% of participants at follow-up (6 months after returning home). The experience of very intense stress was a contributor to increased risk for burnout depersonalization [Adjusted Odds Ratio (AOR) 1.5; 95% Confidence Intervals (CI) 1.17–1.83]. Social support was associated with lower levels of depression (AOR 0.9; 95% CI 0.84–0.95), psychological distress (AOR 0.9; CI 0.85–0.97), burnout lack of personal accomplishment (AOR 0.95; 95% CI 0.91–0.98), and greater life satisfaction ($p = 0.0213$).

More recently, in a prospective observational study among 618 international humanitarian aid workers recruited from 76 countries health changes and ill-health risk factors after mostly short-term (<1 year) medical emergency assignments were assessed. The aid workers were assigned to 27 countries between 2017 and 2020. Humanitarian workers experienced on average, 2.6 experienced and witnessed potential traumatic events, and 4.8 male and 5.6 female assignment-related stressors. Self-report health indicators demonstrated a significant increase in emotional exhaustion, loss of vitality, decreased social functioning and emotional well-being. However, in this study it looks that humanitarian work is highly stressful but most internation humanitarian aid workers remained healthy [14].

It is evident that the choice of the right organization and of its offered pre-, in-, and post-deployment services are crucial for the following stay in at-risk areas. At the beginning of the recent West African Ebola epidemic, a consortium of Boston-based hospitals, on the basis of experiences from international agencies, developed the following recommendations to guide humanitarian aid workers to assess the ability of an international aid organization to ensure volunteer safety [10]. These represent the minimum set of operational standards that a professional organization must have in place to ensure the health and security of humanitarian aid workers, and must be adapted also to other emergencies as follows:

1. Proven experience in humanitarian crisis response, particularly in case of quick and complex medical interventions in contexts with scarce resources. The organization should have an efficient system including logistics, administration, funding, and infrastructures to support a successful response.
2. Comprehensive pre-deployment orientation programmes. Risk acknowledgment, appropriate individual information and clear definitions of roles and responsibilities at individual and organization level should be provided.
3. Provision of comprehensive response training that addresses site-specific safety, health, and security concerns. For diseases requiring the use of personal protective equipment (PPE) prior to providing clinical care or other supportive activity, specific training on proper donning and doffing is required.
4. Ensuring all supplies, medical and other, for complex medical field operations. In case of highly transmissible infections, i.e. Ebola, Marburg, etc. an adequate supply of PPE, as recommended by international agencies, should be provided.
5. Clear contingency plans for medical evacuation or treatment of sick or injured personnel. Contingency plans should also include the management of security threats such as civil unrest, natural disasters, or other large-scale outbreaks. Also clear plans for the return of aid workers back at home should be provided including, in case, management of aid workers on isolation at home after deployment, according to nation and international regulations.

The geographical areas where humanitarian aid workers are deployed often present high concentrations of potentially infectious human vectors (patients, healthcare workers, households of infected individuals, etc.…) and healthcare facilities where a proper protection, i.e. engineering control, personal protective equipments, etc.…, is often inadequate, placing them at greater risk for infections. These factors should be well addressed and mitigated before deployment. At pre-deployment, humanitarian aid workers should be provided with prophylaxis by ordinary vaccines (diphtheria, pertussis, tetanus, hepatitis A and B, influenza, measles, mumps, rubella, polio, typhoid, varicella), vaccines for particular situations, i.e. rabies—if animal exposure is highly significant, Japanese encephalitis virus—if works is in some parts of South and Southeast Asia, meningococcal (meningitis belt of Africa) and Yellow fever (parts of Africa and South America) [15]. Advice for providing with medications to be administered during the stay should be given: geographically appropriate malaria chemoprophylaxis, self-treatment for diarrhoea, and antiretrovirals for blood or other body fluids exposures [15]. Finally, at pre-departure personal protection should be prepared or be warranted by the organization to be eventually used during the stay: dietiltoluamide (DEET) and permethrin for preventing mosquito and tick bites; caps, gowns, gloves, surgical and N-95 masks, facemasks or protective eyewear, alcohol hand rub, and needles for personal use in case of any parenteral treatment [15].

Humanitarian aid workers are likely to work in difficult, crowded, rushed and unfamiliar conditions, with a potential risk for needlesticks or sharp injuries. Epidemiology of infections transmitted by blood-borne route should be aware to aid workers, i.e. HIV, hepatitis viruses but also dengue and haemorrhagic fever viruses, malaria, syphilis, trypanosomiasis, etc.… [15, 16]. Before deployment advice for preventing and managing sharp injuries should be given. Particularly, the use of sharp container or the use of substitutes, i.e. bottles, if they are not available, should be emphasized.

In case of needlesticks or sharp injuries, post-exposure management includes detailed patient's history, HIV test (possibly rapid test) or obtain a blood sample from the patient for later testing. The injury site should be thoroughly cleaned with warm water and soap, avoiding caustic antiseptics that can cause local tissue damage and increase the risk of infection [17]. Plans for follow-up assessment should be available to all aid workers.

Finally, at pre-deployment a more extensive travel health kit than the typical kit used by travellers should be prepared, with basic first aid to self-treat any injury until medical attention can be obtained. The kit should include disinfectants also for water and high-energy food for emergency use. For aid workers with underlying diseases, prescriptions and medications sufficient for the duration of their job are advised. In addition to a basic travel health kit, humanitarian aid workers should consider bringing other potential necessary items, including menstrual supplies, long pants, shorts covering the shoulders, boots if travelling to rudimental settings, leather gloves, safety googles, sunglasses and sunscreen, headlamp, sewing kit, insecticide impregnated bed net if travelling in malaria endemic areas, money belt, cash, and cellular phone that can work internationally, and personal items including documents, extra passport-style photos, photocopies of documents such as passports and credit cards, as well as copies of their medical, nursing, or other license if applicable. Moreover humanitarian aid workers should bring with them medical information such as immunization records and blood type, and should ensure that these documents are securely stored and available in a cloud storage service. An emergency contact is appropriate [5].

4.3 On-site Measures to Prevent Transmission of Pathogens: The Case of Ebola

Infection prevention measures to be taken at the deployment site depend on the specific geographical area and on the endemic infection there occurring, the type of individuals that will come in contact with aid workers, the type of engineering controls in healthcare facilities where they will work, and by the conditions of the work itself, i.e. crowding, overworking, understaffing, etc.… A review of medical files of 652 volunteers from New Zealand with assignment length on average of 2 years evidenced dengue seroconversion at a rate of 3.4 per 1000 person months (pm) on assignment in Southeast Asia, where the risk for dengue is very high. Tuberculosis conversion rate was 1.4 per 1000 pm. No HIV or HCV infections were detected. Of note, 9.8% of aid workers reported a potential exposure to blood and/or blood products [18].

Humanitarian aid workers should be advised by home organization of all infectious risk in the area where they are working, for example in area where fresh water is infested with *Schistosome* parasites they should avoid swimming, wading, or any other aquatic activity in bodies of water. Indeed, contact with infested fresh water exposes the skin to possible penetration by the cercariae [17]. For preventing malaria, humanitarian aid workers should follow all the recommendations given at pre-deployment, including the correct intake of proper antimalarial medications and the measures to avoiding mosquito bites. Several guidelines are available on these issues [19, 20].

Ebola represents another illustrative example. In an area where Ebola virus infection has been reported recently, humanitarian aid workers should follow basic precautions, including avoiding contact with ill or dead people unless wearing appropriate personal protective equipment (PPE), avoiding contact with ill or dead animals—especially primates and bats—and avoiding consumption of "bushmeat". Moreover, they should adhere to safe sex practices. In case of direct involvement in medical care of Ebola virus-infected individuals, infection control practices should be maintained at any time including hand hygiene (soap and water or waterless alcohol-based hand rubs), wearing gloves, and proper disposal of needles and sharps. Furthermore, strict barrier techniques should be followed by aid workers when they are in close contact with suspected or known Ebola virus-infected individuals. Humanitarian aid workers should strictly follow infection control and personal protective equipment protocols given by deploying organizations. Even though a pre-deployment training on PPE donning and doffing has already been done, on-site training on the correct use and removal of PPE is essential before direct contact with infected patients [21].

Humanitarian aid workers may experience an exposure to Ebola virus during their care to infected patients. First of all they should contact their organization immediately. In case they become unwell, the organization's sickness management protocol should be strictly followed. Of note, symptoms of Ebola virus disease are non-specific and other causes of illness, including malaria, should be ruled out. Travelling is allowed only for seeking medical care.

At the end of deployment, a pre-return in-country screening should be done [7]. The purpose of the screening is to assess their exposure risk category [9], to discuss anticipated monitoring and movement restriction on return, and to plan for any contingencies that may rise en route.

4.4 Post-deployment Advice

After deployment, humanitarian aid workers should be advised to seek medical care and to inform their physicians of the recent travel and work, if they sustained injuries or infectious exposures or become ill after returning. If they were directly involved in healthcare of infected individuals and especially in outbreaks' situations post-deployment monitoring is advisable [5]. In the case of aid workers taking direct care of Ebola virus-infected patients, the relevant public health authority will conduct post-arrival procedures, including screening, assessment of risk, assignment of public health officer, and determination of required public health actions [7]. For these aid workers a 21-day personal quarantine and active fever and symptom watch is required before returning to work. In case symptoms develop, an action plan should be available with direct communication with the Occupational Health Service and National Health Agencies. Clinical evaluation, disease testing, and isolation, if required should be warranted to humanitarian aid workers.

Finally, psychological support should be provided to aid workers who witnessed or were involved in situations of mass casualties, deaths, or serious injuries or who have been victims of violence (assault, kidnapping, or serious road traffic crash), and to all of them who report depression shortly after returning home [5].

4.5 Conclusions

Humanitarian aid workers are a valuable asset in developing countries; they deliver much-needed help to those in need, and are often essential to ensure basic health levels. They work in multicultural, multi-country settings every day, and they often face emergencies and work in conflict zones. All of these conditions require well training and excellent communication skills, in order not to become a liability to both and to those they are caring for. Their work often poses them at risk for danger, both physical and psychological. In countries where infectious outbreaks are spreading, they should be aware of the risks and the ways to minimize them; some practical tips are summarized in Table 4.1.

Table 4.1 Practical advice for humanitarian aid workers

Prior deployment
– Be sure of your choice to become humanitarian aid worker
– Choose the organization that guarantees you a good and safe stay
– Require and do training
– Know geo-political factors and local epidemiology of infectious diseases of the country/ area where you will be deployed
– Vaccinate and prepare the necessary for prophylaxis
– Prepare a basic travel health kit and all the items necessary during your stay
On-site
– For highly transmissible infections (i.e. Ebola) on-site training on the correct use and removal of personal protective equipment is essential before direct contact with infected patients
– Personal and hand hygiene should be ensured at any time
– Avoid prepare or eat bushmeat
– Avoid unprotected sexual intercourses
– Avoid bathing in fresh infested (schistosomiasis) body waters
– Respect recommendations/guidelines provided at the pre-deployment
– Take medical prophylaxis when indicated
– In case of injuries or needlestick/sharp injury or mucous membrane exposure by blood or body fluids refer to your organization and their recommendations
Post-deployment
– If directly involved in healthcare of infected individuals and especially in outbreaks' situations post-deployment monitoring is advisable and should be ensured
– Seek medical care and inform your provider of the recent travel and work, if you sustained injuries or infectious exposures or become ill after returning
– In case symptoms develop, an action plan should be available with direct communication with the Occupational Health Service and National Health Agencies
– Ask for psychological support when needed

Conflict of Interests   None declared.

References

1. Gulland A. More health staff are needed to contain Ebola outbreak, warns WHO. BMJ. 2014;349:g5485.
2. https://www.ecdc.europa.eu/sites/portal/files/media/en/publications/Publications/Ebola-west-africa-13th-update.pdf. Accessed 6 Dec 2022.
3. World Health Organization. Ebola virus disease democratic Republic of Congo. https://www.who.int/news-room/fact-sheets/detail/ebola-virus-disease?gclid=Cj0KCQiA7bucBhCeARIs AIOwr-9E_Wc0eUYIfg4pc4wTHzsqG_sTx4aPWBm_BLJlJtq2EmzNhyn-IucaAtivEALw_ wcB. Accessed 6 Dec 2022.
4. https://www.ecdc.europa.eu/en/news-events/ebola-outbreak-uganda#:~:text=According%20 to%20the%20World%20Health,infected%2C%20of%20whom%20seven%20died. Accessed 6 Dec 2022.
5. https://wwwnc.cdc.gov/travel/yellowbook/2020/travel-for-work-other-reasons/humanitarian-aid-workers. Accessed 6 Dec 2022.

6. Guisolan SC, Ambrogi M, Meeussen A, Althaus F, Eperon G. Health and security risks of humanitarian aid workers during field missions: experience of the International Red Cross. Travel Med Infect Dis. 2022;46:102275.

7. Cranmer H, Aschkenasy M, Wildes R, Kayden S, Bangsberg D, Niescierenko M, Kemen K, Hsiao KH, VanRooyen M, Burkle FM Jr, Biddinger PD. Academic Institutions' critical guidelines for health care workers who deploy to West Africa for the Ebola response and future crises. Harvard Health Policy Rev. 2015;14(2):22–4.

8. https://travelhealthpro.org.uk/. Accessed 6 Dec 2022.

9. https://assets.publishing.service.gov.uk/government/uploads/system/uploads/attachment_data/file/837629/Ebola_Information_for_workers_in_at_risk_countries.pdf. Accessed 6 Dec 2022.

10. Wildes R, Kayden S, Goralnick E, Niescierenko M, Aschkenasy M, Kemen KM, Vanrooyen M, Biddinger P, Cranmer H. Sign me up: rules of the road for humanitarian volunteers during the Ebola outbreak. Disaster Med Public Health Prep. 2015;9(1):88–9.

11. Costa M, Oberholzer-Riss M, Hatz C, Steffen R, Puhan M, Schlagenhauf P. Pre-travel health advice guidelines for humanitarian workers: a systematic review. Travel Med Infect Dis. 2015;13(6):449–65.

12. Perry DJ. Effective purpose in transnational humanitarian healthcare providers. Am J Disaster Med. 2013;8:157–68.

13. Lopes Cardozo B, Gotway Crawford C, Eriksson C, Zhu J, Sabin M, Ager A, Foy D, Snider L, Scholte W, Kaiser R, Olff M, Rijnen B, Simon W. Psychological distress, depression, anxiety, and burnout among international humanitarian aid workers: a longitudinal study. PLoS One. 2012;7(9):e44948.

14. De Jong K, Martinmäki SE, Te Brake H, Haagen JFG, Kleber RJ. Mental and physical health of international humanitarian aid workers on short-term assignments: findings from a prospective cohort study. Soc Sci Med. 2021;285:114268.

15. Kortepeter MG, Seaworth BJ, Tasker SA, Burgess TH, Coldren RL, Aronson NE. Health care workers and researchers traveling to developing-world clinical settings: disease transmission risk and mitigation. Clin Infect Dis. 2010;51(11):1298–305.

16. Tarantola A, Abiteboul D, Rachlinec A. Infection risks following accidental exposure to blood or body fluids in health care workers: a review of pathogens transmitted in published cases. Am J Infect Control. 2006;34:367–75.

17. US Public Health Service. Updated U.S. Public Health Service guidelines for the management of occupational exposures to HBV, HCV, and HIV and recommendations for postexposure prophylaxis. MMWR Recomm Rep. 2001;50(RR-11):1–52.

18. Visser JT, Edwards CA. Dengue fever, tuberculosis, human immunodeficiency virus, and hepatitis C virus conversion in a group of long-term development aid workers. J Travel Med. 2013;20(6):361–7.

19. https://assets.publishing.service.gov.uk/government/uploads/system/uploads/attachment_data/file/1102955/guidelines-for-malaria-prevention-in-travellers-from-the-UK-2021.pdf. Accessed 6 Dec 2022.

20. https://www.nicd.ac.za/wp-content/uploads/2017/09/Guidelines-South-African-Guidelines-for-the-Prevention-of-Malaria-2017-final.pdf. Accessed 6 Dec 2022.

21. Public Health England. Ebola: information for humanitarian aid and other workers intending to work in Ebola affected countries in Africa. PHE gateway number 2018158 PDF, 95.7KB, 8 pages. https://assets.publishing.service.gov.uk/government/uploads/system/uploads/attachment_data/file/1033157/ukhsa-ebola-Information-for-humanitarian-aid-and-other-workers.pdf. Accessed 6 Dec 2022.

Health Tourism and Infectious Diseases

5

Diego Viasus and Jordi Carratalà

Abstract

Health tourism is an old concept, but in recent years it has gained enormously in popularity. Health tourists are individuals who leave their local communities and travel to another country for non-emergency medical care. Common procedures performed abroad include dental work, arthroplasty, bariatric, cosmetic and cardiac surgery, reproductive care and organ transplant. At present, complete and accurate data on the volume of health tourism, destination, services, and procedures are unavailable. Similarly, little information is available regarding the risks facing health tourists, such as the infectious diseases associated with surgery or the problems inherent in travelling to other regions. Most reports suggest that procedures carried out abroad are associated with higher rates of infections, but there is no system-wide database currently tracking procedures and outcomes. Transplant tourists are more likely to develop cytomegalovirus, hepatitis B virus, human immunodeficiency virus (HIV), and wound infections, and cosmetic tourists more frequently have wound infections caused by *Mycobacterium absces-*

D. Viasus
Faculty of Medicine, Division of Health Sciences, Universidad del Norte and Hospital Universidad del Norte, Barranquilla, Colombia
e-mail: dviasus@uninorte.edu.co

J. Carratalà (✉)
Infectious Disease Department, Hospital Universitari de Bellvitge and Institut d'Investigació Biomèdica de Bellvitge (IDIBELL), Barcelona, Spain

Faculty of Medicine, Clinical Sciences Department, University of Barcelona, Barcelona, Spain

Centro de Investigación Biomédica en Red de Enfermedades Infecciosas (CIBERINFEC), Instituto de Salud Carlos III, Madrid, Spain
e-mail: jcarratala@ub.edu; jcarratala@bellvitgehospital.cat

H. Leblebicioglu et al. (eds.), *Emerging and Re-emerging Infections in Travellers*, https://doi.org/10.1007/978-3-031-49475-8_5

sus. Nosocomial infections caused by resistant pathogens have also been reported in health tourism patients. Importantly, the delay in the identification of patients with resistant pathogens may potentially result in an outbreak of disease. More research into the health and safety risks in health tourism is urgently needed, and all medical centres should have a predefined approach to the management of patients who have seek medical care abroad.

5.1 Background

5.1.1 Definition

Health tourism is an old concept which has gained great popularity in recent years. Although there is no universally agreed definition of health tourism, essentially the practice refers to individuals leaving their local communities and travelling to another country for non-emergency medical care [1]. Other names for this activity are "cross-border healthcare", "transnational medical travel", "medical-health-wellness tourism" and "medical tourism".

5.1.2 A Brief History of Health Tourism

Before the advent of medical technology, health tourism mostly consisted of mineral thermal springs and baths [2–4]. It was thought that the therapeutic powers of mineral waters were connected with their specific location and that they would lose their effect if they were transferred to another site; therefore, people had to travel to them. With the intention of attracting persons from afar, these places also offered leisure activities where music, dance, theatre and even gambling became part of the healing experience [2]. Archaeological evidence shows that the Greeks and Romans appreciated the value of natural curative springs and thermal baths and built numerous establishments throughout their empires.

Closer to our times, the use of mineral waters remained popular well into the nineteenth century. Hydrotherapy was thought to be beneficial in a wide range of ailments such as pimples, gonorrhoea, rheumatic diseases, and nervous conditions. In France, an entire academic discipline on "medicalized thermalism" was established to promote the spa industry by giving it a scientific veneer [3]. Persia and China also had a long historical tradition in medical tourism, and were visited by a constant stream of travellers in search of medical alternatives.

As the medical advances of the twentieth century generated more effective treatments, the interest in spa healing declined. However, the notion of medical tourism endured, particularly among patients travelling to other countries in pursuit of healthcare that was not available domestically (for example, abortion, euthanasia, or experimental treatments). In modern times, with the removal of most of the physical, economic and cultural barriers and the growing accessibility of international travel [4], other motivations for medical tourism have emerged, such as the lower cost (possibly the main driver of medical tourism), the avoidance of long waiting times (the clearest example being organ transplant for patients who want to avoid long waiting lists in their home countries), incentives offered by employers or insurers, and possibly also the attraction of an exotic vacation combined with a medical procedure [4, 5]. In other cases, patients are motivated by the offer of highly-qualified medical services, or occasionally by religious beliefs or family ties in the country of destination [4].

5.1.3 Importance of Health Tourism

Complete and accurate data on the volume of health tourism, destinations, services, and procedures are currently unavailable [5]. Similarly, the evidence regarding the risks facing health tourists is limited. One report estimated that nearly 11 million patients go abroad annually for medical treatment [6]. The health tourism industry is believed to have generated a turnover of more than 50 billion US dollars, with an annual growth of about 20% between 2005 and 2007 [5]. The main destinations of health tourists include India, Thailand, China, Mexico, Latin America (mainly Brazil), the Caribbean, Europe, Singapore and the Middle East [6]. Common procedures include dental work, arthroplasty, bariatric, cosmetic and cardiac surgery, and reproductive care and organ transplant [6]. Some professional associations and international organizations have developed quality-of-care standards and have established accreditation procedures [7, 8]. Moreover, the provision of health services to foreign patients is considered by some authorities as an opportunity for economic development; indeed, many low- or middle-income countries have chosen to develop traditional and alternative medicine services in order to capitalize on the lower costs, lower insurance requirements, and also the local traditions [4].

5.2 Health Tourism and Infectious Diseases

Research into health tourism and infectious diseases is in its infancy. Most data suggest that procedures performed abroad are associated with higher rates of infections and complications, but at present there is no system-wide database tracking procedures and outcomes. Health tourists are at risk of infectious diseases, either related to their surgical procedure or inherent in the practice of travelling to other regions. In addition, many countries with robust medical tourism programmes are located in tropical and subtropical regions with the presence of malaria, dengue fever, enteric fever, and other endemic infections. Similarly, many have high background rates of tuberculosis, antibiotic resistance, hepatitis B and C, and human immunodeficiency virus (HIV). The consequences may be greater if pathogens or resistance determinants spread during the patients' care or after their return home [6]. Evidence suggests that patients who travel abroad to receive treatment often experience complications on their return and represent a significant cost for their local health systems [9]. A study evaluated the crude costs of treating the infectious complications in medical tourists requiring hospital admission or outpatient home parenteral therapy. The estimated mean costs for the operative procedures required ranged from $6288 to $20,741 [10].

5.2.1 Transplantation

Transplant tourism, defined as travel with the intent of receiving or donating a transplanted organ, has grown tremendously in the past decade [11]. An estimated 10% of organ transplants worldwide on 2007 were the result of transplant tourism [12]. Of course, transplanted organs can be a source of infection and complications [13]. Some transplant-associated infections are geographically restricted, including human T-lymphotropic virus types 1 and 2, West Nile virus, rabies, malaria, Leishmania, *Trypanosoma cruzi*, and several fungi [14]. Many of these organ transplants are not recorded in databases and, as consequence, the incidence of infection is unknown [11].

One meta-analysis concluded that transplant tourists had lower 1-year graft and survival than domestic kidney transplant recipients and were more likely to develop cytomegalovirus, hepatitis B virus, HIV, and wound infections [15]. Several institutions have described their experience with transplant tourism and the subsequent risk of infection. Choon et al. [16] performed a study to evaluate trends and outcomes of Korean patients receiving kidney and liver transplantation overseas between 1999 and 2005. They found that the number of kidney and liver transplants had increased over the years, and that complications occurred in 42.5% of patients, mainly infections (21.5%). The principal infections developed by kidney transplant patients were cytomegalovirus, pneumonia (including tuberculosis), urinary tract infection, and wound infection. In liver transplant patients, the authors reported bacterial infection in 4.9%. Another study [17] compared outcomes of 93 patients who received kidney transplant abroad compared with local transplantation, finding higher rates of cytomegalovirus infection (15.1% vs 5.6%) and hepatitis C seroconversion (7.5% vs 0%) in transplant tourists. Interestingly, a series from Turkey documented that the post-transplant course in commercial transplant recipients was more complicated with infections caused by malaria, invasive fungal infection, tuberculosis and pneumonia due to various opportunistic pathogens [18]. Moreover, 13 of 142 (9%) patients who underwent commercial kidney transplantation in Pakistan developed invasive fungal infection due to ubiquitous organisms (Aspergillus species, followed by Zygomycetes). Of these patients, 77% required transplant nephrectomy and 23% died due to septic shock [19]. Likewise, Allam et al. [20] reported that sepsis and acquired HBV infection were significantly more frequent in patients who received liver transplantation abroad compared to those transplanted in local hospitals. Similar findings were recorded by Cha et al. [21], who found that patients with overseas kidney transplantation had a higher risk of serious infectious diseases requiring hospitalization. Interestingly, pre- and post-transplant management of overseas transplant patients is of a lower standard than that provided to those undergoing liver transplantation in their country [22]. A study found that screening for hepatitis B and C was not performed, and patients received inadequate valganciclovir, co-trimoxazole, antifungal therapy, and hepatitis B immunoglobulins [23].

Because of the practice of transplant tourism in endemic areas of parasitic infections, these infections must be considered in the differential diagnosis of post-transplant complications [24]. Donor-derived parasitic infections are rare, but have been reported with *Tripanosoma cruzi*, *Strongyloides*, *Schistosoma*, malaria and *Babesia*. Rates of morbidity and mortality are high. Appropriate epidemiological screening and diagnostic testing are necessary in patients with risk factors for these infectious complications [11].

5.2.2 Cosmetic Surgery and Arthroplasty

"Cosmetic tourism", the process of travelling overseas for cosmetic procedures, is an expanding global phenomenon. A study of 12 patients who had undergone cosmetic surgery abroad, which evaluated the number and type of complications and the cost incurred [25], found that breast augmentation was the most common procedure, and that infection prosthesis was the most common complication. The infective pathogens found were mainly Streptococci and Staphylococci species. Fungus and multi-resistant organisms were isolated in one patient each. The study showed that these complications incurred a notable financial burden. Other complications reported included pulmonary embolism and penile necrosis. Moreover, a cluster of wound infections caused by *Mycobacterium abscessus* following cosmetic surgery (including abdominoplasty, breast surgery and liposuction) in the Dominican Republic was reported in the United States [26]. Similarly, a literature review by Cai et al. [27] found 14 case reports of *M. abscessus* surgical site infection after cosmetic surgery abroad, with patients typically presenting complications 8 weeks after the procedure. The most frequent cosmetic operations included abdominoplasty, liposuction, breast augmentation, breast reduction, and rejuvenation surgery. The infections were managed with antibiotics and surgical intervention. Another study found that, between October 2012 and August 2014, several Swiss patients developed severe soft tissue infections due to rapidly growing mycobacteria after cosmetic surgery in the Dominican Republic, Ecuador and Mexico. The infections were caused by *M. abscessus*, *Mycobacterium* sp. and *M. conceptionense* [28]. Finally, Miyagi et al. [29] found that the principal complications among cosmetic tourists that return to Cambridge were wound infection or dehiscence. No aetiology of infections was reported.

Regarding arthroplasty tourism, one study described a case of a total knee arthroplasty performed overseas [30] in which the surgical site become infected with a *Mycobacterium fortuitum* organism. Management of the complication on the patient's return to Australia incurred a significant cost.

5.2.3 Resistant Organisms

Nosocomial infections caused by resistant pathogens have been reported in health tourism patients. Medical tourism is accompanied by the risk of transmission of multi-resistant superbugs from the patient's country of origin or from the country where the procedure is performed [31]. Furthermore, the delay in the identification of patients with resistant pathogens may potentially result in an outbreak.

Resistance patterns of nosocomial pathogens vary from country to country. In addition, healthcare-associated infection prevalence in low- and middle-income countries is substantially higher than in Europe and the United States. A meta-analysis revealed that the infection rate in ICUs in developing countries was at least three times higher than those reported in the US [32]. Some of the potential risk factors responsible for the higher rates of hospital-acquired infections in developing countries are inappropriate environmental hygienic conditions, poor infrastructure, insufficient equipment that could lead to reuse of globes or needles, understaffing, overpopulated hospitals, deficient knowledge and implementation of basic infection-control measures and the paucity of local and national guidelines and policies [32].

In 2008, there was an outbreak of carbapenem-resistant *Klebsiella pneumoniae* at a Colombian hospital. The index case was a patient who had travelled from Israel to Colombia for a liver transplant [33]. Moreover, another study reported an uri-noma in a kidney transplant patient operated upon abroad who died within 24 h of admission due to *Acinetobacter baumannii* sepsis [34]. In another study, a patient with acute lymphoblastic leukaemia who travelled from Dhaka (Bangladesh) to Singapore for further treatment presented a bacteraemia due to carbapenem-resistant *Escherichia coli* [31]. Polymerase chain reaction detection performed on the cultures was positive for the New Delhi metallo-beta-lactamase (NDM-1) gene. Similarly, Adler et al. [35] documented carbapenemase OXA-48-producing Enterobacteriaceae in foreign patients who were referred for medical care to Israel.

5.2.4 Other Concerns

Medical tourism has been associated with other serious problems facing health systems in both destination and home countries. Many organizations oppose the widespread promotion of medical tourism in third world countries, on the grounds that the medical infrastructure available in these countries is unable to meet even the domestic demand [4]. In addition, medical tourists run the risk of contracting insufficiently verified services or may encourage secret unethical practices [4]. Moreover, the individual choices of medical tourists may have significant public consequences if the healthcare facilities in their home countries are obliged to devote resources to treating post-operative complications [36]. It has been proposed that patients who choose to travel abroad for surgery must have full travel and medical insurance coverage so that, in the event of complications, the state is not left to carry the costs [37].

5.3 Prevention and Advice for Healthcare Workers and Travellers

The following recommendations are proposed for tackling infections among patients travelling abroad for medical care:

- There is a need for more research into health and safety risks in medical tourism.
- All medical centres should have a predefined approach to the management of patients who seek medical attention abroad. When these patients return, it is sensible to consider screening them for blood-borne pathogens, including HIV, HBV, HCV, as well as bacteraemia, urinary tract infection, and other pathogens depending on their site of medical care (for example, malaria, tuberculosis or Chagas disease) [11]. Patients should be evaluated by an infectious disease specialist as soon as possible after returning home.
- Patients contemplating medical tourism should be advised of both procedure-related and typical travel-associated risks. The public should be informed of the risks of potential infectious disease associated with overseas hospital care, including the endemic and tropical infections that can occur in some countries [6].
- Improved communication is essential to optimize continuity of care of medical tourists in different countries.
- Medical tourists may bring home unusually resistant microbial pathogens. Travellers returning from high-risk destinations should be placed in isolation and cultured for resistant organisms [6]. Similarly, medical tourists may run the risk of transmitting resistant pathogens from their country of origin.
- Patients should make sure that the location and facilities where the treatment and recovery will take place (as well as the medical staff involved) are approved by local medical regulatory authorities and meet all safety standards [37].
- Patients should receive advice regarding the prevention of travel-related infections. All routine and travel-related vaccines should be updated as needed before travel [11].

5.4 Gaps in Knowledge that Need to Be Addressed

Health tourists are at risk of infectious diseases, either related to their surgical procedure or inherent in the practice of travelling to other regions. However, there are clear limits in the current knowledge and areas where the need for further research using appropriately designed studies and standardized outcome variables is evident, in order to determine (a) the frequency of infectious complications, even those related to the different types of procedures, (b) short- and long-term health outcomes associated with the development of infectious diseases among medical tourists, (c) optimal strategies to prevent infectious complications in these patients, and (d) the cost of these complications to the health system.

Box Key Websites for Travellers and Healthcare Workers

Centers for Disease Control and Prevention (CDC)	wwwnc.cdc.gov/travel/yellowbook/2014/chapter-2-the-pre-travel-consultation/medical-tourism.htm
Centers for Disease Control and Prevention (CDC): Travellers' Health	https://wwwnc.cdc.gov/travel/
World Health Organization. International travel and health	https://www.who.int/ith/en/
National Travel Health Network and Centre (NaTHNaC)	https://travelhealthpro.org.uk/
European Commission. Cross-border care policy	https://ec.europa.eu/health/cross_border_care/overview_en
Joint Commission International list of its accredited facilities	https://www.worldhospitalsearch.org/
World Health Organization. Guiding principles on human cell, tissue and organ transplantation	https://www.who.int/transplantation/Guiding_PrinciplesTransplantation_WHA63.22en.pdf
American College of Surgeons. Statement on Medical and Surgical Tourism	https://www.facs.org/about-acs/statements/65-surgical-tourism

Declarations of Conflict of Interest The authors declare that they have no conflict of interest related to this chapter.

References

1. Centers for Disease Control and Prevention. Medical tourism. https://www.cdc.gov/features/medicaltourism/index.html.
2. Weisz G. Historical reflections on medical travel. Anthropol Med. 2011;18(1):137–44. https://doi.org/10.1080/13648470.2010.525880.
3. Li H, Cui W. Patients without borders: the historical changes of medical tourism. UWOMJ. 2014;83(2):20–2. https://doi.org/10.5206/uwomj.v83i2.4434.
4. Badulescu D, Badulescu A. Medical tourism: between entrepreneurship opportunities and bioethics boundaries: narrative review article. Iran J Public Health. 2014;43(4):406–15.
5. MacReady N. Developing countries court medical tourists. Lancet. 2007;369:1849–50. https://doi.org/10.1016/S0140-6736(07)60833-2.
6. Chen LH, Wilson ME. The globalization of healthcare: implications of medical tourism for the infectious disease clinician. Clin Infect Dis. 2013;57(12):1752–9. https://doi.org/10.1093/cid/cit540.
7. Helble M. The movement of patients across borders: challenges and opportunities for public health. Bull World Health Organ. 2011;89(1):68–72. https://doi.org/10.2471/BLT.10.076612.
8. Joint Commission International. www.jointcommissioninternational.org.
9. Hanefeld J, Smith R, Horsfall D, Lunt N. What do we know about medical tourism? A review of the literature with discussion of its implications for the UK National Health Service as an example of a public health care system. J Travel Med. 2014;21(6):410–7. https://doi.org/10.1111/jtm.12147.

10. Robinson PD, Vaughan S, Missaghi B, Meatherall B, Pattullo A, Kuhn S, Conly J. A case series of infectious complications in medical tourists requiring hospital admission or outpatient home parenteral therapy. J Assoc Med Microbiol Infect Dis Can. 2022;7(1):64–74. https://doi.org/10.3138/jammi-2021-0015.

11. Kotton CN, Hibberd PL, AST Infectious Diseases Community of Practice. Travel medicine and transplant tourism in solid organ transplantation. Am J Transplant. 2013;13 Suppl 4:337–47. https://doi.org/10.1111/ajt.12125.

12. World Health Organization. WHO proposes global agenda on transplantation, 2007. http://www.who.int/mediacentre/news/releases/2007/pr12/en/index.html.

13. Torres Soto M, Kotton CN. Infectious disease complications of transplant tourism. Expert Rev Anti Infect Ther. 2021;19(6):671–3. https://doi.org/10.1080/14787210.2020.1851196.

14. Martín-Dávila P, Fortún J, López-Vélez R, Norman F, Montes de Oca M, Zamarrón P, González MI, Moreno A, Pumarola T, Garrido G, Candela A, Moreno S. Transmission of tropical and geographically restricted infections during solid-organ transplantation. Clin Microbiol Rev. 2008;21(1):60–96. https://doi.org/10.1128/CMR.00021-07.

15. Anker AE, Feeley TH. Estimating the risks of acquiring a kidney abroad: a meta-analysis of complications following participation in transplant tourism. Clin Transplant. 2012;26(3):E232–41. https://doi.org/10.1111/j.1399-0012.2012.01629.x.

16. Kwon CH, Lee SK, Ha J. Trend and outcome of Korean patients receiving overseas solid organ transplantation between 1999 and 2005. J Korean Med Sci. 2011;26(1):17–21. https://doi.org/10.3346/jkms.2011.26.1.17.

17. Alghamdi SA, Nabi ZG, Alkhafaji DM, Askandrani SA, Abdelsalam MS, Shukri MM, Eldali AM, Adra CN, Alkurbi LA, Albaqumi MN. Transplant tourism outcome: a single center experience. Transplantation. 2010;90(2):184–8. https://doi.org/10.1097/TP.0b013e3181e11763.

18. Sever MS, Kazancioğlu R, Yildiz A, Türkmen A, Ecder T, Kayacan SM, Celik V, Sahin S, Aydin AE, Eldegez U, Ark E. Outcome of living unrelated (commercial) renal transplantation. Kidney Int. 2001;60(4):1477–83. https://doi.org/10.1046/j.1523-1755.2001.00951.x.

19. Al Salmi I, Metry AM, Al Ismaili F, Hola A, Al Riyami M, Khamis F, Al-Abri S. Transplant tourism and invasive fungal infection. Int J Infect Dis. 2018;69:120–9. https://doi.org/10.1016/j.ijid.2018.01.029.

20. Allam N, Al Saghier M, El Sheikh Y, Al Sofayan M, Khalaf H, Al Sebayel M, Helmy A, Kamel Y, Aljedai A, Abdel-Dayem H, Kenetman NM, Al Saghier A, Al Hamoudi W, Abdo AA. Clinical outcomes for Saudi and Egyptian patients receiving deceased donor liver transplantation in China. Am J Transplant. 2010;10(8):1834–41. https://doi.org/10.1111/j.1600-6143.2010.03088.x.

21. Cha RH, Kim YC, Oh YJ, Lee JH, Seong EY, Kim DK, Kim S, Kim YS. Long-term outcomes of kidney allografts obtained by transplant tourism: observations from a single center in Korea. Nephrology (Carlton). 2011;16(7):672–9. https://doi.org/10.1111/j.1440-1797.2011.01480.x.

22. Neupane R, Taweesedt PT, Anjum H, Surani S. Current state of medical tourism involving liver transplantation—the risk of infections and potential complications. World J Hepatol. 2021;13(7):717–22. https://doi.org/10.4254/wjh.v13.i7.717.

23. Kerr Winter B, Odedra A, Green S. A questionnaire-based assessment of numbers, motivation and medical care of UK patients undergoing liver transplant abroad. Travel Med Infect Dis. 2016;14:599–603. https://doi.org/10.1016/j.tmaid.2016.09.004.

24. Muñoz P, Valerio M, Eworo A, Bouza E. Parasitic infections in solid-organ transplant recipients. Curr Opin Organ Transplant. 2011;16(6):565–75. https://doi.org/10.1097/MOT.0b013e32834cdbb0.

25. Livingston R, Berlund P, Eccles-Smith J, Sawhney R. The real cost of "cosmetic tourism" cost analysis study of "cosmetic tourism" complications presenting to a public hospital. Eplasty. 2015;15:e34.

26. Centers for Disease Control and Prevention (CDC). Nontuberculous mycobacterial infections after cosmetic surgery—Santo Domingo, Dominican Republic, 2003-2004. MMWR Morb Mortal Wkly Rep. 2004;53(23):509.

27. Cai SS, Chopra K, Lifchez SD. Management of Mycobacterium abscessus infection after medical tourism in cosmetic surgery and a review of literature. Ann Plast Surg. 2016;77(6):678–82. https://doi.org/10.1097/SAP.0000000000000745.
28. Maurer F, Castelberg C, von Braun A, Wolfensberger A, Bloemberg G, Bottger E, Somoskovi A. Postsurgical wound infections due to rapidly growing mycobacteria in Swiss medical tourists following cosmetic surgery in Latin America between 2012 and 2014. Euro Surveill. 2014;19(37):20905. https://doi.org/10.2807/1560-7917.es2014.19.37.20905.
29. Miyagi K, Auberson D, Patel AJ, Malata CM. The unwritten price of cosmetic tourism: an observational study and cost analysis. J Plast Reconstr Aesthet Surg. 2012;65(1):22–8. https://doi.org/10.1016/j.bjps.2011.07.027.
30. Cheung IK, Wilson A. Arthroplasty tourism. Med J Aust. 2007;187(11–12):666–7. https://doi.org/10.5694/j.1326-5377.2007.tb01467.x.
31. Chan HL, Poon LM, Chan SG, Teo JW. The perils of medical tourism: NDM-1-positive Escherichia coli causing febrile neutropenia in a medical tourist. Singapore Med J. 2011;52(4):299–302.
32. Allegranzi B, Bagheri Nejad S, Combescure C, Graafmans W, Attar H, Donaldson L, Pittet D. Burden of endemic health-care-associated infection in developing countries: systematic review and meta-analysis. Lancet. 2011;377(9761):228–41. https://doi.org/10.1016/S0140-6736(10)61458-4.
33. Lopez JA, Correa A, Navon-Venezia S, Correa AL, Torres JA, Briceño DF, Montealegre MC, Quinn JP, Carmeli Y, Villegas MV. Intercontinental spread from Israel to Colombia of a KPC-3-producing Klebsiella pneumoniae strain. Clin Microbiol Infect. 2011;17(1):52–6. https://doi.org/10.1111/j.1469-0691.2010.03209.x.
34. Polcari AJ, Hugen CM, Farooq AV, Holt DR, Hou SH, Milner JE. Transplant tourism—a dangerous journey? Clin Transplant. 2011;25(4):633–7. https://doi.org/10.1111/j.1399-0012.2010.01325.x.
35. Adler A, Shklyar M, Schwaber MJ, Navon-Venezia S, Dhaher Y, Edgar R, Solter E, Benenson S, Masarwa S, Carmeli Y. Introduction of OXA-48-producing Enterobacteriaceae to Israeli hospitals by medical tourism. J Antimicrob Chemother. 2011;66(12):2763–6. https://doi.org/10.1093/jac/dkr382.
36. Crooks VA, Turner L, Cohen IG, Bristeir J, Snyder J, Casey V, Whitmore R. Ethical and legal implications of the risks of medical tourism for patients: a qualitative study of Canadian health and safety representatives' perspectives. BMJ Open. 2013;3(2):e002302. https://doi.org/10.1136/bmjopen-2012-002302.
37. Niechajev I, Frame J. A plea to control medical tourism. Aesthetic Plast Surg. 2012;36(1):202–6. https://doi.org/10.1007/s00266-011-9766-0.

Emergence and Spread of Resistant Microorganisms, Related to Travel

6

Ingeborg Fiane, Ernst Kristian Rødland, and Truls M. Leegaard

Abstract

Antimicrobial-resistant microorganisms do not recognise international borders. We acquire bacteria with antimicrobial resistance so easily that it makes this the most prevalent "souvenir" in modern travel. Any kind of travel will contribute to this spread, whether it is because of tourism, business or migration. Travellers will become colonised with the bacterial flora prevalent in the area where they travel which upon returning to their home country can be disseminated.

I. Fiane
Department of Microbiology and Infection Control, Akershus University Hospital, Lørenskog, Norway
e-mail: ingeborg.fiane@ahus.no

E. K. Rødland
Department of Climate and Environmental Health, Norwegian Institute of Public Health, Oslo, Norway
e-mail: ernstkristian.rodland@fhi.no

T. M. Leegaard (✉)
Department of Microbiology and Infection Control, Akershus University Hospital, Lørenskog, Norway

Division of Medicine and Laboratory Sciences, University of Oslo, Oslo, Norway
e-mail: tlee@ahus.no

H. Leblebicioglu et al. (eds.), *Emerging and Re-emerging Infections in Travellers*, https://doi.org/10.1007/978-3-031-49475-8_6

6.1   Background

6.1.1   Brief History

I shall be gone and live or stay and die (Shakespeare)

Since the beginning of mankind, humans have been travelling. The reason could be to find new places to live or to trade. Increasingly travel is also done for one's own sake, just for leisure or to see and learn. Conflict has always caused displacement of humans and war-displaced migrants are still a major problem. Travel is closely linked with a novel problem, antimicrobial resistance (AMR).

When we talk about antimicrobial resistance in this chapter we mean resistance to antimicrobial drugs to which the microorganism used to be susceptible. Over the last decades there has been such an increase in infections caused by antimicrobial-resistant bacteria that it represents one of the greatest threats to global health [1]. The driving factors behind the emergence of antimicrobial-resistant bacteria include the use, and abuse, of antibiotics in patients, livestock, or food production. Antibiotics are not only used in modern medicine but are also used extensively in agriculture and veterinary medicine. Poor control over wastewater and release of antibiotics into the environment contributes further to the emergence and spread of multidrug-resistant bacteria. International travel, international trade and even migrant animals and birds, contributes to its spread globally.

From young tourists backpacking their way through the world, to people fleeing war and conflict, more people are travelling than ever before. This implies that more and more people are carrying bacteria with antimicrobial resistance mechanisms with them and increasing the risk of global dissemination. As a response, many countries have made recommendations for screening and rules for contact isolation for patients who have recently been hospitalised or travelled to countries with a high incidence of antimicrobial resistance. In order to create effective health interventions and national recommendations, it is essential to understand the importance of international travel for the spread of antimicrobial resistance, and its mechanisms.

6.1.1.1 Importance of the Disease

Antibiotics are fundamental to modern medicine. Without antibiotics many of modern medicines achievements like transplantations, advanced surgery or cancer cures will no longer be possible. As travel is an important part in spreading antimicrobial resistance, it is important to understand the consequences.

The increase in the number of bacterial pathogens resistant to multiple bacterial agents is affecting people all over the globe. The global spread of these pathogens related to movement of people may possess a major public health problem causing both personal costs and healthcare-related costs. Multidrug-resistant bacteria are now considered as an emerging global disease, and the risk of spread of multidrug-resistant bacteria is estimated to be higher than the risk of acquisition of other emerging infectious diseases, related to travel [2].

6.2   Aetiology

In this overview we will concentrate on bacteria and antibiotic resistance, but antimicrobial resistance is equally important, and on the rise in many other microbes, like malaria, HIV and fungi, just to mention a few.

We will focus on bacterial pathogens and/or particular strains that have a history of clinical treatment-failure due to their multidrug-resistant status. First, we look at the international distribution and mobility of resistant Gram-negative rods, as these resistant microbes are widely distributed and their prevalence is increasing. This is probably the most clinically important antibiotic resistance and associated with high morbidity and mortality. The mechanisms that will be discussed includes extended-spectrum β-lactamase (ESBL)-producing *Enterobacterales* (ESBL-E) and carbapenemase-producing *Enterobacterales*, *Pseudomonas* and *Acinetobacter*. We will also address colistin resistance, as colistin is considered the last resort when there is resistance to all other antimicrobials, and hence resistance to this drug is of international importance. We then consider the role of travel in the spread of methicillin-resistant *Staphylococcus aureus* (MRSA) and vancomycin-resistant enterococci (VRE). We will also look at resistance in *Neisseria gonorrhoea*, by many considered to have the potential to become the next "superbug", resistant to all known active drugs. Finally, we will look at *Mycobacterium tuberculosis*.

We present a number of maps to illustrate the spread of certain resistance traits. Reference to the websites where the maps are found are given. The level of antimicrobial resistance in the various areas will change from year to year, but the overall trend has been stable for quite some years.

6.2.1   Gram-Negative Rods

Gram-negative rods are among the most important causes of serious hospital-acquired and community-onset bacterial infections in humans, and resistance to antimicrobial agents in these bacteria has become an increasingly relevant problem. International travel and tourism are important modes for the acquisition and spread of antimicrobial-resistant *Enterobacterales*, *Pseudomonas,* and *Acinetobacter*, all abundant in the environment and a cause of serious infections, especially in vulnerable patients. An overview of the most important resistance mechanisms in Gram-negative rods is given in Table 6.1. The mechanisms will be discussed more in detail after the table.

6.2.1.1 ESBL
Extended-spectrum β-lactamases (ESBLs) are a group of β-lactamases enzymes that share the ability to hydrolyse third-generation cefalosporins and aztreonam. The group of enzymes are constantly evolving and new enzymes are regularly being recognised. The first ESBLs were detected in 1983 in Germany [3]. The incidence of ESBL remained low for many years but has been steadily increasing over the last two decades, and is now found worldwide [4]. See Fig. 6.1 (the world) and Fig. 6.2

Table 6.1 The most important resistance mechanisms in Gram-negative rods

Mechanism	Gives resistance to	Common mechanisms	Mainly found in
ESBL	Penicillins, second- and third-generation cefalosporins	CTX-M	*Enterobacterales*
Carbapenemases	Carbapenems	MBL KPC OXA	*Enterobacterales,* *Pseudomonas,* *Acinetobacter* *K. pneumoniae* *Enterobacterales,* *Acinetobacter,* *Pseudomonas*
Colistin resistance	Colistin	crm1	*Enterobacterales*

MBL Metallo-beta-lactamases, *KPC* Klebsiella pneumoniae carbapenemase, *OXA* Oxacillinases

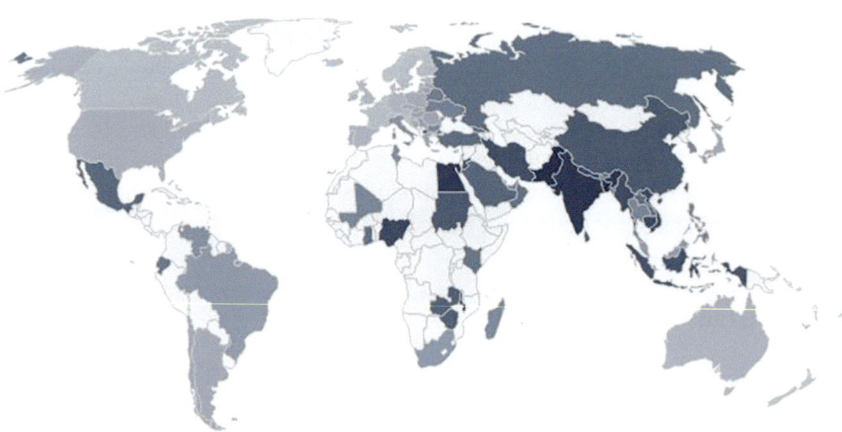

Fig. 6.1 World map: *E. coli* third-generation cefalosporins. OneHealthTrust. ResistanceMap: Antibiotic resistance. 2022. https://resistancemap.onehealthtrust.org/AntibioticResistance.php. Date accessed: December 14, 2022

(Europe) for the spread of *E. coli* resistant to third-generation cefalosporins (indicator for ESBL).

Extended-spectrum β-lactamase-producing *Enterobacterales* (ESBL-E) are often observed in community-acquired infections and in the intestine of healthy volunteers, in contrast to many other multidrug-resistant organisms (MDROs), for which expansion predominantly has occurred in hospitals [5–8]. Clinically, the most important ESBL-Es are ESBL-producing *Escherichia coli* and *Klebsiella pneumoniae* but ESBLs have been found in most *Enterobacterales*.

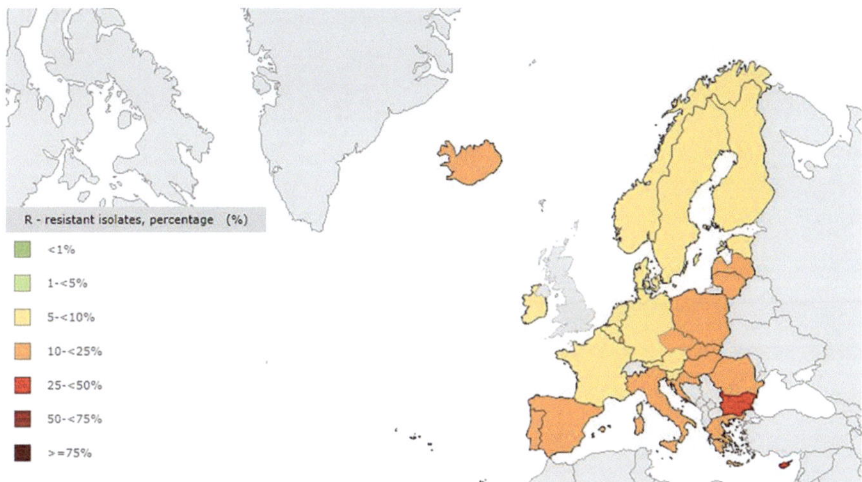

Fig. 6.2 Resistance of *E. coli* to third-generation cefalosporins. Surveillance Atlas of Infectious Diseases, European Centre for Disease Control: https://atlas.ecdc.europa.eu/public/index.aspx?Dataset=27&HealthTopic=4. Date accessed: December 14, 2022

The most common ESBL-E is *E. coli* producing an enzyme with the name CTX-M (named after their activity against cefotaxime and the place of isolation, Munich, Germany), but many other mechanisms are known [9]. Invasive infections caused by ESBL-E are associated with higher mortality rates than those caused by susceptible counterparts, probably because appropriate therapy is more frequently delayed, highlighting the importance of these pathogens [10, 11].

6.2.1.2 Carbapenemases

Carbapenemases confer the largest antibiotic resistance spectrum because they can hydrolyse not only carbapenems but also broad-spectrum penicillins, cefalosporins, and cephamycins. There are several known mechanisms; *Klebsiella pneumoniae* carbapenemase (KPC), OXA and metallo-beta-lactamases. See Fig. 6.3 for the spread of *E. coli* resistant to carbapenems and Fig. 6.4 for the spread of *K. pneumoniae* resistant to carbapenems, both figures show the whole world. See Fig. 6.5 for the spread of *K. pneumoniae* resistant to carbapenems in Europe.

KPC

The KPC enzymes were initially reported from *K. pneumoniae* isolates in several outbreaks in north-eastern USA. KPC enzymes are now found worldwide in multiple other Gram-negative species, such as *E. coli*, *Citrobacter*, *Enterobacter*, *Salmonella*, *Serratia*, and *P. aeruginosa* [12]. KPC is a β-lactamase that confers resistance to virtually all β-lactam antibiotics including carbapenems [13].

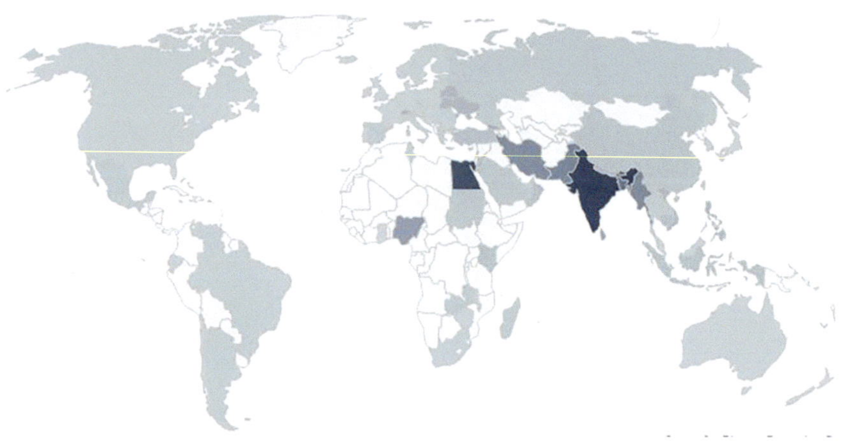

Fig. 6.3 World map: *E. coli* carbapenems

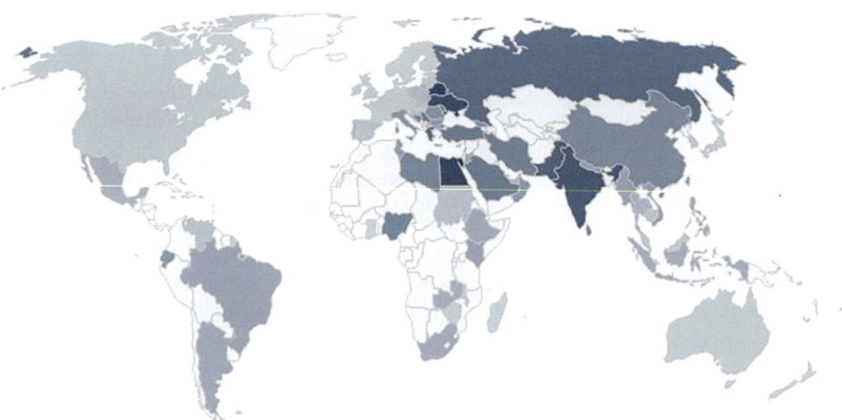

Fig. 6.4 World map: *K. pneumoniae* carbapenems. OneHealthTrust. ResistanceMap: Antibiotic resistance. 2022. https://resistancemap.onehealthtrust.org/AntibioticResistance.php. Date accessed: December 14, 2022

OXA

The OXA β-lactamases were among the earliest β-lactamases detected. In the beginning they were relatively rare and of little clinical consequence. OXA β-lactamases were originally mainly found in *Acinetobacter baumannii*. In the 1980s carbapenem-resistant *Acinetobacter baumannii* emerged and these carbapenemases were categorised as OXA enzymes because of their sequence similarity to earlier OXA

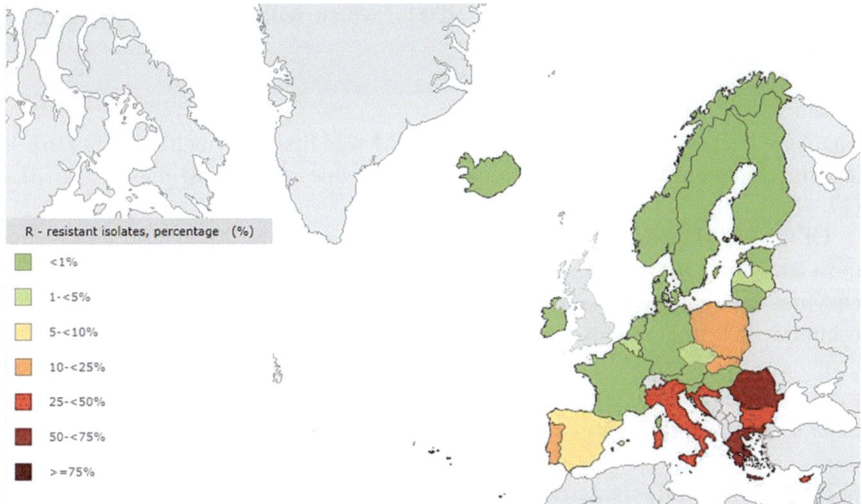

Fig. 6.5 European map: *K. pneumoniae* carbapenems. Surveillance Atlas of Infectious Diseases, European Centre for Disease Control: https://atlas.ecdc.europa.eu/public/index.aspx?Dataset=27 &HealthTopic=4. Date accessed: December 14, 2022

β-lactamases. Later, these OXA enzymes were found in *Enterobacterales* and have become a significant cause of carbapenem resistance. The emergence of OXA enzymes that can confer resistance to carbapenems, particularly in *A. baumannii*, has transformed these OXA- β-lactamases from a minor hindrance into a major problem set to undermine the clinical efficacy of the carbapenems [14].

OXA-carbapenemases have no significant effect on cefalosporins, but isolates with OXA enzymes frequently harbour ESBL as well, increasing the problem.

Metallo-Beta-Lactamases

Metallo-beta-lactamases (MBLs) are enzymes that rapidly hydrolyse most β-lactam agents, especially the carbapenems, but not the monobactams (e.g. Aztreonam), and are resistant to β-lactamase inhibitors. Chromosomally encoded MBLs are primarily found in environmental bacteria like *Aeromonas*, *Chryseobacterium*, and *Stenotrophomonas* spp. and usually has a low pathogenic potential, and as they are encoded chromosomally, they have little potential of dissemination. Later MBLs were identified on plasmids, which have the potential to spread, found in *Bacteroides fragilis*, *Serratia marcescens*, *Klebsiella pneumoniae* and *Pseudomonas aeruginosa*. Bacterial strains with MBLs are now identified in almost any part of the world. Most clinically important MBLs belong to six different families (imipenem [IMP], Verona integron-encoded metallo-β-lactamase [VIM], Sao Paulo metallo-β-lactamase [SPM], German imipenemase [GIM], Seoul imipenemase [SIM]), and New Delhi metallo-β-lactamase (NDM), typically transmitted by mobile gene elements inserted into integrons and spread through *P. aeruginosa*, *Acinetobacter*, and *Enterobacterales* [15].

In this chapter we will focus on NDMs, which will serve as an example of the MBLs.

NDM

The New Delhi metallo-beta-lactamases NDM was first described in 2009 [16]. It has since spread all over the world and become one of the most prevalent MBLs [17, 18].

Of the NDMs the New Delhi metallo-β-lactamase-1 (NDM-1) has received the most attention. Originally described in a *K. pneumoniae* isolate from India, NDM-1 enzymes have since been reported in a number of other countries, primarily in connection with travel to India or Pakistan. Most metallo-β-lactamases reside on mobile gene cassettes inserted into integrons that harbour additional antibiotic resistance genes to other antimicrobial classes; this multidrug resistance can be transferred to other species, severely limiting therapeutic options in serious infections.

6.2.1.3 Colistin Resistance

Colistin, also known as polymyxin E is effective against most Gram-negative bacilli. Colistin resistance is of concern as this is a drug of last resort to which organisms that are highly resistant to other antibiotic classes are often susceptible. It is one of the few drugs available still effective against some carbapenem-resistant *Enterobacterales*, including NDM-1 producers.

The first colistin resistance gene in a plasmid which can be transferred between bacterial strains, was first described in China, and was isolated from animals and raw meat [19]. Bacteria carrying the colistin resistance gene mcr-1 are capable of colonising humans without prior exposure to colistin, including healthy volunteers, and even in the environment in countries with little antibiotic resistance. The presence of this plasmid-borne *mcr*-1 gene has now been found in many areas of the world, including South-East Asia, several European countries and the United States [20–24].

6.2.2 MRSA

Methicillin-resistant *Staphylococcus aureus* (MRSA) was described for the first time in the United Kingdom in 1961, shortly after the introduction of the methicillin [25].

Methicillin resistance is caused by the formation of an extra penicillin binding protein (PBP2). PBP2 has a low affinity for methicillin and hence give resistance to all β-lactam antibiotics except the newly introduced class of anti-MRSA cefalosporins. Even though we use other penicillinase stable penicillin's such as (di-)cloxacillin and the drug methicillin is no longer in use, the name has remained in MRSA, as the abbreviation is so well known.

In the beginning, MRSA was usually found in hospitals and healthcare environments, but the epidemiology of MRSA has gradually changed, and MRSA is now

Resistance of *Staphylococcus aureus* to Oxacillin (MRSA)

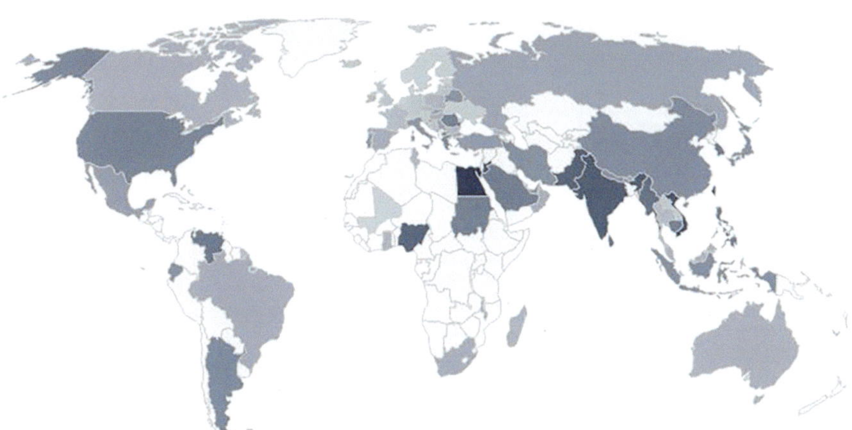

Fig. 6.6 World map: *S. aureus* oxacillin. OneHealthTrust. ResistanceMap: Antibiotic resistance. 2022. https://resistancemap.onehealthtrust.org/AntibioticResistance.php. Date accessed: December 14, 2022

widely disseminated in the community. In low prevalence countries, immigration and importation from countries with a higher level of MRSA represent important factors for the increasing notification rate of MRSA infections [26]. See Fig. 6.6 for the spread of *S. aureus* resistant to oxacillin in the world.

6.2.3 Vancomycin-Resistant Enterococci (VRE)

Vancomycin has been in use since the 1940s, but vancomycin-resistant enterococci (VRE) were not reported in the UK and France until the late 1980s [27]. The emergence of vancomycin resistance has been associated with the extensive use of vancomycin to treat MRSA and *C. difficile* infections. There are two predominant genes carried by strains of VRE, *van*A and *van*B. *van*A normally mediates high-level vancomycin and teicoplanin resistance. *van*B-positive isolates are vancomycin-resistant, but susceptible to teicoplanin in vitro, but teicoplanin is not recommended as monotherapy for *van*B VRE due to reported selection of teicoplanin resistance in vivo.

The spread of VRE is an example of how rapidly resistance can spread if not effectively contained. Ten years after VRE was first identified in Europe, more than 25% of enterococci associated with bloodstream infections were VRE in US hospitals [28]. Most hospital-derived strains of VRE found in Europe, USA, South America and Asia are part of a single clonal lineage, suggesting importation and spread through transfer of humans, livestock and animal products. See Fig. 6.7 for the spread of *E. faecium* resistant to vancomycin in the world.

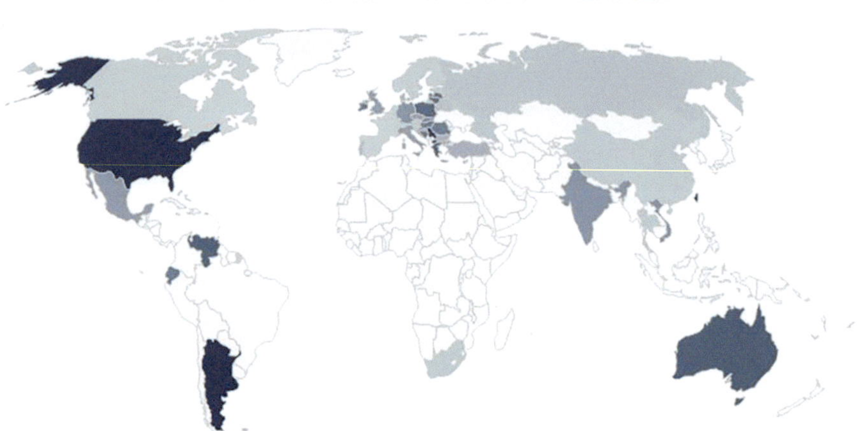

Fig. 6.7 World map: *E. faecium* vancomycin. OneHealthTrust. ResistanceMap: Antibiotic resistance. 2022. https://resistancemap.onehealthtrust.org/AntibioticResistance.php. Date accessed: December 14, 2022

6.2.4 *Neisseria gonorrhoeae*

In all societies, sexual transmitted diseases are said to have been imported from somewhere else. In earlier years syphilis was named "the English disease" in France, and contrary "the French disease" in England. The name given depends on which country the speaker wishes to disparage. *N. gonorrhoeae*, the cause of gonorrhoea, is one of the most common sexually transmitted diseases worldwide and this bacterium is often resistant to many classes of antibiotics traditionally used to treat the disease, including sulfonamides, penicillins, tetracyclines, fluoroquinolones, erythromycin and cefuroxime. Current recommended first-line therapy is ceftriaxone, often combined with azithromycin [29].

Multi-resistant *gonorrhoea* is on the rice, and in 2018 reached the headlines in various newspapers all over Europe when a British man and two Australians picked up the infection after sexual encounters in South-East Asia [30]. The strains found were resistant to ceftriaxone and high-level resistance to azithromycin. The reason for the headlines is the fear that *Neisseria gonorrhoeae* could eventually become untreatable by any antibiotic, thereby becoming the first true "super-bug" [31]. Due to AMR, gonorrhoea has been defined as a global public health threat. In order to avoid the emergence of untreatable gonorrhoea, novel, commonly accessible, cost-effective and nontoxic therapeutics are needed [32].

6.2.5 TBC

Multidrug-resistant (MDR) *Mycobacterium tuberculosis*, causing tuberculosis that does not respond to at least isoniazid and rifampicin, is becoming increasingly prevalent worldwide. Even more worrisome is the emergence of extensively drug-resistant (XDR) *Mycobacterium tuberculosis*, bacterial strains that are resistant to isoniazid and rifampicin, any fluoroquinolone, and at least one of three injectable second-line drugs (i.e. amikacin, kanamycin, or capreomycin). The emergence of MDR and XDR tuberculosis is caused by incorrect use of antimicrobial drugs, use of ineffective formulations of drugs, or failure to complete the full course of treatment. Person-to-person transmission rates are especially high in crowded settings such as hospitals and prisons.

XDR *Mycobacterium tuberculosis* is estimated to cause about 10% of cases of MDR tuberculosis and has been reported in 117 countries [33]. The numbers might be even higher given the fact that there is a lack of validated standards for drug-susceptibility testing in low-resource settings.

The possibility to acquire tuberculosis during travel is increasing, although the definitive attribution is difficult due to the wide range of latency periods [34].

6.3 Dissemination

One Health is the acknowledgement that the health of humans is closely interconnected with the health of the environment, including all living creatures, domestic and wild. AMR develops in the microbial biosphere when bacteria are exposed to naturally occurring or man-made antimicrobials. The spread of AMR happens between different bacteria, one example being through exchange of mobile genetic elements. Thus, development of AMR in any ecological niche may spread to other, meaning that the dissemination of antibiotic-resistant genes between various bacteria should be addressed with a One Health approach.

There is a crude estimation of one billion migrants worldwide, of whom approximately 3/4 migrates within their home country, while 1/4, or approximately 250 million people, migrate across borders. Meanwhile, the UNWTO World Tourism Barometer registered almost 1.2 billion international tourist arrivals in 2015, and the number of international flights performed by the global airline industry has steadily increased and reached almost 40 million in 2018 [35]. The total movement of people globally is not exactly known, but it is estimated that around 2 billion people cross international borders every year.

Travel is a well-established route of acquisition of antimicrobial-resistant organisms. Depending on the region visited, more than 70% of travellers to AMR high-endemic areas risk colonisation with multidrug-resistant *Enterobacterales*, although with a duration of colonisation in most cases of less than 3 months after returning to their home countries [36]. A study from Canada demonstrated a relative risk of community-onset infections with ESBL-producing *E. coli* in returning travellers of 145.6 after travel to the Indian subcontinent, 7.7 after travel to Africa and 18.1 after travel to the Middle East [37].

The prevalence of ESBL-E infections has reached 70–80% in some regions of the world. Some of these regions are tourism hotspots, which mean that many travellers visiting these areas are at risk of acquiring ESBL-E and subsequently spreading them in their country of origin upon return. Multiple ESBL-E colonisation studies indicate that travel is a risk factor for developing infections caused by multidrug-resistant organisms [37–41]. The prevalence of ESBL-E colonisation was the highest in visitors returning from high prevalence areas. These includes the Indian subcontinent (29–88%), China and Southeast Asia (18–67%), Middle East (13–52%), Northern Africa (0–57%) and Central and South America (0–49%), whereas the risk of colonisation is lower in North America and Europe [7, 42, 43]. In another study, 75.1% of visitors to Southern Asia, 40–50% of those to central, eastern, or western Asia and northern Africa and 44.4% of those to Uganda acquired ESBL-E while travelling. The highest acquisition rate was seen in India at 88.6% [44].

Aside from destination, other factors associated with ESBL-E acquisition include antibiotic consumption, traveller's diarrhoea or other abdominal complaints, contact with orphan children, staying in rural areas and consumption of street food [36, 41, 44, 45].

Carriage of bacteria with resistance mechanisms is often limited to the first 3 months after return from travel but persistent colonisation of up to 36 months has been observed in some studies [36, 44, 46]. Factors associated with persistence are not fully understood, but risk factors found for prolonged carriage are various, such as urinary catheter use, immobility and infection with *E. coli* strains belonging to certain phylogroups [47–50].

The speed of the spread of resistant microorganisms is well exemplified with the carbapenemase New Delhi metallo-β-lactamase (NDM). The gene encoding this enzyme was first described in *Enterobacterales* in 2009 and was in less than 10 years present globally [17]. Similar findings have been documented for the emergence and dissemination of resistance to colistin, which has been reintroduced in clinical practice as a last resort antibiotic to treat infections with carbapenem-resistant Gram-negative bacteria. The first mobile gene encoding resistance to colistin, the mcr-1, was first discovered in a pig-population in China in 2011, and was within a few years present all over the world [20].

Millions of migrants have entered Europe over the last years, which have imposed challenges to the social and healthcare systems in the countries of arrival [51]. Around 70% of migrants arriving in Europe originate from Ukraine, Syria, Afghanistan, Iraq, Eritrea and Nigeria, all countries without any functioning AMR surveillance programmes [52]. It is nevertheless reasonable to assume that these countries have a high burden of AMR, as the prevalence of drug-resistant organisms in neighbouring countries is high. So, especially during the refugee-crisis following the civil war in Syria, concerns were raised whether refugees and asylum-seekers from potential high endemic regions brought with them drug-resistant bacteria to the countries of arrival. Studies have shown that 20–60% of asylum seekers and refugees are colonised with resistant bacteria [53–55]. However, most of these studies are done in hospital settings, and data from primary healthcare settings, refugee camps, reception centres, etc. is scarce.

The term "migrant" covers a huge variety of people, as there are many causes for people to move from one country to another. There is evidence for differences in the prevalence of colonisation with resistant bacteria depending on the reasons for migration. A recently published review article and meta-analysis conclude with a pooled prevalence of colonisation or infection with antibiotic-resistant bacteria in refugees and asylum-seekers of 33%, as compared to 6.6% in other migrant groups [56].

Many refugees and asylum-seekers are admitted to, and spend some time in, refugee-camps and reception centres characterised by overcrowding, lack of access to healthcare facilities and poor hygienic conditions. In addition, humans from low- and middle-income countries often do not have recommended vaccinations. All these factors increase the risk for contracting infections, and for the spread of drug-resistant bacteria. In contrast, people who migrate for economic reasons or for family reunion, rarely spend time in reception centres or camps, but travel directly from their country of origin to their destination. Thus, the poor conditions in several arrival centres and refugee-camps are not only of concern to each and every person who stays in these camps but may contribute to transmission of drug-resistant organisms in the population on site followed by further dissemination to the receiving countries.

Another fact, which has to be considered, is that the European countries to which most migrants arrive in Europe are themselves AMR high-prevalent countries. This means that the transmission dynamics of drug-resistant organisms may actually be of greater concern for the migrant him- or herself, than for people living in the country of arrival.

6.4 Epidemiology

6.4.1 Geographic Distributions

The prevalence of antimicrobial-resistant bacteria is in general higher in developing countries. Over-crowding, improper sewage disposal and poor control in the use of antimicrobial agents are among the factors that select for antimicrobial resistance genes and encourage their dissemination. Many of the tourist destinations are also in low-income countries where poor sanitation and sewage systems facilitate the spread of resistant microorganisms in the communities.

There is a higher antibiotic selection pressure in the tropics. The reason for this is multifactorial. Improper use of antimicrobials, lack of microbiological diagnostic services, poor sanitation, shortage of clean water and interpersonal spread are key factors in the development and dissemination of resistant bacterial strains. All these factors are common in resource-limited countries.

Low- and middle-income countries (LMIC) in general have less control of the use of antimicrobial agents due to over-the-counter distribution. The lack of a solid diagnostic infrastructure in LMIC contributes further to the misuse of antibiotics and emergence of drug resistance. Lack of diagnostic opportunities and poor hospital facilities also increase the risk of hospital-acquired infections and spread of multi-resistant bacteria. To achieve effective resistance control it is necessary to have well-functioning clinical microbiology laboratories [57].

6.4.2 Recent Epidemics/Outbreaks

The spread of AMR is epidemic. Regularly outbreaks with AMR organisms occur, which is often a prerequisite for resistant microbes to become endemic in a region. We will mention a few recent outbreaks as examples.

Extensively drug-resistant *Salmonella typhi* is spreading in Pakistan. The outbreak is attributed to poor sewage and water systems, causing contamination of drinking water, in combination with low vaccination rates and overcrowded city centres. In less than a year, 800 cases of extensively drug-resistant *Salmonella* were detected by the health authorities in Pakistan in the city of Hyderabad alone. It is essential to get control of the outbreak by securing clean drinking water and provide vaccination [58, 59].

The potential of extensively drug-resistant *Salmonella typhi* to spread globally is raising fears beyond the borders of Pakistan [60, 61]. *Salmonella typhi* is endemic in many areas, and extensively drug-resistant typhoid may spread globally by replacing less-resistant strains. There are still antibiotic treatment options, azithromycin and carbapenems, but further genetic mutation could make typhoid fever untreatable and give death-rates that has not been seen since the pre-antibiotic era.

Several travel-related cases are reported. One travel-associated case was reported from the United Kingdom in 2018 [62]. In the United States, enhanced surveillance identified five patients with extensively drug-resistant *Salmonella typhi* who had travelled to or from Pakistan [63].

In Europe, there has recently been a regional outbreak of New Delhi metallo-beta-lactamase-producing carbapenem-resistant *Enterobacterales* in Italy [64]. The affected area in Italy is a major tourist destination making it highly likely that cross-border transmission will occur and that further spread to other European countries will happen.

6.4.3 Risk Factors

Hospitalisation abroad is a major risk factor for acquisition of multidrug-resistant organisms. International travel is easy accessible to nearly all groups of the society. Data from Eurostat show that more than half of the EU population in all age groups (15 and over) made tourism trips for personal purposes in the course of 2016, except those aged 65 or over, where it dropped to 49%. Still this age group represents nearly 48 million tourists [65]. One can imagine that the risk of hospitalisation while travelling might be higher in the older age groups with higher prevalence of chronic illness. Older travellers are more likely to have clinically significant coexisting conditions and consequently increased morbidity from infections [66].

Medical tourism emerges as people are seeking faster medical services at a lower cost. Cost-consciousness, and also availability of accredited facilities delivering medical service of high quality, have led to a growth in medical tourism in countries like Singapore, Thailand, India, Malaysia, Taiwan, Mexico and Costa Rica. In 2015 alone, 500,000 foreign nationals visited India for medical care. Most of these originating from other Asian countries, but medical tourism from other areas of the world is also increasing.

Studies show that suffering from travellers' diarrhoea and taking antibiotics while travelling are two of the main risk factors associated with becoming colonised with drug-resistant organisms [67]. The use of antibiotics, in particular quinolone use, during travel is shown to be a strong predictor for ESBL-acquisition [44]. Prophylactic use of antibiotics should thus be discouraged.

Travel, even without additional risk factors, increases the risk of colonisation with drug-resistant organisms. It is described that changes in the gut microbiome while travelling can reduce the resistance against colonisation with multidrug-resistant organisms, and thus making acquisition of resistant bacteria possible [68].

Whether staying with friends and relatives is a risk factor or protects against acquisition of drug-resistant organisms remains unclear as different studies show contradictive results. Increased length of stay however, is identified as a risk factor for becoming colonised [69, 70].

Personal hygiene, the standard of drinking water and toilet facilities, as well as living by the rule "boil it, cook, it, peel it or forget it" will all play a role in determining the risk of acquisition of against colonisation with multidrug-resistant organisms.

6.5 Clinical Findings

As infections caused by drug-resistant organisms has the same symptoms as infections caused by susceptible organisms, any patient seeking healthcare due to infections should be asked about their recent travels, meaning travels during the last 12 months. Hospitalisation in endemic regions should lead to screening for colonisation as well as being taken in to consideration when choosing the appropriate antibiotic treatment. The importance of thoroughly addressing travel history to identify individuals at risk of carrying multidrug-resistant microbes that can cause illness must be stressed. As it has been shown that much of the transmission of drug-resistant organisms occurs in households, and household members' travel histories should preferably be included.

6.6 Laboratory Diagnosis

Detecting antimicrobial resistance requires close cooperation with the medical/ clinical microbiology laboratory. In order for the analysis of potential AMR to be valuable for clinical decisions, there is a need for rapid detection of resistance mechanisms. The need for speed in laboratory methods has been the focus of attention for some years. Rapid methods for the detection of resistant bacteria have recently become more available, as both automated commercial methods using molecular techniques and new ways of using traditional methods more rapidly have been developed [71].

To be able to support clinicians with relevant and important information about resistance and resistance mechanisms, authorities must be encouraged to staff and finance the laboratories sufficiently to be able to provide such knowledge. Most new and rapid methods, including automated commercial methods using molecular techniques, are expensive, and few laboratories will be able to tell the mechanisms behind AMR without sufficient funding.

6.7 Differential Diagnosis and Diagnostic Hints

For all patients information on travel history and contact with healthcare facilities in high-risk areas the last 12 months should be obtained on admission to hospital. It is also advisable to ask your patients about diarrhoea or use of antibiotics while travelling.

Although being hospitalised abroad in a high prevalence area is a particular risk factor for acquiring AMR microbes, travellers may be colonised with MDR strains without having been in contact with healthcare facilities. Any travel to high-risk countries or areas should be considered. Travellers to all endemic regions are potential carriers of resistant bacteria. One study has even noted a 12% risk of transmitting ESBL-E to another household member after travel [17].

The prevalence of colonisation with drug-resistant organisms and type of resistance mechanism acquired varies according to the destination. The risk of acquiring ESBL-E colonisation is in several studies found to be highest in visitors returning from the Indian subcontinent. The risk is lower in developed countries [72]. However, the recent outbreak of NDM in Italy shows that even travel in Europe may represent a risk of infection or colonisation with multidrug-resistant strains.

6.8 Management

In order to manage patients with infections caused by multidrug-resistant organisms it is necessary to have knowledge about those at risk, who therefore should be treated with broad-spectrum antibiotics.

Similarly, and maybe even more important, knowledge about whom that can be treated with old narrow spectrum antibiotics is essential. As antibiotic treatment, and especially broad-spectrum antibiotic treatment, is considered to be the major driver of AMR, this makes it essential to know how to treat without unnecessarily contributing to the problem. We must be aware that the presence of multidrug-resistant microbes will in turn lead to the use of more broad-spectrum antibiotics that will further drive resistance development.

This problem can be illustrated by the case of VRE, were, as already mentioned, the use of vancomycin to treat MRSA and *Clostridium difficile* infections has led to the acquisition of van genes in *Enterococci*, thereby becoming VRE.

Vaccination and Infection Prevention and Control (IPC) measures are other possible ways to limit further development and spread for AMR. Vaccination reduces the burden of cases that need to be treated with antibiotics, thus reducing the risk of developing drug resistance. The spread of multidrug-resistant *Salmonella typhi* can be limited by providing vaccine for travellers to endemic or epidemic regions. IPC measures have been shown to remain an important tool in managing infections, and which in our opinion has not received the acknowledgement it deserves in hindering infections and therefore, lower the need for antibiotic use.

6.9   Public Health Responses

Many national and international organisations and public health authorities are beginning to make procedures for how to contain development and spread of AMR. As a response to the outbreak of New Delhi metallo-beta-lactamase (NDM) producing carbapenem-resistant *Enterobacterales* (CRE) in Italy in 2018/2019, ECDC (European Centre for Disease Control) has developed a rapid risk assessment that stress the importance of collecting a detailed history of travels and hospitalisations for every patient at hospital admission. Pre-emptive isolation and screening for carriage of CRE in patients who are directly transferred from, or hospitalised in, countries, areas, or hospitals with known high prevalence in the 12 months before admission, should be considered.

In order to be able to deal with the problem of AMR, there is a need of improved surveillance systems, both nationally and internationally. Without proper understanding of the problem and its magnitude, it is impossible to plan and design counteractions. Most of what is known about AMR today is knowledge produced in a limited number of countries, although the surveillance systems are improving. Global efforts to improve surveillance are needed in order to identify carriers of multi-resistant microbes, treat accordingly in the case of an infection, prevent further spread and address the effects of efforts to contain AMR.

Diagnostic tools that allow laboratory results to become more readily available to clinicians is a prerequisite to tackle the problem of AMR. If crucial information, such as an organism's susceptibility to various antibiotics, is delayed, the patient might experience a significantly prolonged period of illness, or in the most severe cases death may be the final outcome. Over the last decade many companies, and scientists, have come up with solutions to increase the speed of diagnostics. Much can be achieved by just working smarter, improve logistics and extending the working hours for the laboratory staff, but still improved and affordable diagnostic tools are needed. Some of the better commercial solutions today are far too expensive, maybe with the exception of the richest countries.

The role of tourism in spreading bacteria with AMR became clear by the travel restrictions imposed by the COVID-19 pandemic. In many AMR low-prevalence countries a significant decrease in ESBL-E was observed in 2020–2022, while recent data show a return to pre-pandemic national numbers.

6.10   Prevention and Advice for Travellers

All bacteria can develop resistance to various types of antibiotics, and we have learned that the presence of resistant bacteria varies widely between countries and regions of the world.

The overall aim must be to prevent resistant bacteria from spreading to vulnerable patients in healthcare institutions. Limiting spread from AMR high prevalence areas to regions with lower prevalence is a prerequisite to achieve this goal.

The share of resistant bacteria in the microbial biosphere is significantly increased most places around the world. In Europe, there is a higher prevalence in countries in the south and east. Outside Europe, many countries have a high prevalence, including countries that are popular tourist destinations for Europeans. Although the risk of getting an infection with resistant bacteria is higher for those treated in healthcare institutions, the transmission of resistant bacteria also occurs by regular contact between humans or through food. General measures, such as good hand and kitchen hygiene, are important in preventing being colonised or infected during travel and vacation abroad. Immigrants visiting their home country after having lived in their new country over a period is an important subgroup of travellers. Migrants is another subgroup of travellers also at risk for acquiring resistant bacteria during the process of migrating.

There are no existing vaccines specifically for resistant bacteria. It is nevertheless very wise to follow the vaccine-recommendations to reduce the overall risk of contracting an infection. We recommend travellers to follow the existing national guidelines. This reduces the risk of getting other infectious diseases and thereby reduces the need for healthcare and potential need of antibiotics while travelling.

If possible, one should avoid contact with healthcare institutions abroad. Health tourism, including dentistry, is associated with a significant risk for acquiring resistant bacteria. Even though the greatest risk is related to hospitalisation, there is also an increased risk associated with outpatient procedures.

Travel advice to patients before travelling can prevent the likelihood of becoming infected or colonised, and therefore reduce the number of infections that needs to be treated. Travel advice should include advice on methods of preventing and treating travellers' diarrhoea, the use of antibiotics, personal hygiene, food and drinking advice, safe sexual practices including condom use, and how to prevent skin infections and injuries. Such advice will largely also prevent infections with resistant bacteria. Most national authorities will have such information available to the public and to healthcare personnel.

Self-treatment with antibiotics occurs more often in travellers. One obvious reason is that medication, including antibiotics, is available over the counter without prescription in some countries. Another possibility is that the traveller has brought medication from home [73]. Travellers should therefore be discouraged to buy antibiotics not prescribed by a doctor while travelling.

For physicians or other healthcare workers, obtaining the patients' travel history is essential. This should include information on where the patient has been and for how long, which will give information on the risk that the sick is being colonised or infected with resistant bacteria. This is especially important when patients have received healthcare or dental treatment abroad, or have stayed in a country with a high incidence of resistant bacteria for a long time. Such information may be necessary to treat infections properly, and to prevent spread of resistant microbes.

In many countries there are guidelines that inform healthcare workers whom to screen for drug-resistant organisms. The ECDC has also developed guidelines [74]. Recommendations usually implies screening patients on admittance to a healthcare institutions, personnel who has previously been colonised with antibiotic-resistant bacteria without documented remediation, people who live with colonised persons or who over the last 12 months has been admitted to or undergone extensive treatment or examination in a foreign health institution or a refugee-camp. It is not recommended to screen people merely returning after travelling to high-endemic areas or asylum-seekers who have not lived in refugee-camps.

There are reasons for not screening for drug-resistant organisms. For example, there exists no means of remediation if colonised with multidrug-resistant *Enterobacterales* or VRE, and a positive test could lead to stigmatisation. Poor patient care, long, stays, and increased costs due to isolation practices and nursing barriers have been described for individuals colonised with resistant organisms [75].

6.11   Gaps in Knowledge that Need to Be Addressed

There is still a lack of knowledge about the clinical impact of AMR. How long do colonisation last? What are the increases in morbidity and mortality? Most of what is known today originate from hospital studies, while most of the carriers of AMR microbes are in the community. Most incidence and prevalence data for AMR cannot be linked with relevant epidemiological, clinical, or outcome data. This shows that studies on the impact of having infections with AMR microbes is a priority [76].

Declarations of Conflict of Interest   The authors declare no conflict of interest.

References

1. World Health Organisation (WHO). https://www.who.int/drugresistance/activities/wha66_side_event/en/.
2. Vignier N, Bouchaud O. Travel, migration and emerging infectious diseases. eJIFCC. 2018;29:175–9.
3. Knothe H, Shah P, Krcmery V, Antal M, Mitsuhashi S. Transferable resistance to cefotaxime, cefoxitin, cefamandole and cefuroxime in clinical isolates of Klebsiella pneumoniae and Serratia marcescens. Infection. 1983;11:315–7.
4. Woerther PL, Andremont A, Kantele A. Travel-acquired ESBL-producing Enterobacteriaceae: impact of colonization at individual and community level. J Travel Med. 2017;24(Suppl 1):S29–34.
5. Pitout JD, Nordmann P, Laupland KB, Poirel L. Emergence of Enterobacteriaceae producing extended-spectrum beta-lactamases (ESBLs) in the community. J Antimicrob Chemother. 2005;56:52–9.

6. van Duin D, Paterson DL. Multidrug-resistant bacteria in the community: trends and lessons learned. Infect Dis Clin North Am. 2016;30:377–90.

7. Woerther PL, Burdet C, Chachaty E, Andremont A. Trends in human fecal carriage of extended-spectrum beta-lactamases in the community: toward the globalization of CTX-M. Clin Microbiol Rev. 2013;26:744–58.

8. Coque TM, Baquero F, Canton R. Increasing prevalence of ESBL-producing Enterobacteriaceae in Europe. Euro Surveill. 2008;13(47):19044.

9. Naseer U, Sundsfjord A. The CTX-M conundrum: dissemination of plasmids and Escherichia coli clones. Microb Drug Resist. 2011;17:83–97.

10. Barbier F, Pommier C, Essaied W, Garrouste-Orgeas M, Schwebel C, Ruckly S, et al. Colonization and infection with extended-spectrum beta-lactamase-producing Enterobacteriaceae in ICU patients: what impact on outcomes and carbapenem exposure? J Antimicrob Chemother. 2016;71:1088–97.

11. Schwaber MJ, Carmeli Y. Mortality and delay in effective therapy associated with extended-spectrum beta-lactamase production in Enterobacteriaceae bacteraemia: a systematic review and meta-analysis. J Antimicrob Chemother. 2007;60:913–20.

12. Yigit H, Queenan AM, Anderson GJ, Domenech-Sanchez A, Biddle JW, Steward CD, et al. Novel carbapenem-hydrolyzing beta-lactamase, KPC-1, from a carbapenem-resistant strain of Klebsiella pneumoniae. Antimicrob Agents Chemother. 2001;45:1151–61.

13. Queenan AM, Bush K. Carbapenemases: the versatile beta-lactamases. Clin Microbiol Rev. 2007;20:440–58.

14. Evans BA, Amyes SG. OXA beta-lactamases. Clin Microbiol Rev. 2014;27(2):241–63.

15. Bush K. Other β-lactam antibiotics. In: Finch RG, Greenwood D, Whitley RJ, Norrby R, editors. Antibiotic and chemotherapy. 9th ed. Philadelphia: W. B. Saunders; 2010. p. 226–44.

16. Yong D, Toleman MA, Giske CG, Cho HS, Sundman K, Lee K, et al. Characterization of a new metallo-beta-lactamase gene, bla(NDM-1), and a novel erythromycin esterase gene carried on a unique genetic structure in Klebsiella pneumoniae sequence type 14 from India. Antimicrob Agents Chemother. 2009;53:5046–54.

17. Johnson AP, Woodford N. Global spread of antibiotic resistance: the example of New Delhi metallo-beta-lactamase (NDM)-mediated carbapenem resistance. J Med Microbiol. 2013;62:499–513.

18. Dortet L, Poirel L, Nordmann P. Worldwide dissemination of the NDM-type carbapenemases in Gram-negative bacteria. Biomed Res Int. 2014;2014:249856.

19. Liu YY, Wang Y, Walsh TR, Yi LX, Zhang R, Spencer J, et al. Emergence of plasmid-mediated colistin resistance mechanism MCR-1 in animals and human beings in China: a microbiological and molecular biological study. Lancet Infect Dis. 2016;16:161–8.

20. Wang Y, Tian GB, Zhang R, Shen Y, Tyrrell JM, Huang X, et al. Prevalence, risk factors, outcomes, and molecular epidemiology of mcr-1-positive Enterobacteriaceae in patients and healthy adults from China: an epidemiological and clinical study. Lancet Infect Dis. 2017;17:390–9.

21. von Wintersdorff CJ, Wolffs PF, van Niekerk JM, Beuken E, van Alphen LB, Stobberingh EE, et al. Detection of the plasmid-mediated colistin-resistance gene mcr-1 in faecal metagenomes of Dutch travellers. J Antimicrob Chemother. 2016;71:3416–9.

22. Nakayama T, Kumeda Y, Kawahara R, Yamaguchi T, Yamamoto Y. Carriage of colistin-resistant, extended-spectrum beta-lactamase-producing Escherichia coli harboring the mcr-1 resistance gene after short-term international travel to Vietnam. Infect Drug Resist. 2018;11:391–5.

23. Bernasconi OJ, Kuenzli E, Pires J, Tinguely R, Carattoli A, Hatz C, et al. Travelers can import Colistin-resistant Enterobacteriaceae, including those possessing the plasmid-mediated mcr-1 gene. Antimicrob Agents Chemother. 2016;60:5080–4.

24. Jørgensen SB, Søraas A, Arnesen LS, Leegaard T, Sundsfjord A, Jenum PA. First environmental sample containing plasmid-mediated colistin-resistant ESBL-producing Escherichia coli detected in Norway. APMIS. 2017;125:822–5.

25. Barber M. Methicillin-resistant staphylococci. J Clin Pathol. 1961;14:385–93.

26. Di Ruscio F, Bjørnholt JV, Leegaard TM, Moen AEF, de Blasio BF. MRSA infections in Norway: a study of the temporal evolution, 2006-2015. PLoS One. 2017;12:e0179771.
27. Leclercq R, Derlot E, Duval J, Courvalin P. Plasmid-mediated resistance to vancomycin and teicoplanin in Enterococcus faecium. N Engl J Med. 1988;319:157–61.
28. Willems RJ, Top J, van Santen M, Robinson DA, Coque TM, Baquero F, et al. Global spread of vancomycin-resistant Enterococcus faecium from distinct nosocomial genetic complex. Emerg Infect Dis. 2005;11:821–8.
29. Unemo M, Ross J, Serwin AB, Gomberg M, Cusini M, Jensen JS. 2020 European guideline for the diagnosis and treatment of gonorrhoea in adults. Int J STD AIDS. 2020:956462420949126.
30. Man has 'world's worst' super-gonorrhoea. BBC world news. 2018. Man has 'world's worst' super-gonorrhoea—BBC News.
31. Unemo M, Bradshaw CS, Hocking JS, de Vries HJC, Francis SC, Mabey D, et al. Sexually transmitted infections: challenges ahead. Lancet Infect Dis. 2017;17:e235–79.
32. Unemo M, Seifert HS, Hook EW 3rd, Hawkes S, Ndowa F, Dillon JR. Gonorrhoea. Nat Rev Dis Primers. 2019;5:79.
33. World Health Organisation (WHO). What is multidrug-resistant tuberculosis (MDR-TB) and how do we control it? https://www.who.int/features/qa/79/en/.
34. Salazar-Austin N, Ordonez AA, Hsu AJ, Benson JE, Mahesh M, Menachery E, et al. Extensively drug-resistant tuberculosis in a young child after travel to India. Lancet Infect Dis. 2015;15:1485–91.
35. Number of flights performed by the global airline industry from 2004 to 2019 (in millions): Statista. https://www.statista.com/statistics/564769/airline-industry-number-of-flights/.
36. Ruppe E, Armand-Lefevre L, Estellat C, Consigny PH, El Mniai A, Boussadia Y, et al. High rate of acquisition but short duration of carriage of multidrug-resistant Enterobacteriaceae after travel to the tropics. Clin Infect Dis. 2015;61:593–600.
37. van der Bij AK, Pitout JD. The role of international travel in the worldwide spread of multiresistant Entcrobacteriaceae. J Antimicrob Chemother. 2012;67:2090–100.
38. Jørgensen SB, Samuelsen Ø, Sundsfjord A, Bhatti SA, Jørgensen I, Sivapathasundaram T, et al. High prevalence of faecal carriage of ESBL-producing Enterobacteriaceae in Norwegian patients with gastroenteritis. Scand J Infect Dis. 2014;46:462–5.
39. Laupland KB, Church DL, Vidakovich J, Mucenski M, Pitout JD. Community-onset extended-spectrum beta-lactamase (ESBL) producing Escherichia coli: importance of international travel. J Infect. 2008;57:441–8.
40. Angue M, Allou N, Belmonte O, Lefort Y, Lugagne N, Vandroux D, et al. Risk factors for colonization with multidrug-resistant bacteria among patients admitted to the intensive care unit after returning from abroad. J Travel Med. 2015;22:300–5.
41. Kantele A, Laaveri T, Mero S, Vilkman K, Pakkanen SH, Ollgren J, et al. Antimicrobials increase travelers' risk of colonization by extended-spectrum betalactamase-producing Enterobacteriaceae. Clin Infect Dis. 2015;60(6):837–46.
42. Ruppe E, Andremont A, Armand-Lefevre L. Digestive tract colonization by multidrug-resistant Enterobacteriaceae in travellers: an update. Travel Med Infect Dis. 2018;21:28–35.
43. Hassing RJ, Alsma J, Arcilla MS, van Genderen PJ, Stricker BH, Verbon A. International travel and acquisition of multidrug-resistant Enterobacteriaceae: a systematic review. Euro Surveill. 2015;20(47).
44. Arcilla MS, van Hattem JM, Haverkate MR, Bootsma MCJ, van Genderen PJJ, Goorhuis A, et al. Import and spread of extended-spectrum beta-lactamase-producing Enterobacteriaceae by international travellers (COMBAT study): a prospective, multicentre cohort study. Lancet Infect Dis. 2017;17:78–85.
45. Kantele A, Mero S, Kirveskari J, Laaveri T. Increased risk for ESBL-producing bacteria from co-administration of Loperamide and antimicrobial drugs for travelers' diarrhea. Emerg Infect Dis. 2016;22:117–20.
46. Jørgensen SB, Søraas A, Sundsfjord A, Liestol K, Leegaard TM, Jenum PA. Fecal carriage of extended spectrum beta-lactamase producing Escherichia coli and Klebsiella pneu-

moniae after urinary tract infection—a three year prospective cohort study. PLoS One. 2017;12:e0173510.

47. Papst L, Beovic B, Seme K, Pirs M. Two-year prospective evaluation of colonization with extended-spectrum beta-lactamase-producing Enterobacteriaceae: time course and risk factors. Infect Dis (Lond). 2015;47:618–24.

48. Feldman N, Adler A, Molshatzki N, Navon-Venezia S, Khabra E, Cohen D, et al. Gastrointestinal colonization by KPC-producing Klebsiella pneumoniae following hospital discharge: duration of carriage and risk factors for persistent carriage. Clin Microbiol Infect. 2013;19:E190–6.

49. Titelman E, Hasan CM, Iversen A, Naucler P, Kais M, Kalin M, et al. Faecal carriage of extended-spectrum beta-lactamase-producing Enterobacteriaceae is common 12 months after infection and is related to strain factors. Clin Microbiol Infect. 2014;20:O508–15.

50. Overdevest I, Haverkate M, Veenemans J, Hendriks Y, Verhulst C, Mulders A, et al. Prolonged colonisation with Escherichia coli O25:ST131 versus other extended-spectrum beta-lactamase-producing E. coli in a long-term care facility with high endemic level of rectal colonisation, the Netherlands, 2013 to 2014. Euro Surveill. 2016;21(42):30376.

51. EU Migrant. Refugee arrivals by land and sea approach one million in 2015. https://www.iom.int/news/eu-migrant-refugee-arrivals-land-and-sea-approach-one-million-2015.

52. UNHCR (United Nations High Commissioner for Refugees). Refugees/migrants emergency response—Mediterranean 2016. http://data.unhcr.org.

53. de Smalen AW, Ghorab H, Abd El Ghany M, Hill-Cawthorne GA. Refugees and antimicrobial resistance: a systematic review. Travel Med Infect Dis. 2017;15:23–8.

54. Reinheimer C, Kempf VA, Gottig S, Hogardt M, Wichelhaus TA, O'Rourke F, et al. Multidrug-resistant organisms detected in refugee patients admitted to a University Hospital, Germany JuneDecember 2015. Euro Surveill. 2016;21(2).

55. Heudorf U, Albert-Braun S, Hunfeld KP, Birne FU, Schulze J, Strobel K, et al. Multidrug-resistant organisms in refugees: prevalences and impact on infection control in hospitals. GMS Hyg Infect Control. 2016;11:Doc16.

56. Nellums LB, Thompson H, Holmes A, Castro-Sanchez E, Otter JA, Norredam M, et al. Antimicrobial resistance among migrants in Europe: a systematic review and meta-analysis. Lancet Infect Dis. 2018;18:796–811.

57. Okeke I. Poverty and root causes of resistance in developing countries. In: Antimicrobial resistance in developing countries. Springer; 2009. p. 27–36.

58. Rasheed MK, Hasan SS, Babar ZU, Ahmed SI. Extensively drug-resistant typhoid fever in Pakistan. Lancet Infect Dis. 2019;19:242–3.

59. Qamar FN, Yousafzai MT, Khalid M, Kazi AM, Lohana H, Karim S, et al. Outbreak investigation of ceftriaxone-resistant Salmonella enterica serotype Typhi and its risk factors among the general population in Hyderabad, Pakistan: a matched case-control study. Lancet Infect Dis. 2018;18:1368–76.

60. Dalton J. Typhoid superbug in Pakistan raises fears of global antibiotic failure. The Independent; 2018. https://www.independent.co.uk/news/world/asia/typhoid-superbug-pakistan-global-antibiotic-failure-a8307836.html.

61. Baumgaertner E. 'We're out of options': doctors battle drug-resistant typhoid outbreak. The New York Times; 2018. https://www.nytimes.com/2018/04/13/health/drug-resistant-typhoid-epidemic.html.

62. Klemm EJ, Shakoor S, Page AJ, Qamar FN, Judge K, Saeed DK, et al. Emergence of an extensively drug-resistant Salmonella enterica Serovar Typhi clone harboring a promiscuous plasmid encoding resistance to fluoroquinolones and third-generation cephalosporins. mBio. 2018;9:e00105–18.

63. Chatham-Stephens K, Medalla F, Hughes M, Appiah GD, Aubert RD, Caidi H, et al. Emergence of extensively drug-resistant Salmonella typhi infections among travelers to or from Pakistan—United States, 2016-2018. MMWR Morb Mortal Wkly Rep. 2019;68:11–3.

64. Rapid risk assessment: regional outbreak of New Delhi metallo-betalactamase-producing carbapenem-resistant Enterobacteriaceae, Italy, 2018–2019. European Centre for Disease Prevention and Control (ECDC); 2019. https://ecdc.europa.eu/en/publications-data/RRA-new-delhi-metallo-beta-lactamase-producing-CRE.
65. Eurostat. Share of EU population (aged 15 and over) participating in tourism. https://ec.europa.eu/eurostat/statistics-explained/index.php?title=Tourism_statistics_-_participation_in_tourism.
66. Thwaites GE, Day NPJ. Approach to fever in the returning traveler. N Engl J Med. 2017;376:1798.
67. Tängden T, Cars O, Melhus A, Löwdin E. Foreign travel is a major risk factor for colonization with Escherichia coli producing CTX-M-type extended-spectrum beta-lactamases: a prospective study with Swedish volunteers. Antimicrob Agents Chemother. 2010;54:3564–8.
68. Kuenzli E. Antibiotic resistance and international travel: causes and consequences. Travel Med Infect Dis. 2016;14:595–8.
69. Kuenzli E, Jaeger VK, Frei R, Neumayr A, DeCrom S, Haller S, et al. High colonization rates of extended-spectrum beta-lactamase (ESBL)-producing Escherichia coli in Swiss travellers to South Asia—a prospective observational multicentre cohort study looking at epidemiology, microbiology and risk factors. BMC Infect Dis. 2014;14:528.
70. Schaumburg F, Sertic SM, Correa-Martinez C, Mellmann A, Kock R, Becker K. Acquisition and colonization dynamics of antimicrobial-resistant bacteria during international travel: a prospective cohort study. Clin Microbiol Infect. 2019;25:1287.e1–7.
71. European Comittee on Antimicrobial Susceptibility Testing (EUCAST). Rapid AST directly from blood culture bottles. http://www.eucast.org/rapid_ast_in_blood_cultures/.
72. Frost I, Van Boeckel TP, Pires J, Craig J, Laxminarayan R. Global geographic trends in antimicrobial resistance: the role of international travel. J Travel Med. 2019;26:taz036.
73. Laxminarayan R, Matsoso P, Pant S, Brower C, Rottingen JA, Klugman K, et al. Access to effective antimicrobials: a worldwide challenge. Lancet. 2016;387:168–75.
74. ECDC. Directory of online resources for the prevention and control of antimicrobial resistance (AMR) and healthcare-associated infections (HAI). https://ecdc.europa.eu/en/publications-data/directory-online-resources-prevention-and-control-antimicrobial-resistance-amr.
75. Fatkenheuer G, Hirschel B, Harbarth S. Screening and isolation to control meticillin-resistant Staphylococcus aureus: sense, nonsense, and evidence. Lancet. 2015;385:1146–9.
76. Tacconelli E, Sifakis F, Harbarth S, Schrijver R, van Mourik M, Voss A, et al. Surveillance for control of antimicrobial resistance. Lancet Infect Dis. 2018;18:e99–e106.

Filovirus Infections in Travellers

Tom E. Fletcher

Abstract

Filovirus disease (FVD) outbreaks present significant public health challenges when they occur in West and Central Africa. FVD includes Ebola and Marburg disease that carry high case fatality rates and significant nosocomial risk, with limited proven antiviral treatment options. African fruit bats are highly likely to be the reservoir host and whilst travellers are rarely infected, they are most at risk through exposure to bat's natural habitat or as healthcare workers responding to an FVD outbreak. Basic precautionary measures will mitigate this risk as will vaccination that is available for Ebola virus disease.

7.1 Background

The filovirus infections include Ebola and Marburg disease and are the most feared of all the viral hemorrhagic fevers due to their high case fatality rates, limited treatment options and high nosocomial risk. They are RNA viruses that are endemic in sub-Saharan Africa, with increasing numbers of outbreaks reported in the last 20 years, with the largest to date being the West African Ebola Virus Disease outbreak in 2013–2015, that resulted in almost 30,000 cases and over 11,000 deaths.

T. E. Fletcher (✉)
Department of Clinical Sciences, Liverpool School of Tropical Medicine, Liverpool, UK
e-mail: Tom.fletcher@lstmed.ac.uk

H. Leblebicioglu et al. (eds.), *Emerging and Re-emerging Infections in Travellers*, https://doi.org/10.1007/978-3-031-49475-8_7

7.2   Etiology

Ebolaviruses were first discovered in 1976 when two consecutive outbreaks of fatal hemorrhagic fever occurred in Africa. The first outbreak occurred in the Democratic Republic of Congo near the Ebola River [1], which gave the virus its name and the second outbreak occurred in South Sudan [2]. There are four *Ebolaviruses* and one species of *Marburgvirus* that can cause illness in people. Ebola virus (species Zaire ebolavirus) causes Ebola virus disease, Sudan virus (species Sudan ebolavirus) causes Sudan virus disease, Tai Forest virus (species Taï Forest ebolavirus, formerly Côte d'Ivoire ebolavirus) causes Taï Forest virus disease and Bundibugyo virus (species Bundibugyo ebolavirus) causes Bundibugyo virus disease [3]. Marburg virus was first recognized in 1967, following laboratory outbreaks in Marburg and Frankfurt, Germany and in Belgrade, Serbia [4]. Initial cases were linked to African green monkeys imported from Uganda, with subsequent transmission to their close contacts and healthcare workers, resulting in a total of thirty-one cases and seven deaths.

7.3   Transmission

Human-to-human transmission of filoviruses usually occurs through direct contact with infected blood or body fluids with a very low viral infective dose/inoculum required [5]. Transmission is predominantly through mucous membrane exposure whilst providing care in the community or in a healthcare setting, with additional risk posed by funeral activities that are often the first signal of an FVD outbreak, along with nosocomial amplification. As patients become more unwell with FVD they present increased risk of transmission as a result of increased diarrhoea and bleeding, with viral levels remaining high in severe cases through to death. There is no evidence of pre-symptomatic transmission. Aerosol transmission can occur as a result of aerosol generating procedures, and is a potential risk when in close contact during forceful vomiting or diarrhoea [6].

7.4   Epidemiology

Filoviruses are endemic to central and West Africa with the Democratic Republic of Congo (DRC) reporting the highest number of outbreaks (Fig. 7.1). Filovirus outbreaks appear to be occurring more frequently since the mid-1990s, possibly as result of enhanced surveillance and diagnostic capacity, but may also indicate more frequent spillover event due to anthropological and climate change. African fruit bats are highly likely to be involved in the spread of filoviruses and may be the reservoir host. Like in other VHFs, the reservoir host likely remains asymptomatic with the virus maintained in the environment by spreading from host to host or through intermediate hosts or vectors. Infected animals carrying the virus can transmit it to other animals, with severe illness seen in non-human primates (NHPs) and

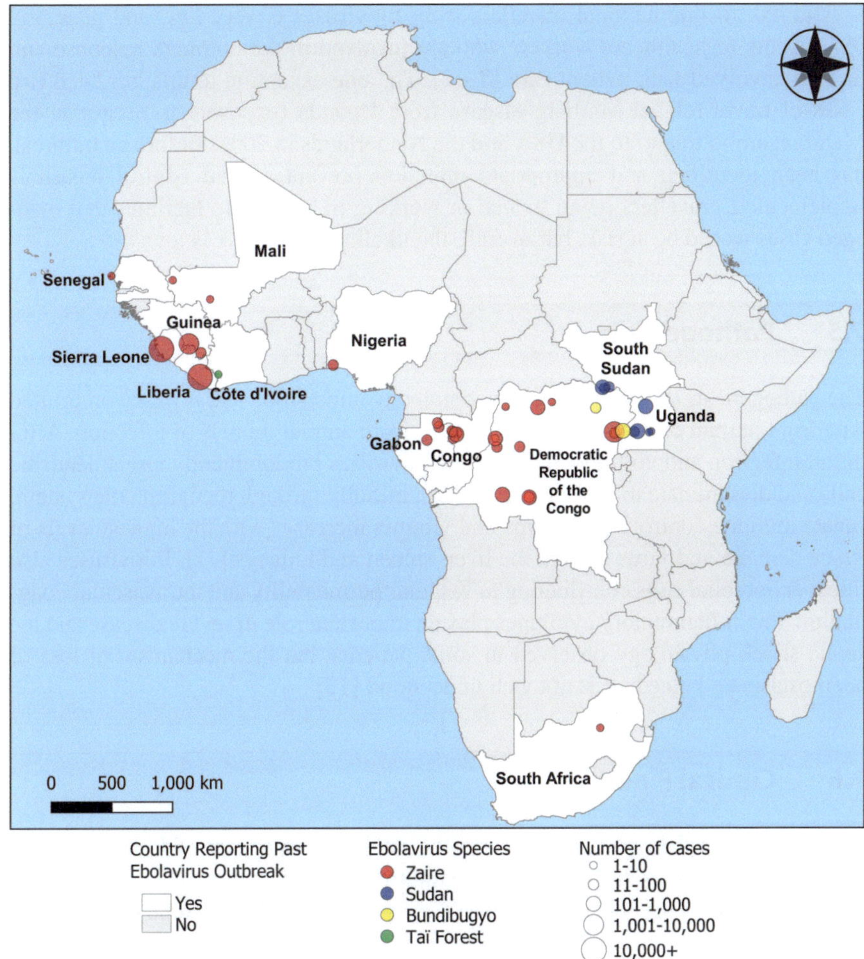

Fig. 7.1 Ebola disease outbreaks by species and size since 1976. (Source: Reference to specific commercial products, manufacturers, companies, or trademarks does not constitute its endorsement or recommendation by the U.S. Government, Department of Health and Human Services, or Centers for Disease Control and Prevention; https://www.cdc.gov/vhf/ebola/history/distribution-map.html; available free of charge)
Ebola https://www.cdc.gov/vhf/ebola/history/distribution-map.html

humans. The first humans can become infected through exposure to bat excreta/saliva, or through contact with blood or bodily fluids of infected NHPs. Risk factors include certain occupations such as miners, forestry worker and hunters. After generally a single zoonotic introduction human-to-human transmission predominates during outbreaks with nosocomial transmission to healthcare workers and patients regularly reported [7].

The risk to international travellers from filoviruses is very low, and generally only occurs to healthcare workers who are involved in the outbreak response and directly involved with patient care [8–10]. The one exception to this has been two cases of travel-related Marburg disease from Uganda (exposure to a cave in the Maramagambo forest) to the USA and the Netherlands in 2008. Before an outbreak has been identified and appropriate infection prevention and control measures implemented, travellers being treated or working in healthcare facilities that managed cases would be at risk, but overall, the likelihood and risk is low.

7.5 Pathogenesis

The pathogenesis of FVD remains incompletely understood and is based on limited data from human outbreaks and that gained from animal models of infection. After initial infection and viral inoculation, the filoviruses predominantly target dendritic cells and disseminate to virtually all organs, initially through the lymphatic system. Innate immune control is overcome and viremia increases with the highest levels of tissue damage and virus seen in the liver, spleen and kidneys [11]. Filoviruses also infect endothelial cells contributing to vascular permeability and intravascular coagulation. Pro-inflammatory cytokines play an important role in severe disease and the septic shock physiology observed in some patients, but the mechanism of loss of haemostasis and bleeding is not well understood [12].

7.6 Clinical Findings

There is limited data on differences in the clinical phenotypes of Ebolavirus and Marburg virus species, but all have a maximum incubation period of 21 days (generally 7–10 days). A spectrum of disease severity is observed with some patients having mild or even asymptomatic infection [13]. The most clinical data is available for EVD, that initially manifests as non-specific febrile illness including fever, headache, myalgia and progressive malaise [14, 15]. The malaise/asthenia is progressive and a characterizing feature of FVD progressing to severe vomiting and diarrhoea in the majority of cases. This is characterized by progressive organ dysfunction including acute kidney injury, significant electrolyte imbalance and viral hepatitis. Severe FVD includes patients who develop bleeding (generally from mucous membranes, the gastrointestinal tract and intravenous line sites), encephalopathy/seizures and irreversible renal failure, all of which often lead to fatal outcomes. The case fatality rates differ between Ebola species and Marburg disease. Ebola virus disease (species Zaire ebolavirus) has the highest case fatality rates of 80–90% without treatment, reducing to around <35% with optimized supportive care and access to monoclonal antibody therapies.

7.7   Laboratory Diagnosis

Diagnosis of acute infection is by reverse transcription polymerase chain reaction (RT-PCR) on blood or oral swabs in suspected fatal cases. Advances since the west African EVD outbreak in 2013—205 include availability of cartridge-based near-patient PCR platforms for some species that facilitates rapid diagnosis and treatment [16]. Serology can be utilized after viremia has cleared and whilst rapid diagnostic tests such as lateral flow assays have been developed none are yet in routine use. Standard haematology and biochemistry assays can only be done under strict laboratory containment, and show leucopenia, thrombocytopenia, transaminitis and electrolyte imbalance predominantly hypo/hyperkalemia and hypoglycemia, with raised urea and creatinine levels almost universal [15].

7.8   Differential Diagnosis

The initial presentation of FVD is non-specific and resembles many undifferentiated febrile illnesses observed in west and central Africa [17]. The most important differential diagnosis in febrile returning travellers that requires rapid diagnosis and treatment is malaria. This commonly occurs as a co-infection in endemic populations during Ebola disease outbreaks but in traveller a positive malaria test effectively excludes FVD unless there has been a high-risk exposure. Severe bacterial infections such as meningococcus and dysentery should be considered, as should rickettsial infection that is often missed. The key component to enable diagnosis of FVD in a traveller is an appropriate risk assessment and detailed travel and exposure history [9]. This should include identifying at-risk occupations such as miners/healthcare workers and contact with sick people or attending funerals (Fig. 7.2).

- Is there an ongoing FVD outbreak (Ebola or Marburg disease) in the country the patient has travelled from?
- Has the patient developed symptoms including fever or had a fever measured >37.5 °C within 21 days of leaving that country?
- Has the patient cared for/come into contact with body fluids of/handled clinical specimens from an individual or laboratory animal known or strongly suspected to have FVD?
- Has the patient visited any caves in Africa where bats may be present?

Fig. 7.2 Key questions to be answered for risk assessment of filovirus disease (FVD) in travelers

7.9 Treatment

The mainstay of case management for patients with FVD is focused on the provision of optimized supportive care, including fluid and electrolyte replacement and treatment of co-infections [18–20]. This is challenging in all settings due to the nosocomial risk and infection prevention and control requirements, combined with the high likelihood of the patient becoming critically unwell. For EVD there are two monoclonal antibody therapeutics targeting the Ebola virus glycoprotein (REGN-EB3, a co-formulated cocktail of three human monoclonal antibodies and mab114, a recombinant human IgG1) licensed by the U.S. FDA that have demonstrated survival benefit in randomized clinical trials in the DRC [21]. Both were more effective in reducing the case fatality rate in patients who sought treatment early after symptom onset, who had low viral loads, and who had lower baseline creatinine or alanine aminotransferase levels [22].

Critical care admission including provision of renal replacement therapy and mechanical ventilation should be considered for severe cases when the capability including infection prevention and control requirements is available. In a case series of 27 patients with EVD who were cared for in the United States or Europe during the 2013–2015 west African outbreak, close monitoring and aggressive supportive care that included intravenous fluid hydration, correction of electrolyte abnormalities, nutritional support, and critical care management for respiratory and renal failure was provided; resulting in 81.5% of the patients surviving. Patients, including travellers who have recovered from confirmed FVD, need careful follow-up to manage complications and longer-term sequelae, including psychological [23]. Male survivors should also encourage to use barrier methods of contraception until their semen has tested negative by RT-PCR.

7.10 Prevention and Advice for Travellers

For travellers working in or visiting an area where filoviruses are potentially present, there are a number of basic protective measures that they can be recommended to take. These include avoiding contact with:

- Blood and body fluids, or items contaminated with them, especially from people who are sick.
- Body or fluids of someone at a funeral or burial practice who was suspected or confirmed to have had FVD.
- Semen from a patient who has recovered from FVD until it has tested negative.
- Bats, forest antelopes, non-human primates and the blood, bodily fluids, or raw meat of these animals.

Healthcare workers in FVD endemic areas should focus on good adherence to universal and transmission-based precautions; being ready to identify alert cases of FVD; and on being trained to utilize appropriate personal protective equipment. The

U.S. FDA and European Medical Agency (EMA) approved the first Ebola vaccine raves-ZEBOV (called Ervebo®) in 2019, that is protective against Ebola virus (species Zaire ebolavirus) [24]. Since then, Burundi, Central African Republic, the Democratic Republic of the Congo, Ghana, Guinea, Rwanda, Uganda, and Zambia have also approved the vaccine. Pre-exposure vaccination can be considered for those who are at potential occupational risk, including people responding or an outbreak or laboratory staff working with live virus. In 2020 the EMA recommended to grant marketing authorization to a second new vaccine delivered in two doses called Zabeen (Ad26.ZEBOV) and Mvabea (MVA-BN-Filo) for individuals 1 year and older. Although no post-exposure prophylaxis has been proven for filovirus disease, a range of therapeutics have been utilized on compassionate grounds and should be considered based on an individual risk assessment and availability [25].

Conflict of Interest I declare no conflict of interest.

References

1. Burke J, Declerq R, Ghysebrechts G. Ebola haemorrhagic fever in Zaire, 1976. Report of an international commission. Bull World Health Organ. 1978;56(2):271–93.
2. Report of a WHO/International Study Team. Ebola haemorrhagic fever in Sudan, 1976. Bull World Heal Organ. 1978;56:247–70. https://doi.org/10.1021/ie000475z.
3. Kuhn JH, et al. New filovirus disease classification and nomenclature. Nat Rev Microbiol. 2019;17(5) https://doi.org/10.1038/s41579-019-0187-4.
4. Siegert GMR, Shu HL, Slenczka HL, Peters D. The aetiology of an unknown human infection transmitted by monkeys (preliminary communication). Ger Med Mon. 1968;13(1):1–2.
5. Bausch DG, et al. Assessment of the risk of Ebola virus transmission from bodily fluids and fomites. J Infect Dis. 2007;196(Suppl. 2):S142–7. https://doi.org/10.1086/520545.
6. Osterholm MT, et al. Transmission of Ebola viruses: what we know and what we do not know. MBio. 2015;6(2):1–9. https://doi.org/10.1128/mBio.00137-15.Editor.
7. Jain S, Khaiboullina S, Martynova E, Morzunov S, Baranwal M. Epidemiology of Ebolaviruses from an etiological perspective. Pathogens. 2023;12(2) https://doi.org/10.3390/pathogens12020248.
8. Isaäcson M. Viral hemorrhagic fever hazards for travelers in Africa. Clin Infect Dis. 2001;33(10):1707–12. https://doi.org/10.1097/00006454-200203000-00027.
9. Beeching NJ, Fletcher TE, Wijaya L. Returned travellers. In: Zuckerman JN, editor. Principles and practice of travel medicine (Chapter 15). 2nd ed. John Wiley & Sons; 2013. p. 260–86.
10. Beeching NJ, Fletcher T, Hill DR, Thomson GL. Travellers and viral haemorrhagic fevers—what are the risks? Int J Antimicrob Agents. 2010;36:S26–39. https://doi.org/10.1016/j.ijantimicag.2010.06.017. [Epub ahead of print 10 Aug 2010]. http://www.ijaaonline.com/article/S0924-8579%2810%2900258-X/fulltext
11. Baseler L, Chertow DS, Johnson KM, Feldmann H, Morens DM. The pathogenesis of Ebola virus disease. Annu Rev Pathol Mech Dis. 2017;12:387–418. https://doi.org/10.1146/annurev-pathol-052016-100506.
12. Fletcher TE, Fowler RA, Beeching NJ. Understanding organ dysfunction in Ebola virus disease. Intensive Care Med. 2014;40(12):1936–9. https://doi.org/10.1007/s00134-014-3515-1.
13. WHO Ebola Response Team. Ebola virus disease in West Africa—the first 9 months of the epidemic and forward projections. Engl New J Med. 2014:1–15. https://doi.org/10.1056/NEJMoa1411100.

14. Schieffelin JS, et al. Clinical illness and outcomes in patients with Ebola in Sierra Leone. N Engl J Med. 2014;371(22):2092–100. https://doi.org/10.1056/NEJMoa1411680.
15. Hunt L, et al. Clinical presentation, biochemical, and haematological parameters and their association with outcome in patients with Ebola virus disease: an observational cohort study. Lancet Infect Dis. 2015;15(11) https://doi.org/10.1016/S1473-3099(15)00144-9.
16. Semper AE, et al. Performance of the GeneXpert Ebola assay for diagnosis of ebola virus disease in Sierra Leone: a field evaluation study. PLoS Med. 2016;13(3):1–15. https://doi.org/10.1371/journal.pmed.1001980.
17. O'Shea MK, Clay KA, Craig DG, Matthews SW, Kao RL, Fletcher TE, Bailey MS, Hutley E. Diagnosis of febrile illnesses other than ebola virus disease at an Ebola treatment unit in Sierra Leone. Clin Infect Dis. 2015;61(5):795–8. https://doi.org/10.1093/cid/civ399.
18. Dickson SJ, et al. Enhanced case management can be delivered for patients with EVD in Africa: Experience from a UK military Ebola treatment centre in Sierra Leone. J Infect. 2018; https://doi.org/10.1016/j.jinf.2017.12.006.
19. Brett-Major DMDM, et al. Being ready to treat Ebola virus disease patients. Am J Trop Med Hyg. 2015;92(2):233–7. https://doi.org/10.4269/ajtmh.14-0746.
20. Lamontagne F, et al. Evidence-based guidelines for supportive care of patients with Ebola virus disease. Lancet. 2017; https://doi.org/10.1016/S0140-6736(17)31795-6.
21. Mulangu S, et al. A randomized, controlled trial of Ebola virus disease therapeutics. N Engl J Med. 2019;381(24):2293–303. https://doi.org/10.1056/nejmoa1910993.
22. Levine MM. Monoclonal antibody therapy for Ebola virus disease. N Engl J Med. 2019;381(24):2365–6. https://doi.org/10.1056/nejme1915350.
23. Jagadesh S, et al. Disability among Ebola survivors and their close contacts in sierra leone: a retrospective case-controlled cohort study. Clin Infect Dis. 2018;66(1) https://doi.org/10.1093/cid/cix705.
24. Henao-Restrepo AM, et al. Efficacy and effectiveness of an rVSV-vectored vaccine in preventing Ebola virus disease: final results from the Guinea ring vaccination, open-label, cluster-randomised trial (Ebola Ça Suffit!). Lancet. 2017;389(10068):505–18. https://doi.org/10.1016/S0140-6736(16)32621-6.
25. Jacobs M, et al. Post-exposure prophylaxis against Ebola virus disease with experimental antiviral agents: a case-series of health-care workers. Lancet Infect Dis. 2015;15(11):1300–4. https://doi.org/10.1016/S1473-3099(15)00228-5.

Crimean-Congo Haemorrhagic Fever in Travellers

8

Resat Ozaras and Hakan Leblebicioglu

Abstract

Crimean-Congo haemorrhagic fever (CCHF) is a tick-borne viral disease caused by the CCHF virus. It is transmitted to humans through the bites of infected ticks and the direct contact with the infected animals or humans. It is endemic in many countries in Africa, Asia, the Middle East, and South-Eastern Europe, and it has been reported in many others since the infected ticks are introduced into new areas through movement and transport of wildlife and livestock and sick people visiting the endemic regions carry the virus to their home countries. Clinical findings range from asymptomatic or mild febrile illness to severe disease characterized by severe haemorrhagic manifestations, multi-organ failure and shock. The laboratory diagnosis of CCHF depends on the detection of the virus or viral antigens in clinical samples of the patients. The management includes supportive care and treatment of complications.

Travelling is increasing all over the world and there have been reported cases of CCHF among travellers. During visit to an area where CCHF is reported, travellers can take some measures to prevent themselves from contracting CCHF including avoiding contact with animals, wearing protective clothing, using insect repellent, staying in screened or air-conditioned places, practicing good hygiene, being aware of the risk, seeking advice from a healthcare provider, avoiding high-risk activities, and seeking medical attention if symptoms develop.

R. Ozaras (✉)
Department of Infectious Diseases, Beylikdüzü Medilife Hospital, Istanbul, Turkey

H. Leblebicioglu
Department of Infectious Diseases, VM Medicalpark Samsun Hospital, Samsun, Turkey

© The Author(s), under exclusive license to Springer Nature Switzerland AG 2024

H. Leblebicioglu et al. (eds.), *Emerging and Re-emerging Infections in Travellers*, https://doi.org/10.1007/978-3-031-49475-8_8

8.1   Introduction

Crimean-Congo haemorrhagic fever (CCHF) is a zoonotic viral disease caused by the CCHF virus. It is a tick-borne disease and primarily transmitted to humans through the bites of infected ticks and also through the direct contact with the blood, tissues, or bodily fluids of infected animals or humans [1]. While the disease is endemic in many countries, it has been also reported in many others since the infected ticks are introduced into new areas through movement and transport of wildlife and livestock and sick people visiting the endemic regions carry the virus to their home countries [2, 3]. This chapter discusses the types of travel-related CCHF cases, the characteristics of cases with CCHF acquired abroad, the number of travel-related CCHF cases, cross-border travel, the outcomes of cases, the source and destination countries, and the risk occupations or activities for travel-related CCHF, as well as the risk for immigrants.

8.2   The Disease

8.2.1   Epidemiology

The geographic range of CCHF virus is wide. CCHF endemic areas are seen in Africa, Asia, the Middle East, and South-Eastern Europe, and it has spread to previously unaffected regions and nations [4–6] (Fig. 8.1).

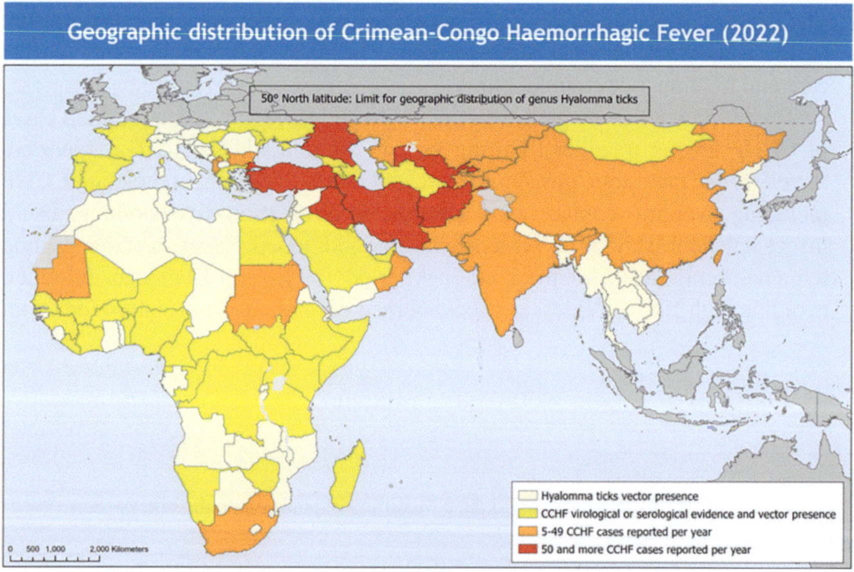

Fig. 8.1 Geographic distribution of Crimean-Congo haemorrhagic fever in 2022 [4]

8.2.1.1 Africa

CCHF is endemic in several African countries, including South Africa, Mauritania, Senegal, Burkina Faso, Niger, Nigeria, Ghana, Uganda, Tanzania, Kenya, Somalia, Sudan, and Egypt. Outbreaks of the disease have also been reported in other African countries such as Congo, Madagascar, and Angola.

8.2.1.2 Asia

CCHF is endemic in many countries in Asia, including Afghanistan, Iran, Iraq, Pakistan, Kazakhstan, Tajikistan, Uzbekistan, Turkmenistan, and China. Outbreaks of the disease have also been reported in other Asian countries such as India, Oman, Saudi Arabia, and Turkey.

8.2.1.3 Europe

CCHF is sporadic in several countries in Europe. Eastern European countries including Bulgaria, Greece, Romania, Russia, and Turkey reported several cases. Outbreaks of the disease have also been reported in other European countries such as Kosovo, Montenegro, and Ukraine.

8.2.1.4 Middle East

CCHF is endemic in many countries in the Middle East, including Yemen, United Arab Emirates, Kuwait, Bahrain, Qatar, Lebanon, and Jordan. Outbreaks of the disease have also been reported in other Middle Eastern countries such as Syria, Iraq, and Iran.

CCHF incidence varies greatly by country and region. Some countries, such as Turkey and Iran, have reported a high number of cases of CCHF each year. In contrast, other countries, such as South Africa and Greece, have reported relatively few cases. In some countries, the disease is more prevalent in rural areas, where tick populations are higher and animal husbandry practices are more common. Overall, the global incidence of CCHF is increasing, and the disease is becoming a growing public health concern.

8.2.2 Clinical Findings

Individuals infected with CCHF virus present with a variety of symptoms, ranging from asymptomatic or mild febrile illness to severe disease characterized by severe haemorrhagic manifestations, multi-organ failure and shock [1].

The incubation period of the disease is 3–7 days (range 1–14 days), after which symptoms begin to appear. The incubation period can be shorter when the viral load is high.

The initial symptoms of CCHF are non-specific and can include fever, headache, muscle aches, malaise, dizziness, neck pain and stiffness, backache, fatigue, sore eyes and photophobia. Some patients describe nausea, vomiting, diarrhoea, abdominal pain and sore throat. Two to four days of sharp mood swings, agitation and confusion are followed by sleepiness, depression and lassitude. The abdominal pain may localize to the upper right quadrant with detectable liver enlargement.

As the illness progresses, patients may develop more severe symptoms, including haemorrhagic symptoms such as petechiae, ecchymoses, uncontrolled bleeding at injection sites and mucosal bleeding beginning on about the fourth day of illness and lasting for about 2 weeks. Bleeding from the gums, nose, and gastrointestinal tract is common in severe cases. The disease can also cause liver and kidney dysfunction, and pulmonary problems.

8.2.3 Laboratory Diagnosis

Early and accurate diagnosis of CCHF is needed for appropriate treatment and management of the disease. Laboratory diagnosis of CCHF requires specialized facilities and expertise, and samples must be handled in a Biosafety Level 4 (BSL-4) laboratory to ensure the safety of laboratory personnel.

The laboratory diagnosis of CCHF depends on the detection of the virus or viral antigens in clinical samples of the patients. In the convalescent phase of the disease, the diagnosis is confirmed by demonstration of an antibody response. Various laboratory techniques can be used to detect the virus, including polymerase chain reaction (PCR), antigen detection assays, and virus isolation in cell culture [7].

Serological testing can be used to detect the presence of antibodies against the virus in patient serum. Antibody tests include enzyme-linked immunosorbent assays (ELISAs) and indirect immunofluorescence assays (IFAs).

The type of assay to use is closely related with the duration of time elapsed since symptom onset and the validity of the test for the CCHFV strains found in the suspected region of exposure [8]. In a nonfatal human case, the studies that directly assess for the infection, such as viral culture, nucleic acid amplification tests, and viral antigen detection studies are most useful during the first week of the disease. Viremia vanes over the first week of the disease, the time when the anti-CCHFV antibodies develop. Serological response consistent with acute infection (anti-CCHFV IgM antibodies or a fourfold increase in anti-CCHFV IgG titers between serial blood samples) is possible following the first week of the disease [7].

8.2.4 The Pathogenesis

CCHF pathogenesis is mainly derived from the interaction between the virus and the host [9]. The CCHF virus (CCHFV) replicates in various cells and tissues of the human body. The virus targets cells of the mononuclear phagocyte system, including macrophages and dendritic cells, replicates in these cells and leads to the release of large amounts of virus into the bloodstream. It also infects endothelial cells lining the blood vessels. Infection of endothelial cells lead to damage to the vascular walls and increased vascular permeability. This can cause haemorrhages in various organs, including the skin, the liver, spleen, and kidneys.

The entry of the virus into the body stimulates an immune response, including the activation of innate and adaptive immune cells. High levels of the pro-inflammatory cytokines (IL-6, IL-8, IL-10, and TNFα) are secreted by endothelial cells, CCHFV-infected macrophages and dendritic cells [10]. CCHFV leads to haemorrhagic complications through multiple factors including vascular endothelial damage, disseminated intravascular coagulation, thrombocytopenia, liver dysfunction, and decreased levels of coagulation factors [11].

Liver is a target organ of the virus. Kupffer cells, hepatic endothelial cells, and hepatocytes are affected [12]. The necrosis of hepatocytes is responsible from the increase in liver enzymes [13]. The AST/ALT ratio is reported higher in patients with severe disease than for those with mild disease [14].

Leukopenia is likely derived from an increased myeloperoxidase expression in leukocytes leading to increased leukocyte lysis. Thus, leukopenia in patients with CCHF may be attributed to leukocyte lysis [15].

The virus can evade the immune response through several mechanisms, including the inhibition of interferon production and the suppression of antigen presentation by infected cells. This allows the virus to continue to replicate and spread throughout the body.

The viral load is associated with the severity and prognosis of the disease; a load of $>10^8$ viral copies /ml in plasma is associated with fatal outcome [16, 17].

8.2.5 The Differential Diagnosis

The clinical findings of CCHF can be similar to other viral haemorrhagic fevers (VHFs) and some other infectious diseases, which can make the differential diagnosis challenging. VHFs are often difficult to discriminate only by clinical findings. Initial symptoms are nonspecific including fever, fatigue, dizziness, myalgia, weakness, and exhaustion.

Viruses other than CCHF virus causing VHFs include: Arenaviridae (Lassa fever, Lujo haemorrhagic fever (HF), Chapare HF, Junin HF, Machupo HF and Sabia HF), Filoviridae (Ebola virus (EBOV) disease and Marburg virus disease), Flaviviridae (Alkhurma HF, Dengue fever, Kyasanur Forest disease, Omsk HF and yellow fever), Hantaviridae (HF with renal syndrome and hantavirus pulmonary syndrome), and Phenuiviridae (Rift Valley fever) [9].

Some of the diseases that can be considered in the differential diagnosis of CCHF include:

Ebola virus disease (EVD): EVD is another viral haemorrhagic fever that can cause similar symptoms to CCHF, including fever, haemorrhage, and multi-organ failure. It caused an outbreak in West Africa in 2014–2016. EVD is typically characterized by a more severe clinical course and a higher case fatality rate.

Dengue fever: Dengue fever is a viral disease transmitted by mosquitoes that can cause fever, headache, and muscle and joint pain. However, dengue fever typically does not cause haemorrhagic symptoms, which can help differentiate it from CCHF. It is seen worldwide, mainly in tropics and subtropics.

Malaria: Malaria is a parasitic disease transmitted by mosquitoes that can cause fever, headache, and muscle aches, similar to CCHF. However, malaria typically does not cause haemorrhagic symptoms, and it can be diagnosed using blood smears or rapid diagnostic tests. The disease is seen worldwide, especially in tropical and subtropical areas.

Typhoid fever: Typhoid fever is a bacterial infection that can cause fever, headache, and gastrointestinal symptoms. Typhoid fever typically does not cause haemorrhagic symptoms, and it can be diagnosed using blood culture or serological tests. It is seen in Eastern and Southern Asia (especially Pakistan, India, and Bangladesh), Africa, the Caribbean, Central and South America, and the Middle East.

Rickettsial infections: Rickettsial infections, such as Rocky Mountain spotted fever and Mediterranean spotted fever, can cause fever, headache, and rash, similar to CCHF. However, these infections typically do not cause haemorrhagic symptoms, and they can be diagnosed using serological tests or PCR. Rocky Mountain spotted fever is seen in southeastern and south central U.S. and Mediterranean spotted fever is endemic in the Mediterranean basin.

Brucellosis: Brucellosis is a zoonotic disease transmitted mainly through infected dairy products. It can cause fever, headache, and muscle aches. It is seen worldwide, particularly Mediterranean basin, the Arabic peninsula, the Indian subcontinent, and in Central America, and South America. It can be diagnosed using serological tests or blood culture.

It is important for healthcare providers to consider these other diseases in the differential diagnosis of CCHF, especially in non-endemic areas, and to use appropriate diagnostic tests to differentiate between them.

8.2.6 The Management

The management of CCHF requires specialized facilities and expertise, and patients with suspected or confirmed CCHF should be managed in a specialized hospital with appropriate facilities and trained personnel.

In addition to supportive care and antiviral treatment, infection control measures are also important for preventing the spread of CCHF. Patients with suspected or confirmed CCHF should be isolated and healthcare workers should follow appropriate infection control precautions, including the use of personal protective equipment (PPE).

There is no specific treatment for CCHF and the management mainly involves supportive care [1].

Fluid and electrolyte management: Patients with CCHF may experience dehydration due to vascular leaks, fever, vomiting, and diarrhoea, and require intravenous fluids to maintain hydration and electrolyte balance.

Management of haemorrhagic symptoms: Patients with severe CCHF may experience haemorrhagic symptoms, and may require blood transfusions or other interventions to manage bleeding.

Treatment of complications: Patients with CCHF may experience complications such as liver or kidney failure, and may require additional treatments to manage these complications.

8.2.7 Antiviral Treatment

Antiviral treatment may be considered for patients with CCHF, especially those with severe disease or those who are at high risk of developing severe disease. The antiviral drug ribavirin has been used in the treatment of CCHF. However, the evidence for its effectiveness is not definitive, and there are concerns about the potential for adverse effects including anaemia, liver toxicity, and teratogenicity. Because of the uncertain effectiveness and potential risks of ribavirin, there is ongoing debate among healthcare providers and public health officials about its use for the treatment of CCHF. Some experts recommend considering ribavirin on a case-by-case basis, particularly in patients with early disease and no contraindications for its use. Others recommend against the routine use of ribavirin for CCHF, given the lack of definitive evidence for its effectiveness and the potential for harm. Systematic reviews and meta-analyses showed insufficient efficacy of ribavirin for CCHF patients [18]. Further research is needed to better understand the role of ribavirin and other potential treatments for CCHF, and to identify the most effective and safe treatment strategies for this serious disease.

8.2.8 CCHF as an Emerging and/or Reemerging Disease

CCHF is classified as an emerging and/or reemerging infectious disease, since it has showed the ability to spread to new geographic areas and populations recently, and it continues to cause outbreaks and epidemics in some parts of the world.

CCHF was first identified in the Crimean Peninsula in 1944, and subsequently in the Congo in 1956. For many years, it was considered to be a relatively rare disease confined to a limited geographic area. However, in recent decades, CCHF has been spreading to new regions and populations, and has become recognized as an important emerging infectious disease [1].

The reasons for the emergence and reemergence of CCHF are complex and multifactorial. Some contributing factors include:

Environmental changes: Changes in the environment, such as deforestation, urbanization, and climate change, can create new opportunities for the transmission of CCHF.

Global travel and trade: Increased global travel and trade can facilitate the spread of CCHF to new geographic areas, and can increase the risk of importation of the disease to non-endemic countries.

Changes in animal populations: Changes in the populations and movements of the animal reservoirs of CCHF, such as ticks and livestock, can increase the risk of human exposure to the virus.

Lack of effective surveillance and control measures: In some regions, there may be limited capacity for surveillance, diagnosis, and control of CCHF, which can contribute to the spread of the disease.

As a result of these factors, CCHF is now considered to be an important emerging and reemerging infectious disease. Ongoing efforts are needed to improve surveillance, diagnosis, and control of CCHF, and to better understand the complex factors that contribute to its emergence and spread.

8.3 Travel and CCHF

Travelling is increasing all over the world and developing regions represent nearly half of all travel destinations. Travellers visiting developing regions become ill during their journey in more than half of the cases [19]. The travellers may return to their home country with a febrile illness and the causes of febrile illness imported by travellers vary with their travel destination and occupational and recreational exposures [20]. CCHF is among the disease of travellers with a diagnostic challenge. The travellers may return to their home country in which CCHF is not prevalent. There have been reported cases of CCHF among travellers (Table 8.1) [21–34].

8.3.1 Types of Travel-Related CCHF Cases

There are two main types of travel-related CCHF cases: imported and autochthonous. Imported cases are those in which an individual acquires the disease while travelling to a CCHF-endemic region and then returns to their home country with the disease. Autochthonous cases are those in which an individual acquires the disease within their home country, but the disease was initially introduced to the country by someone who had acquired the disease while travelling abroad. Conger et al. [26] and Ölschläger et al. [27] reported a US soldier infected with CCHF virus in Afghanistan, was carried to Germany for treatment. During care of this patient, nosocomial transmission to two persons was reported.

8.3.2 Characteristics of Cases with CCHF Acquired Abroad

CCHF cases acquired abroad tend to be more severe than cases acquired within a person's home country. This is likely due to several factors, including the fact that individuals may be exposed to a more virulent strain of the virus, may delay seeking medical attention due to language barriers or unfamiliarity with local healthcare systems, and may be exposed to other illnesses while travelling that weaken their immune systems. Healthcare providers in the non-endemic area may be unfamiliar with the disease and may not consider CCHF in the differential diagnosis.

Table 8.1 A review of CCHF cases acquired abroad

Authors (reference)	Year	Source of origin	Country of importation	Route of transmission	Occupation/reason for travel	Secondary infection	Outcome
Swanepoel et al. [21]	1985	Zaire (DRC)	South Africa	Cattle-farm exposure	ND	ND	Died
Swanepoel et al. [21]	1986	Tanzania	South Africa	Possible tick bites	ND	ND	Survived
Stuart [22]	1997	Zimbabwe	UK	Unknown	Leisure	None	Died
ECDC [23]	2001	Bulgaria	Germany	Unknown	Tourist	ND	Survived
Jaureguiberry et al. [24]	2004	Senegal	France	Unknown	Business (voluntary radiology technician)	None	Survived
Tall et al. [25]	2004	Senegal	France	Unknown	Leisure	None	Died
Conger et al. [26], Ölschläger et al. [27]	2009	Afghanistan	Germany	Frequent outdoor activities, tick bites, and exposure to undercooked goat meat and blood	Soldier (US)	Nosocomial transmission to two persons: Both survived	Died
Barr et al. [28]	2012	Afghanistan	UK	Animal slaughtering, contact with blood and other tissues of infected animal	Leisure	None	Died
ProMED [29]	2013	South Sudan	Uganda	Unknown	Trader	None	Survived
ProMED [30]	2014	Namibia	South Africa	Farmer	Farmer	None	Died
Lumley et al. [31]	2014	Bulgaria	UK	Tick bite and tick crushing	Leisure	None	Survived
Yadav et al. [32]	2017	Oman	India	Unknown	Business	ND	Survived
Papa et al. [33]	2018	Bulgaria	Greece	Tick bite	Business	None	Survived
Thomas et al. [34]	2019	India	UAE	Unknown	Business	None	Survived

DRC Democratic Republic of Congo, *ND* not defined, *UK* United Kingdom, *US* United States, *UAE* United Arab Emirates

8.3.3   Number of Travel-Related CCHF Cases

The number of travel-related CCHF cases is difficult to determine due to underreporting and lack of surveillance in many countries. However, according to the World Health Organization, there have been increasing numbers of travel-related CCHF cases reported in recent years. There have been 14 travel-related CCHF cases in medical literature and databases [21–34].

8.3.4   Cross-Border Travel

Cross-border travel is a significant risk factor for the spread of CCHF. In particular, the border between Afghanistan and Pakistan is a known hotspot for the disease [35]. The region is endemic for the disease, and there are many animal markets and slaughterhouses where the disease can be transmitted to humans. Additionally, there is a high volume of cross-border travel and trade in the region, which increases the risk of transmission.

8.3.5   Outcome of Cases

The outcome of CCHF cases can vary depending on the severity of the disease and the individual's immune response. Some individuals may experience mild symptoms, while others may develop severe haemorrhagic fever, which can lead to death. According to the Centers for Disease Control and Prevention, fatality rates in hospitalized patients have ranged from 9% to as high as 50% varying depending on the outbreak and the population affected [36]. Among the reported travel-associated 16 CCHF cases, 8 has had died.

8.3.6   Source and Destination Countries

CCHF is endemic in many countries, particularly in regions of Africa, Asia, and Europe. The disease is most commonly reported in countries such as Afghanistan, Iran, Pakistan, and Turkey. Travellers to these regions, particularly those who are engaging in outdoor activities or working with animals, are at increased risk of acquiring the disease.

8.3.7   Risk Occupations or Activities for Travel-Related CCHF

Occupations or activities that involve contact with animals, particularly livestock, are at increased risk for CCHF. This includes individuals who work in animal husbandry, agriculture, veterinary medicine, or wildlife management. Additionally, hunters and campers who may come into contact with wild animals or ticks are at increased risk. Travellers who visit animal markets or slaughterhouses are also at increased risk for CCHF.

8.3.8 The Index of Suspicion for CCHF in Non-endemic Countries' Healthcare Services

In CCHF non-endemic areas, healthcare providers may not be familiar with the signs and symptoms of CCHF and may not have encountered the disease previously. Thus, the index of suspicion for CCHF in non-endemic countries may be low, and the disease may not be initially considered as a possible diagnosis.

However, because of the increasing global travel, healthcare providers in non-endemic countries should have a high index of suspicion for CCHF in travellers who have recently visited endemic areas and present with symptoms such as fever, headache, muscle aches, vomiting, and bleeding. A detailed travel history to endemic areas should be obtained from all patients presenting with these symptoms, especially those who have had contact with animals or have participated in outdoor activities or activities that may have put them at risk for exposure to the CCHF virus.

Healthcare providers should consider CCHF in the differential diagnosis of febrile illnesses in travellers returning from endemic areas. Rapid diagnosis and treatment of CCHF are essential not only to improve patient outcomes but also to prevent the spread of the disease. Therefore, healthcare providers should be aware of the risk of CCHF in travellers and should be familiar with the diagnostic and treatment protocols for the disease.

8.3.9 Prevention of Travellers from the Disease

During visit to an area where CCHF is reported, travellers can take some measures to prevent themselves from contracting CCHF including:

- Avoiding contact with animals: Travellers should avoid any contact with animals, especially those known to carry the virus, including ticks, livestock, and rodents. Animal carcasses should not be handled and unpasteurized dairy products should not be consumed.
- Wearing protective clothing: Travellers should wear some protective clothings, such as boots, long-sleeved shirts, pants, especially when they are in CCHF-prevalent areas. Tucking their pants into their socks prevents ticks from crawling up their legs.
- Using insect repellent: To repel ticks and other biting insects, travellers can use insect repellent that contains DEET or another approved active ingredient.
- Staying in screened or air-conditioned place: Travellers should stay in places that are screened or air-conditioned to prevent insects from entering the room.
- Practicing good hygiene: Travellers should practice good hygiene, such as washing their hands frequently with soap and water, especially after handling animals or being in contact with animal fluids.
- Being aware of the risk: Travellers should be aware of the risk of CCHF in the areas they are visiting and should seek medical attention if they experience any symptoms of the disease, such as fever, headache, muscle aches, vomiting, and

bleeding. They should also inform their healthcare provider of their recent travel history.

- Seeking advice from a healthcare provider: Travellers should seek advice from their healthcare provider before traveling to areas whether the area they plan to visit is CCHF-prevalent. Healthcare providers can provide information on the risk of CCHF in the area, recommend preventive measures, and provide guidance on what to do if they develop signs and symptoms.
- Avoiding high-risk activities: Travellers should avoid high-risk activities, such as hunting or handling animals that may increase their risk of exposure to the CCHF virus in CCHF-endemic areas.

In summary, travellers can prevent themselves from contracting CCHF by avoiding contact with animals, wearing protective clothing, using insect repellent, staying in screened or air-conditioned places, practicing good hygiene, being aware of the risk, seeking advice from a healthcare provider, avoiding high-risk activities, and seeking medical attention if symptoms develop.

Declaration of Interest We declare no conflict of interest.

References

1. Leblebicioglu H. Crimean-Congo hemorrhagic fever UpToDate; 2023.
2. Maltezou HC, Andonova L, Andraghetti R, et al. Crimean-Congo hemorrhagic fever in travellers: a systematic review. Travel Med Infect Dis. 2019;27:48–60.
3. Gale P, Estrada-Peña A, Martinez M, Ulrich RG, Wilson A, Capelli G, Phipps P, de la Torre A, Muñoz MJ, Dottori M, Mioulet V, Fooks AR. The feasibility of developing a risk assessment for the impact of climate change on the emergence of Crimean-Congo haemorrhagic fever in livestock in Europe: a review. J Appl Microbiol. 2010;108(6):1859–70.
4. Crimean-Congo haemorrhagic fever. World Health Organization. Available at: https://www.who.int/health-topics/crimean-congo-haemorrhagic-fever#tab=tab_14 (accessed 24 Apr 2023).
5. Shahhosseini N, Wong G, Babuadze G, Camp JV, Ergonul O, Kobinger GP, Chinikar S, Nowotny N. Crimean-Congo hemorrhagic fever virus in Asia, Africa and Europe. Microorganisms. 2021;9(9):1907.
6. Fereidouni M, Apanaskevich DA, Pecor DB, Pshenichnaya NY, Abuova GN, Tishkova FH, Bumburidi Y, Zeng X, Kuhn JH, Keshtkar-Jahromi M. Crimean-Congo hemorrhagic fever virus in central, Eastern, and South-eastern Asia. Virol Sin. 2023; S1995-820X(23)00001-9
7. Turell MJ, Rossi CA, Bailey CL, et al. Detection of Crimean-Congo hemorrhagic fever virus antibodies in human and animal serum samples by indirect ELISA. Vector Borne Zoonotic Dis. 2017;17(6):427–34.
8. Shepherd AJ, Swanepoel R, Leman PA. Antibody response in Crimean-Congo hemorrhagic fever. Rev Infect Dis. 1989;11:S801–6.
9. Hawman DW, Feldmann H. Crimean-Congo haemorrhagic fever virus. Nat Rev Microbiol. 2023:1–15.
10. Connolly-Andersen AM, Moll G, Andersson C, Akerstrom S, Karlberg H, Douagi I, et al. Crimean-Congo hemorrhagic fever virus activates endothelial cells. J Virol. 2011;85(15):7766–74.

11. Chen JP, Cosgriff TM. Hemorrhagic fever virus-induced changes in hemostasis and vascular biology. Blood Coagul Fibrinol. 2000;11(5):461–83.
12. Çevik MA, Erbay A, Bodur H, et al. Clinical and laboratory features of Crimean-Congo hemorrhagic fever: predictors of fatality. Int J Infect Dis. 2008;12(4):374–9.
13. Baskerville A, Satti A, Murphy FA, Simpson D. Congo-Crimean haemorrhagic fever in Dubai: histopathological studies. J Clin Pathol. 1981;34(8):871–4.
14. Vorou R, Pierroutsakos IN, Maltezou HC. Crimean-Congo hemorrhagic fever. Curr Opin Infect Dis. 2007;20:495–500.
15. Guven FM, Aydin H, Yildiz G, et al. The importance of myeloperoxidase enzyme activity in the pathogenesis of CrimeanCongo haemorrhagic fever. J Med Microbiol. 2013;62(3):441–5.
16. Cevik MA, Erbay A, Bodur H, et al. Viral load as a predictor of outcome in Crimean-Congo hemorrhagic fever. Clin Infect Dis. 2007;45:e96–100.
17. Papa A, Drosten C, Bino S, et al. Viral load and Crimean-Congo hemorrhagic fever. Emerg Infect Dis. 2007;13:805–6.
18. Ascioglu S, Leblebicioglu H, Vahaboglu H, Chan KA. Ribavirin for patients with Crimean-Congo haemorrhagic fever: a systematic review and meta-analysis. J Antimicrob Chemother. 2011;66:1215–22.
19. Steffen R, Rickenbach M, Wilhelm U, Helminger A, Schar M. Health problems after travel to developing countries. J Infect Dis. 1987;156(1):84–91.
20. Leblebicioglu H, Ozaras R, Fletcher TE, Beeching NJ. ESCMID Study Group for Infections in Travellers and Migrants (ESGITM)Crimean-Congo haemorrhagic fever in travellers: a systematic review. Travel Med Infect Dis. 2016;14(2):73–80.
21. Swanepoel R, Shepherd AJ, Leman PA, et al. Epidemiologic and clinical features of Crimean-Congo hemorrhagic fever in southern Africa. Am J Trop Med Hyg. 1987;36:120–32.
22. Stuart J. Suspected case of Crimean/Congo haemorrhagic fever in British traveller returning from Zimbabwe. Euro Surveill. 1998;2. pii=1256. Available online: http://www.eurosurveillance.org/ViewArticle.aspx?ArticleId=
23. European Centre for Disease Prevention and Control (ECDC). Consultation on Crimean-Congo Haemorrhagic Fever Prevention and Control; Meeting Report; ECDC: Stockholm, Sweden, 2008. Available online: https://www.ecdc.europa.eu/sites/portal/files/ media/en/publications/Publications/0809_MER_Crimean_Congo_Haemorragic_Fever_ Prevention_and_ Control.pdf (accessed on 8 February 2023).
24. Jaureguiberry S, Tattevin P, Tarantola A, et al. Imported Crimean-Congo hemorrhagic fever. J Clin Microbiol. 2005;43(9):4905–7.
25. Tall A, Diallo M, Faye O, Diab H, Diatta B, Sall AA. Crimean-Congo hemorrhagic fever in Senegal. Med Trop (Mars). 2009;69:18.
26. Conger NG, Paolino KM, Osborn EC, et al. Health care response to CCHF in US soldier and nosocomial transmission to health care providers, Germany, 2009. Emerg Infect Dis. 2015;21:23–31.
27. Olschläger S, Gabriel M, Schmidt-Chanasit J, Meyer M, Osborn E, Conger NG, Allan PF, Günther S. Complete sequence and phylogenetic characterisation of Crimean-Congo hemorrhagic fever virus from Afghanistan. J Clin Virol. 2011;50(1):90–2.
28. Barr DA, Aitken C, Bell DJ, et al. First confirmed case of Crimean-Congo haemorrhagic fever in the UK. Lancet. 2013;382:1458.
29. ProMED-mail 201308261903826 ProMED-mail. Crimean-Congo hem. fever e Uganda (04): clarification. 2013 [updated 26 August 2003, 17 August 2015].
30. ProMED-mail 201409192788764 ProMED-mail. Crimean-Congo hem. fever e South Africa ex Namibia. 2014 [updated 19 September 2014, 17 August 2015].
31. Lumley S, Atkinson B, Dowall S, Pitman J, Staplehurst S, Busuttil J, et al. Non-fatal case of Crimean-Congo haemorrhagic fever imported into the United Kingdom (ex Bulgaria), CCHF and Travel 79 June 2014. Euro Surveill 2014;19(30). piiZ20864. Available from: http://www. eurosurveillance.org/ViewArticle.aspx?ArticleId=20864.

32. Yadav PD, Thacker S, Patil DY, Jain R, Mourya DT. Crimean-Congo hemorrhagic fever in Migrant Worker returning from Oman to India, 2016. Emerg Infect Dis. 2017;23(6):1005–8.
33. Papa A, Markatou F, Maltezou HC, Papadopoulou E, Terzi E, Ventouri S, Pervanidou D, Tsiodras S, Maltezos E. Crimean-Congo haemorrhagic fever in a Greek worker returning from Bulgaria, June 2018. Euro Surveill. 2018;23(35):1800432.
34. Thomas R, Mathew F, Louis EM, Valsan C, Priyanka R, Thomas J, Raphael L. Contact tracing for an imported case of Crimean-Congo hemorrhagic fever—experience from a tertiary care center in Kerala, South India. Indian J Community Med. 2019;44(3):285–7.
35. Atif M, Saqib A, Ikram R, Sarwar MR, Scahill S. The reasons why Pakistan might be at high risk of Crimean Congo haemorrhagic fever epidemic; a scoping review of the literature. Virol J. 2017;14(1):63.
36. Centers for Disease Control and Prevention. Crimean-Congo Hemorrhagic Fever (CCHF). Available at: https://www.cdc.gov/vhf/crimean-congo/symptoms/index.html.

Severe Fever with Thrombocytopenia Syndrome in Travellers

9

Kato Yasuyuki

Abstract

Severe fever with thrombocytopenia syndrome (SFTS) was first recognized in eastern China in 2009. A novel bunyavirus, severe fever thrombocytopenia virus (SFTSV), was identified as the causative agent. Japan, South Korea and Vietnam have also reported domestic SFTS cases since then. SFTS is perceived as a tick-borne viral haemorrhagic fever that has recently emerged in East Asia. Treatment is generally supportive. There are no licensed vaccines available.

As of the end of 2023, there have been no SFTS cases reported in international travellers. Given that SFTS endemic hilly and mountainous areas are geographically limited and far from eastern Asia's urban centers, the risk of contracting the disease is generally low in international travellers.

9.1 Background

Severe fever with thrombocytopenia syndrome (SFTS) was first recognized in eastern China in 2009 [1]. Subsequently, a novel bunyavirus was identified in the patient's blood samples. Japan, South Korea and Vietnam have also reported domestic SFTS cases since then.

The disease shares several characteristics of viral haemorrhagic fevers: zoonotic spillover, high case-fatality rate, and person-to-person transmission potential. Therefore, SFTS is perceived as a tick-borne viral haemorrhagic fever that has recently emerged in East Asia. The UK designates SFTS as a disease of public health importance similar to Crimean-Congo haemorrhagic fever.

K. Yasuyuki (✉)
Department of Infectious Diseases, School of Medicine, International University of Health and Welfare, Narita, Chiba, Japan
e-mail: katoy@iuhw.ac.jp

H. Leblebicioglu et al. (eds.), *Emerging and Re-emerging Infections in Travellers*, https://doi.org/10.1007/978-3-031-49475-8_9

9.2   Aetiology

A novel virus, *Dabie bandavirus,* which belongs to the genus bandavirus in the family *Phenuiviridae*, order *Bunyavirales*, synonymously known as severe fever thrombocytopenia virus (SFTSV), is the causative agent of the disease [2]. The virus is enveloped and has negative-sense, single-stranded RNA as its genome.

The virus is maintained by the interaction of vectors, amplifiers and natural hosts in nature. *Haemaphysalis* and other species of ticks play a pivotal role as vectors and reservoirs of the virus. Transovarial transmission of the virus in ticks is not so efficient that various types of mammals seem to act as amplifiers. Domestic animals like goats seem to be involved in China, while wild deer and boar are in Japan. These animals show only transient viraemia and are considered incidental hosts. The true natural hosts of SFTSV remain unknown.

9.3   Transmission

Tick bite is considered the major transmission route of SFTSV. However, other transmission routes have been identified. Contact with infected animals is the second most common route of transmission. Cats are susceptible to the virus and develop similar symptoms as humans.

Probable person-to-person transmission has also been reported in China and South Korea [3]. Direct contact with blood and body fluids of severe patients, or even dead bodies, can transmit the virus.

9.4   Epidemiology

9.4.1   Geographic Distribution

SFTS endemic countries are widely distributed across eastern Asia, including China, Japan, South Korea and Vietnam. Epidemiologic data on neighbouring countries such as North Korea remains unavailable.

Each country has its own endemic areas (Fig. 9.1). In China, seven coastal provinces, Henan, Shandong, Hubei, Anhui, Zhejiang, Liaoning, and Jiangsu, represent most SFTS cases [4]. In Japan, most cases have occurred in western parts, including Kyusyu and Shikoku islands [5]. In South Korea, SFTS has been higher in the southern region [6]. In Vietnam, a single retrospective study conducted in Hue found just two cases [7]. Hilly and mountainous areas in such regions are the most common places where the transmission of SFTSV likely occurs.

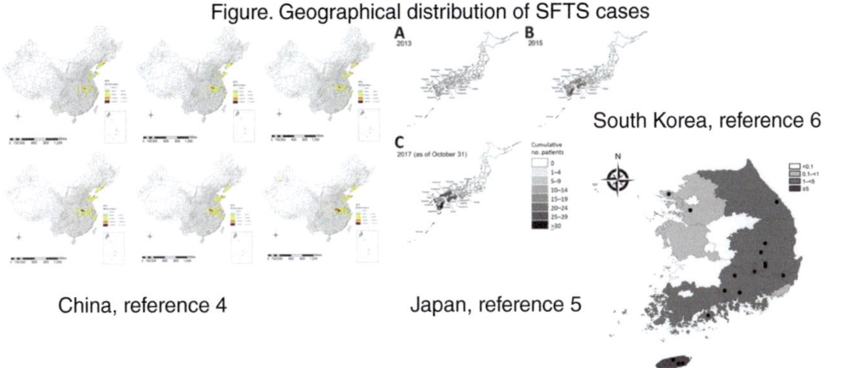

Fig. 9.1 Geographical distribution of SFTS cases

9.4.2 Recent Epidemics/Outbreaks

Most SFTS cases are sporadic, and no large outbreaks with sustained transmission between humans have been reported. China reported 1800 cases, South Korea around 300 cases, and Japan around 100 cases in 2018. The incidence of SFTS clearly shows seasonality in each country. Most cases have been reported in spring and summer (from April to September), which might reflect human behaviour change (increase in outdoor activity) and the increase in tick activity.

9.4.3 Risk Factors

Outdoor activities in hilly and mountainous areas in SFTS endemic regions are a risk factor for contracting the disease. In terms of occupation, farmers are the most vulnerable group to SFTS. The reason is that they have more opportunity to contact infected ticks and animals. Veterinary physicians and nurses caring for domestic animals should also be considered a high-risk group.

Severe symptoms develop almost exclusively in elderly people. Children and young adults have only mild or asymptomatic infections. Any underlying diseases except older age have not been identified as risk factors for severe disease or death.

9.4.4 Risks for International Travellers

As of the end of 2023, there have been no SFTS cases reported in international travellers. Given that SFTS endemic hilly and mountainous areas are geographically limited and far from eastern Asia's urban centers, the risk of contracting the disease is generally low in international travellers. However, a small number of SFTS cases in domestic tourists were identified in Japan. Adventure travel containing profound outdoor activities might expose travellers to infected ticks and animals.

9.4.5 Pathogenesis

The virus infects B cell-lineage lymphocytes [8]. Autopsy series revealed that SFTSV-infected B cells were distributed in both lymphoid and non-lymphoid organs. An excessive inflammatory response through high induction of proinflammatory cytokines and chemokines was demonstrated in fatal cases.

9.4.6 Clinical Findings

The incubation period ranges from 7 to 14 days. Initial symptoms are usually nonspecific, including fever, headache, fatigue and muscle pain. Gastrointestinal symptoms such as nausea, vomiting and diarrhoea commonly follow. Mild cases gradually improve within 7 days. However, usually after the seventh day of illness, organ failures and/or haemorrhagic symptoms develop in severe cases. Neurological symptoms such as delirium and convulsions are not uncommon in elderly patients. The case-fatality rates vary from 5% to 30% among endemic countries.

Depending on tick-bite sites, regional adenopathy can be detected on physical examination [9]. Erythematous rash does not usually appear, which contrasts sharply with rickettsial diseases. However, eschar can be detected in some SFTS cases.

9.4.7 Laboratory Diagnosis

Complete blood count usually shows low white blood cell and platelet counts. Serum transaminases and lactate dehydrogenase are also elevated. Coagulation studies sometimes show prolonged activated partial thromboplastin time. Serum ferritin is usually elevated in severe cases. Some cases fill the definition of virus-induced haemophagocytic syndrome. In comparison, serum C-reactive protein is within the normal range.

Diagnosis is confirmed by the detection of SFTSV in the patient's serum by RT-PCR.

9.4.8 Differential Diagnosis

Other tick-borne diseases such as Japanese spotted fever, scrub typhus, and anaplasmosis are generally more common in SFTS endemic areas. Although symptoms of malaria and dengue are similar to those of SFTS, they have been eliminated in most SFTS endemic areas and are less likely to be diagnosed.

Severe sepsis, virus-induced haemophagocytic syndrome, and viral encephalitis/encephalopathy should be considered for suspected severe SFTS.

9.5 Management

Treatment is generally supportive. Severe cases should be managed in intensive care units. Immunomodulators such as steroids have been tried in severe cases, but their effectiveness remains unclear. Antivirals are under development.

9.6 Public Health Response

Local policy and guidelines in a destination country should guide public health response. Standard precautions must be installed in patient care. Contact and droplet precautions should also be encouraged to manage severe cases. Several clusters of healthcare workers have been reported where aerosol transmission was suspected, and air-borne precaution is recommended for conducting aerosol-generating procedures such as cardiopulmonary resuscitation.

9.7 Prevention and Advice for Travellers

The risk of contracting the disease is extremely low. However, awareness of the disease should be raised, and tick-bite prevention should be encouraged for long-term travellers visiting eastern Asia. Elderly people who have a higher risk of severe disease deserve the main priority.

Healthcare workers and veterinary professionals who plan to work in endemic areas should be informed of the disease and the risk of occupational exposure to SFTS.

There are no licensed vaccines against the virus available.

9.8 Gaps in Knowledge that Need to Be Addressed

It remains unclear what factors drive SFTSV to emerge in eastern Asia and whether neighbouring regions are affected.

Acknowledgements This work was partly supported by a grant, Ministry of Health, Labour and Welfare, HA2002.

Declarations of Conflict of Interest I declare no conflict of interest.

References

1. Xue-Jie Y, Mi-Fang L, Shou-Yin Z, et al. Fever with thrombocytopenia associated with a novel bunyavirus in China. N Engl J Med. 2011;364:1523–32.
2. Casel MA, Park SJ, Choi YK. Severe fever with thrombocytopenia syndrome virus: emerging novel phlebovirus and their control strategy. Exp Mol Med. 2021;53:713–22.
3. Kato Y. Infection control and prevention in hospitals and household. In: Saijo M, editor. Severe fever with thrombocytopenia syndrome. Singapore: Springer; 2019.
4. Jimin S, Liang L, Haixia W, et al. The changing epidemiological characteristics of severe fever with thrombocytopenia syndrome in China, 2011–2016. Sci Rep. 2017:9236.
5. Kobayashi Y, Kato H, Yamagishi T, et al. Severe fever with thrombocytopenia syndrome, Japan, 2013–2017. Emerg Infect Dis. 2020;26:692–9.
6. Shin J, Kwon D, Youn SK, et al. Characteristics and factors associated with death among patients hospitalized for severe fever with thrombocytopenia syndrome, South Korea, 2013. Emerg Infect Dis. 2015;21:1704–10.
7. Tran XC, Yun Y, An LV, et al. Endemic severe fever with thrombocytopenia syndrome, Vietnam. Emerg Infect Dis. 2019;25:1029–31.
8. Suzuki T, Sato Y, Sano K, et al. Severe fever with thrombocytopenia syndrome virus target B cells in lethal human infections. J Clin Invest. 2020;130:799–812.
9. Takahashi T, Maeda K, Suzuki T, et al. The first identification and retrospective study of severe fever with thrombocytopenia syndrome in Japan. J Infect Dis. 2014;209:816–27.

Alkhurma Haemorrhagic Fever in Travellers

10

Jaffar A. Al-Tawfiq and Ziad A. Memish

Abstract

Alkhurma haemorrhagic fever (AHFV) is an important emerging virus and is classified as a variant genotype of Kyasanur Forest disease virus (KFDV). The first report of AHF was in the mid-1990s when the virus was isolated from the blood of a patient admitted with a febrile haemorrhagic illness to a private hospital in the city of Jeddah in the western part of the Kingdom of Saudi Arabia. Later, the virus was recognized in many patients in Saudi Arabia and was rarely reported outside the Kingdom in Egypt and Djibouti. AHFV causes a relatively low case fatality rate of 1%. AHFV is a zoonotic disease, and transmission occurs from livestock animals to humans through direct contact with the blood of slaughtered animals and consumption of raw milk.

J. A. Al-Tawfiq (✉)
Specialty Internal Medicine, Johns Hopkins Aramco Healthcare, Dhahran, Saudi Arabia

Quality and Patient Safety Department, Johns Hopkins Aramco Healthcare, Dhahran, Saudi Arabia

Department of Medicine, Indiana University School of Medicine, Indiana, IN, USA

Department of Medicine, Johns Hopkins University School of Medicine, Baltimore, MD, USA
e-mail: jaffar.tawfiq@jhah.com

Z. A. Memish
College of Medicine, Alfaisal University, Riyadh, Saudi Arabia

Department of Infection Control, King Saud Medical City, Ministry of Health, Riyadh, Saudi Arabia

Hubert Department of Global Health, Rollins School of Public Health, Emory University, Atlanta, GA, USA

H. Leblebicioglu et al. (eds.), *Emerging and Re-emerging Infections in Travellers*, https://doi.org/10.1007/978-3-031-49475-8_10

10.1 Background

(a) **Brief history:** The first report of Alkhurma haemorrhagic fever (AHF) was in the mid-1990s when the virus was isolated from the blood of a patient who was admitted with a febrile haemorrhagic illness to a private hospital in the city of Jeddah in the Western part of the Kingdom of Saudi Arabia [1]. The patient was a 32-year-old butcher who worked in the city of Makkah, 50 miles to the south of Jeddah. He developed haemorrhagic fever and was initially hospitalized with the diagnosis of Crimean Congo haemorrhagic fever (CCHF) based on an immunofluorescence assay (IFA) test. However, IgM against CCHF was not detected using capture enzyme-linked immunosorbent assay (ELISA). This finding was thought to represent a past infection with CCHF, not an acute one.

Further work-up resulted in the inoculation of adult mice with the patient's serum intraperitoneally and into Vero cells. This experiment resulted in the death of the infected mice in 1 week. The brain of the mice was grossly haemorrhagic, and this issue was suspended in a 10% cell culture medium and injected into suckling mice. The second mice also died, and a suspension of the brain resulted in the development of a cytopathogenic effect in Vero cells. Testing of these cells by indirect IFA utilizing monoclonal antibodies specific for Rift Valley fever virus (RFV), CCHF virus, dengue virus (DF), yellow fever virus (YFV), and a pan-flaviviruses monoclonal antibody was negative. A new virus resembling the Kyasanur Forest disease virus (KFDV) was identified and named AHFV [1]. Additionally, the virus was isolated from the blood of 6 butchers, aged 24–39 years, in November and December 1995 [1, 2]. An additional four patients were diagnosed by immunoglobulin M capture enzyme-linked immunosorbent assay [1]. The virus had been labelled as Alkhurma haemorrhagic fever virus in few studies. However, the virus was corrected as Alkhurma haemorrhagic fever virus by the International Committee on Taxonomy of Viruses (ICTV) in 2011 [3].

(b) **Importance of the disease:** Although AHFV causes a relatively low case fatality rate of about 1% [4], AHFV is an important emerging virus due to the geographical distribution of the disease. Most of the cases were reported from Jeddah city, located 50 miles away from the Holy city of Makkah, where millions of Pilgrims perform the annual Hajj and Umrah yearly with the potential spread of the virus [5]. Figure 10.1 shows the geographic location of reported cases [6]. In addition, AHFV occurred as outbreaks and sporadic cases in KSA, and AHF cases were reported among tourists, returning travellers or ticks in Egypt, Djibouti, India, and Europe [7–16].

(c) **Why it is classified as emerging and/or reemerging:** One of the reasons that AHVF classification as reemerging virus is the occurrence of outbreaks and the development of sporadic cases in Saudi Arabia. In addition, there were reports of the virus among travellers in Egypt, Djibouti, India, and Europe [7, 17, 18].

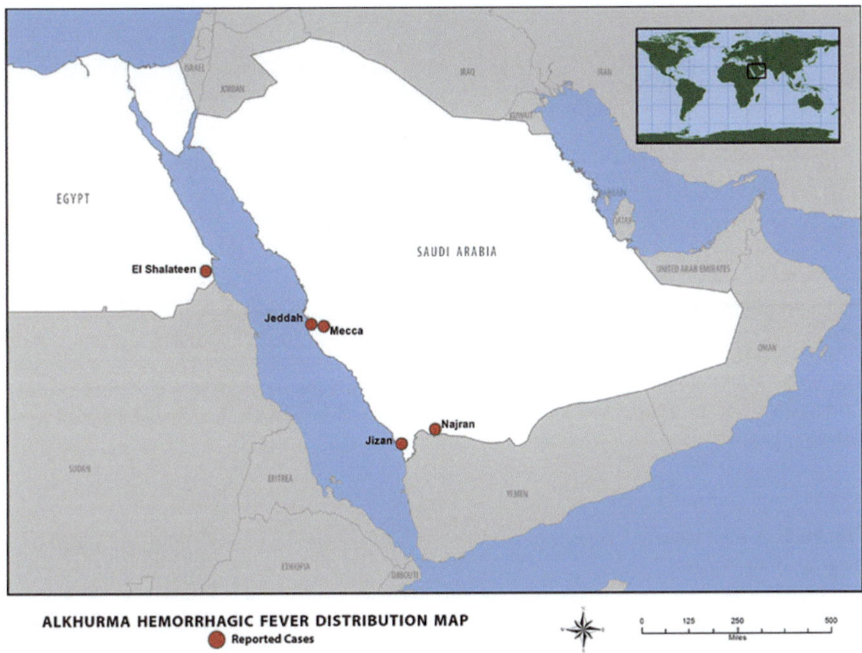

Fig. 10.1 A geographic distribution of Alkhurma haemorrhagic fever, Reproduced from the USA CDC [5] (Source: CDC; Reference to specific commercial products, manufacturers, companies, or trademarks does not constitute its endorsement or recommendation by the U.S. Government, Department of Health and Human Services, or Centers for Disease Control and Prevention; https://www.cdc.gov/vhf/alkhurma/outbreaks/distribution-map.html; available free of charge). From: https://www.cdc.gov/vhf/alkhurma/outbreaks/distribution-map.html

10.2 Aetiology

Alkhurma haemorrhagic fever (AHF) is a tick-borne flavivirus (Fig. 10.2), a member of the family Flaviviridae and the genus Flavivirus with other tick-borne viruses [1], Fig. 10.3. AHFV is closely related genetically to the Kyasanur Forest disease virus (KFDV) [10, 19]. In 2017, a complete coding sequence of AHVF virus was done and the virus was found to be 10,248 nucleotides (nt) long and to have a single ORF encode a single 3416 amino acid polyprotein [20]. This virus sequencing showed that AHFV is closely related to other tick-borne flaviviruses with a genetic distance of 21–24.3% compared to a genetic distance of 57% to non-tick-borne flaviviruses [20]. One study showed that AHFV, KFDV and tick-borne encephalitis virus (TBEV) are very similar in relation to the following: codon frequency, number of transmembrane regions, properties of the polyprotein, RNA-RNA interaction sequences, NS3 protease and NS5 polymerase structures and 5' UTR structure [21].

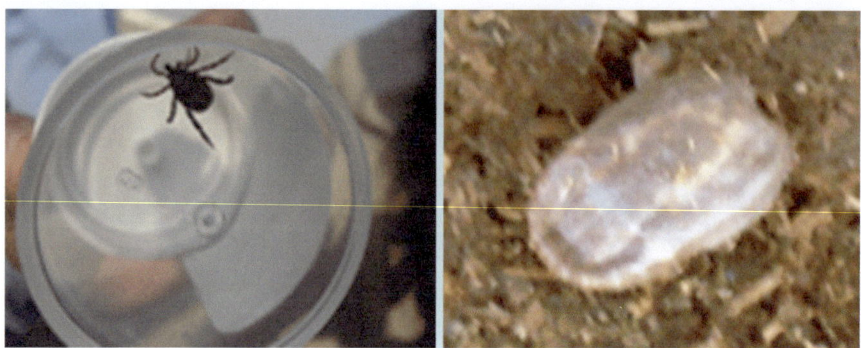

Fig. 10.2 A photograph showing the Tick vector. (The photos were used from the Saudi Ministry of Health website (https://www.moh.gov.sa/en/HealthAwareness/Campaigns/Alkhurma/Pages/default.aspx)

Fig. 10.3 A schematic diagram of the viruses within the Genus Flavivirus

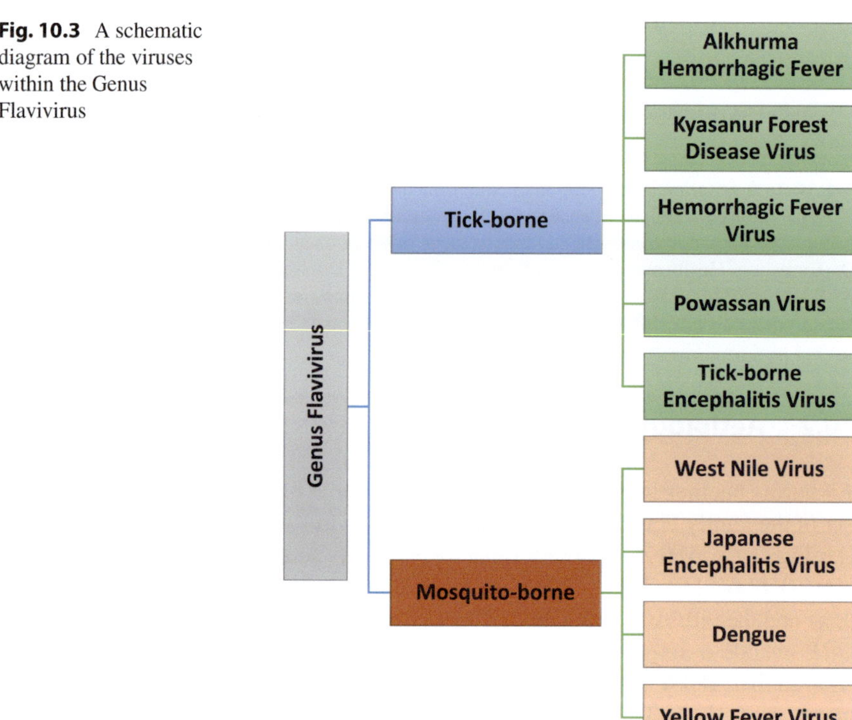

10.3 Transmission

AHFV is a zoonotic disease where transmission from livestock animals to humans mainly through direct contact with the blood of slaughtered animals and consumption of raw milk in addition to indirect contact through tick bites [22]. The data on transmission are derived from epidemiologic studies where 42% of cases of AHFV were among butchers, shepherds, abattoir workers or people who had contacts with the livestock industry [23]. However, it is reported that about one-third of patients with AHFV had no animal contact and about one-third of cases in another study occurred as clusters among families [23]. Mosquito bites were suggested as a possible transmission route but the data on this is limited [24].

10.4 Epidemiology

(a) **Geographic distributions:** The disease seems to be limited to the Kingdom of Saudi Arabia. However, travel-related cases have been reported in Egypt and Djiboti, as indicated above. The total number of reported cases from 1995 to 2017 was 620, with a case fatality rate of 2.3% [25].

(b) **Recent epidemics/outbreaks:** There have been no recent outbreaks of AHFV infection. However, AHF cases had been reported from Jeddah, Makkah, including four cases during the 2001 Hajj, Jizan and Najran in the southern part of Saudi Arabia [8, 17, 18, 26]. In addition, a cluster of 25 cases was reported among five families, accounting for 32.1% of cases reported from Najran, Saudi Arabia [8].

(c) **Risk factors:** The main risk factors for AHFV infection seem to be exposure to livestock animals and among animal handlers [1, 2, 8, 23]. In a study of 28 cases of AHFV infection in Najran, Saudi Arabia, animal contact, neighbouring farms, and tick bites were found to be a risk factor for infection in multivariate analysis with adjusted Odd Ratios of 3.17, 6.2, and 3.63, respectively [18]. In addition, transmission of AHFV was classified based on a questionnaire of admitted patients. The administered questionnaire suggested three different modes of infection: skin wound ($n = 6$), tick bite ($n = 2$), and consumption of unpasteurized raw camel milk ($n = 3$) [22].

(d) **Risks for international travellers:** There are few reported cases of AHFV infection among travellers, including three travellers returning to Italy from Egypt [7, 12]. In 2001, there were four cases during the annual Hajj season, and no other cases were reported [17]. Thus, the risk of AHFV transmission to international travellers remains low.

(e) **Differing issues for migrants and those "visiting friends and relations" (VFR):** The disease had not been reported widely in the Arabian Peninsula and seems to be limited to handling livestock animals; thus, VFR are encouraged not to have direct contact with livestock animals in these areas.

10.5 Pathogenesis

Data on the pathogenesis of AHFV are limited. The whole genome sequence of the virus showed low variability between the different isolates [22]. The virus was estimated to have diverged from KFDV about 66–177 years ago [22]. However, another study utilized a Bayesian coalescent phylogenetic analysis and showed that the divergence of AHFV and KFDV occurred 700 years ago [27]. It was suggested that AHFV, similar to KFDV, causes haemorrhagic disease through molecular determinants within the viral genome and that the E protein is a major determinant of tissue tropism for the flaviviruses [28]. The viral polyprotein associated with the virus-encoded NS2B/NS3 trypsin-like serine protease plays a role in the virus replication cycle and possibly the pathogenesis of the virus [29]. Two studies described the pathogenesis of AHFV in animal models. AHFV infections of C57BL/6 J mice resulted in clinical diseases similar to human cases [30]. However, the propagation of AHFV in the brains of newborn Wistar rats leads to the development of meningo-encephalitis and death [31]. As there are limited experimental data, a computer-generated comparison of ALHVF and KFDV and Tick-borne encephalitis virus (TBEV) showed one conserved major histocompatibility complex (MHC) binding epitope, DRB0401 allele [32].

10.6 Clinical Findings

The majority of identified cases were clinically symptomatic, and more recently subclinical infections were reported [18, 33]. The initial symptoms of AHFV infection may be non-specific and resemble any viral illness, including fever, headache, body ache, arthralgia, and gastrointestinal symptoms such as anorexia and vomiting [1]. The occurrence of these symptoms was reported as follows: fever (95.6–100%), headache (65.6–86%), malaise (59–86%), arthralgia (43–83%), anorexia (20–82%), myalgia (58–82%), backache (35–72%), nausea and vomiting (50–72%), diarrhoea (31–51%), abdominal pain (10–49%), chills (25–60%), retro-orbital pain (5–55%), haemorrhagic manifestations (25.6%), central nervous system manifestations (23.1%) [8, 17, 23]. Other presentations included encephalitis, skin rash, and the development of rhabdomyolysis and severe muscular weakness [1, 12, 17]. The case fatality rate of clinically diagnosed cases reached 25% [8, 17, 22, 34]. However, a low case fatality rate of 1.3% was reported in 281 cases [4]. Figure 10.4 summarizes presenting signs and symptoms based on data from various studies [8, 17, 23].

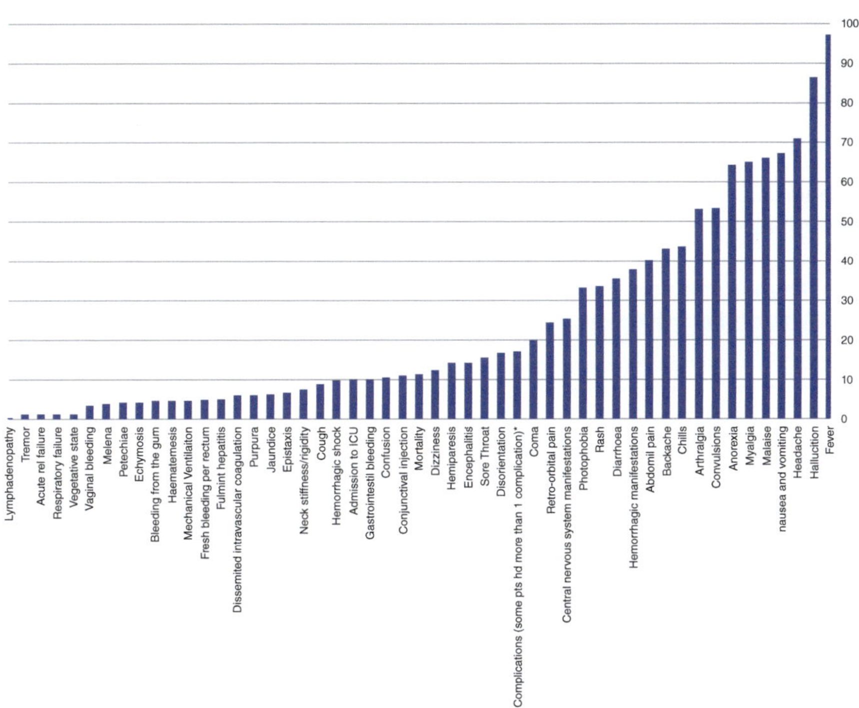

Fig. 10.4 A bar graph showing the rate of signs and symptoms among patients with Alkhurma haemorrhagic fever virus infection. (Data are from Refs. [7, 16, 22])

10.7 Laboratory Diagnosis

Various laboratory findings were reported, including leucopenia, thrombocytopenia, elevated liver transaminase, elevated creatinine phosphokinase, and elevated blood urea [1]. The occurrence of these laboratory findings was reported in one study as follows: leucopenia (87.7%), elevated liver enzymes (85.7%), prolonged partial thromboplastin time (52.6%), thrombocytopenia (46.2%), elevated creatinine kinase level (45.7%), and elevated lactate dehydrogenase (25.0%) [8]. The definite diagnosis of AHFV relies on viral isolation, PCR testing or serology. Early in the disease, viremia develops, and thus, viral culture is rarely used, or a more helpful strategy is based on real-time or conventional RT-PCR [35]. Serology utilizes a four-fold IgM or IgG antibody rise in paired serum samples using ELISA or IFA [18, 26]. Another test that could be used is the neutralization test utilizing plaque reduction of paired sera.

10.8   Differential Diagnosis

The differential diagnosis of patients presenting with hemorrhagic manifestations and epidemiologic link to the Kingdom of Saudi Arabia should include, in addition to AHFV infection, the following viral haemorrhagic fevers: Crimean–Congo haemorrhagic fever (CCHF) [36–38], dengue fever [39], and Rift Valley fever (RVF) [40, 41] and chikungunya [42, 43].

(a) **Diagnostic hints:** The initial clinical presentation is non-specific, and a significant overlap exists between the various hemorrhagic fevers.

10.9   Treatment

To date there are no available vaccines and no approved anti-viral medications. Thus, supportive therapy is the mainstay of the therapy, and patients should receive fluids and blood products.

10.10 Public Health Responses Around the Management of an Individual Case

Such as isolation measures, laboratory safety protocols, contact precautions, advice and management for patient contacts, e.g., healthcare and household and other close contacts.

10.11 Prevention

The prevention of AHFV in primary cases relies on avoiding the risk factors. There are no specific prophylactic agents and no available vaccines. Vector control might be difficult and interruption of the virus cycle within the reservoirs is not possible.

10.12 Advice for Travellers

(a) **General advice pre-travel and during travel**: It is advisable that travellers avoid tick-infected areas and limit their contact with tick-infested livestock and domestic animals. The use of tick repellents on skin and clothes is also recommended. In addition travellers should check their skin for any ticks to remove them.
(b) **Specific advice for healthcare workers**: There have been no reports of healthcare-associated transmission of AHFV. Admitted patients should be cared for using standard infection control.

(c) **Specific advice for special people:** There is no specific recommendations for special populations such as pregnant, immunocompromised, very young, and those >65 years of age.

10.13 Gaps in Knowledge That Need to Be Addressed

The current understanding of AHFV needs to be expanded in the area of the pathogenesis of the disease as well as the treatment and vaccine development.

Box 10.1: Key Websites for Travellers and Healthcare Workers
https://www.cdc.gov/vhf/alkhurma/index.html
https://ecdc.europa.eu/en/alkhurma-haemorrhagic-fever
https://www.moh.gov.sa/en/HealthAwareness/Campaigns/Alkhurma/Pages/
  default.aspx

Box 10.2: Things Commonly Forgotten
- AHFV does not cause dramatic bleeding from orifices.
- AHFV usually causes a mild illness.
- Tick avoidance is an important strategy to prevent AHFV infection.

Box 10.3: Information Resources for Patients
- https://www.cdc.gov/vhf/alkhurma/index.html
- https://ecdc.europa.eu/en/alkhurma-haemorrhagic-fever
- https://www.moh.gov.sa/en/HealthAwareness/Campaigns/Alkhurma/
  Pages/default.aspx

Acknowledgments None.

Declarations of Conflict of Interest None to declare.

References

1. Zaki AM. Isolation of a flavivirus related to the tick-borne encephalitis complex from human cases in Saudi Arabia. Trans R Soc Trop Med Hyg. 1997;91:179–81.

2. Charrel RN, de Lamballerie X, Zaki AM. Human cases of hemorrhagic fever in Saudi Arabia due to a newly discovered flavivirus, Alkhurma hemorrhagic fever virus. In: Lu Y, Essex M, Roberts B, editors. Emerging infections in Asia. Boston, MA: Springer US; 2008. p. 179–92. https://doi.org/10.1007/978-0-387-75722-3_11.

3. Pletnev A, Gould E, Heinz FX, Meyers G, et al. Flaviviridae. In: King AMQ, Adams MJ, Carstens EB, Lefkowitz EJ, et al., editors. Virus taxonomy, ninth report of the International Committee on viruses. Oxford: Elsevier; 2011. pp. 1003–1020.

4. Gaw ZR, Assiri AM, Ali AO, Farhat GN. A newly emergent viral hemorrhagic fever in Saudi Arabia: descriptive epidemiology of Alkhurma Hemorrhagic Fever 2016. http://kingabdul-lahfellowship.com/wp-content/uploads/Zahra-Poster-Final-4-27-16.pdf (accessed December 30, 2016).

5. Al-Tawfiq JA, Memish ZA. Mass gatherings and infectious diseases. Prevention, detection, and control. Infect Dis Clin N Am. 2012;26:725–37. https://doi.org/10.1016/j.idc.2012.05.005.

6. US CDC. Outbreak distribution map | Alkhurma Hemorrhagic Fever (Alkhurma HF) 2014. https://www.cdc.gov/vhf/alkhurma/outbreaks/distribution-map.html (accessed September 16, 2022).

7. Carletti F, Castilletti C, Di Caro A, Capobianchi MR, Nisii C, Suter F, et al. Alkhurma hemorrhagic fever in travelers returning from Egypt, 2010. Emerg Infect Dis. 2010;16:1979–82. https://doi.org/10.3201/eid1612.101092.

8. Madani TA, Azhar EI, Abuelzein E-TME, Kao M, Al-Bar HMS, Abu-Araki H, et al. Alkhumra (Alkhurma) virus outbreak in Najran, Saudi Arabia: epidemiological, clinical, and laboratory characteristics. J Infect. 2011;62:67–76. https://doi.org/10.1016/j.jinf.2010.09.032.

9. Hoffman T, Lindeborg M, Barboutis C, Erciyas-Yavuz K, Evander M, Fransson T, et al. Alkhurma hemorrhagic fever virus RNA in *Hyalomma rufipes* ticks infesting migratory birds, Europe and Asia Minor. Emerg Infect Dis. 2018;24:879–82. https://doi.org/10.3201/eid2405.171369.

10. Tambo E, El-Dessouky AG. Defeating reemerging Alkhurma hemorrhagic fever virus outbreak in Saudi Arabia and worldwide. PLoS Negl Trop Dis. 2018;12:e0006707. https://doi.org/10.1371/journal.pntd.0006707.

11. Ul-Rahman A. Genetic diversity of Alkhurma hemorrhagic fever virus in Western Asia. Infect Genet Evol. 2019;70:80–3. https://doi.org/10.1016/j.meegid.2019.02.012.

12. Ravanini P, Hasu E, Huhtamo E, Crobu MG, Ilaria V, Brustia D, et al. Rhabdomyolysis and severe muscular weakness in a traveler diagnosed with Alkhurma hemorrhagic fever virus infection. J Clin Virol. 2011;52:254–6. https://doi.org/10.1016/j.jcv.2011.08.001.

13. Horton KC, Fahmy NT, Watany N, Zayed A, Mohamed A, Ahmed AA, et al. Crimean Congo hemorrhagic fever virus and Alkhurma (Alkhumra) virus in ticks in Djibouti. Vector Borne Zoonotic Dis. 2016;16:680–2. https://doi.org/10.1089/vbz.2016.1951.

14. Charrel R, Gould EA. Alkhurma hemorrhagic fever in travelers returning from Egypt, 2010. Emerg Infect Dis. 2011;17:1573–4.; author reply 1574. https://doi.org/10.3201/eid1708.101858.

15. Musso M, Galati V, Stella MC, Capone A. A case of Alkhumra virus infection. J Clin Virol. 2015;66:12–4. https://doi.org/10.1016/j.jcv.2015.02.019.

16. Andayi F, Charrel RN, Kieffer A, Richet H, Pastorino B, Leparc-Goffart I, et al. A sero-epidemiological study of arboviral fevers in Djibouti, Horn of Africa. PLoS Negl Trop Dis. 2014;8:e3299. https://doi.org/10.1371/journal.pntd.0003299.

17. Madani T. Alkhumra virus infection, a new viral hemorrhagic fever in Saudi Arabia. J Infect. 2005;51:91–7. https://doi.org/10.1016/j.jinf.2004.11.012.

18. Alzahrani AG, Al Shaiban HM, Al Mazroa MA, Al-Hayani O, Macneil A, Rollin PE, et al. Alkhurma hemorrhagic fever in humans, Najran, Saudi Arabia. Emerg Infect Dis. 2010;16:1882–8. https://doi.org/10.3201/eid1612.100417.

19. Al-Tawfiq JA, Memish ZA. Alkhurma hemorrhagic fever virus. Microbes Infect. 2017;19:305–10. https://doi.org/10.1016/j.micinf.2017.04.004.

20. Charrel RN, Zaki AM, Attoui H, Fakeeh M, Billoir F, Yousef AI, et al. Complete coding sequence of the Alkhurma virus, a tick-borne flavivirus causing severe hemorrhagic fever

in humans in Saudi Arabia. Biochem Biophys Res Commun. 2001;287:455–61. https://doi.org/10.1006/bbrc.2001.5610.

21. Palanisamy N, Akaberi D, Lennerstrand J, Lundkvist Å. Comparative genome analysis of Alkhumra hemorrhagic fever virus with Kyasanur forest disease and tick-borne encephalitis viruses by the in silico approach. Pathog Glob Health. 2018;112:210–26. https://doi.org/10.1080/20477724.2018.1471187.

22. Charrel RN, Zaki AM, Fakeeh M, Yousef AI, de Chesse R, Attoui H, et al. Low diversity of Alkhurma hemorrhagic fever virus, Saudi Arabia, 1994–1999. Emerg Infect Dis. 2005;11:683–8. https://doi.org/10.3201/eid1105.041298.

23. Memish ZA, Fagbo SF, Osman Ali A, AlHakeem R, Elnagi FM, Bamgboye EA. Is the epidemiology of alkhurma hemorrhagic fever changing? A three-year overview in Saudi Arabia. PLoS One. 2014;9:e85564. https://doi.org/10.1371/journal.pone.0085564.

24. Madani TA, Kao M, Azhar EI, Abuelzein E-TME, Al-Bar HMS, Abu-Araki H, et al. Successful propagation of Alkhumra (misnamed as Alkhurma) virus in C6/36 mosquito cells. Trans R Soc Trop Med Hyg. 2012;106:180–5. https://doi.org/10.1016/j.trstmh.2011.11.003.

25. Madani TA, Abuelzein ETME. Alkhumra hemorrhagic fever virus infection. Arch Virol. 2021;166:2357–67. https://doi.org/10.1007/s00705-021-05083-1.

26. Memish ZA, Albarrak A, Almazroa MA, Al-Omar I, Alhakeem R, Assiri A, et al. Seroprevalence of Alkhurma and other hemorrhagic fever viruses, Saudi Arabia. Emerg Infect Dis. 2011;17:2316–8. https://doi.org/10.3201/eid1712.110658.

27. Dodd KA, Bird BH, Khristova ML, Albariño CG, Carroll SA, Comer JA, et al. Ancient ancestry of KFDV and AHFV revealed by complete genome analyses of viruses isolated from ticks and mammalian hosts. PLoS Negl Trop Dis. 2011;5:e1352. https://doi.org/10.1371/journal.pntd.0001352.

28. Lin D, Li L, Dick D, Shope RE, Feldmann H, Barrett ADT, et al. Analysis of the complete genome of the tick-borne Flavivirus Omsk hemorrhagic fever virus. Virology. 2003;313:81–90.

29. Bessaud M, Grard G, Peyrefitte CN, Pastorino B, Rolland D, Charrel RN, et al. Identification and enzymatic characterization of NS2B–NS3 protease of Alkhurma virus, a class-4 flavivirus. Virus Res. 2005;107:57–62. https://doi.org/10.1016/j.virusres.2004.06.015.

30. Dodd KA, Bird BH, Jones MEB, Nichol ST, Spiropoulou CF. Kyasanur Forest disease virus infection in mice is associated with higher morbidity and mortality than infection with the closely related Alkhurma hemorrhagic fever virus. PLoS One. 2014;9:e100301. https://doi.org/10.1371/journal.pone.0100301.

31. Madani TA, Kao M, Abuelzein E-TME, Azhar EI, Al-Bar HMS, Abu-Araki H, et al. Propagation and titration of Alkhumra hemorrhagic fever virus in the brains of newborn Wistar rats. J Virol Methods. 2014;199:39–45. https://doi.org/10.1016/j.jviromet.2013.12.004.

32. Mohabatkar H. Computer-based comparison of structural features of envelope protein of Alkhurma hemorrhagic fever virus with the homologous proteins of two closest viruses. Protein Pept Lett. 2011;18:559–67.

33. Memish ZA, Charrel RN, Zaki AM, Fagbo SF. Alkhurma haemorrhagic fever—a viral haemorrhagic disease unique to the Arabian Peninsula. Int J Antimicrob Agents. 2010;36(Suppl. 1):S53–7. https://doi.org/10.1016/j.ijantimicag.2010.06.022.

34. Charrel RN, Zaki AM, Fagbo S, de Lamballerie X. Alkhurma hemorrhagic fever virus is an emerging tick-borne flavivirus. J Infect. 2006;52:463–4. https://doi.org/10.1016/j.jinf.2005.08.011.

35. Madani TA, Abuelzein E-TME, Azhar EI, Kao M, Al-Bar HMS, Abu-Araki H, et al. Superiority of the buffy coat over serum or plasma for the detection of Alkhumra virus RNA using real time RT-PCR. Arch Virol. 2012;157:819–23. https://doi.org/10.1007/s00705-012-1237-7.

36. Leblebicioglu H, Sunbul M, Memish ZA, Al-Tawfiq JA, Bodur H, Ozkul A, et al. Consensus report: preventive measures for Crimean-Congo hemorrhagic fever during Eid-al-Adha festival. Int J Infect Dis. 2015;38:9–15. https://doi.org/10.1016/j.ijid.2015.06.029.

37. El-Azazy OM, Scrimgeour EM. Crimean-Congo haemorrhagic fever virus infection in the western province of Saudi Arabia. Trans R Soc Trop Med Hyg. 1997;91:275–8.

38. Hassanein KM, El-Azazy OM, Yousef HM. Detection of Crimean-Congo haemorrhagic fever virus antibodies in humans and imported livestock in Saudi Arabia. Trans R Soc Trop Med Hyg. 1997;91:536–7.
39. Alhaeli A, Bahkali S, Ali A, Househ MS, El-Metwally AA. The epidemiology of Dengue fever in Saudi Arabia: a systematic review. J Infect Public Health. 2016;9:117–24. https://doi.org/10.1016/j.jiph.2015.05.006.
40. Balkhy HH, Memish ZA. Rift Valley fever: an uninvited zoonosis in the Arabian peninsula. Int J Antimicrob Agents. 2003;21:153–7.
41. Al-Afaleq AI, Hussein MF. The status of Rift Valley fever in animals in Saudi Arabia: a mini review. Vector Borne Zoonotic Dis. 2011;11:1513–20. https://doi.org/10.1089/vbz.2010.0245.
42. Hussain R, Alomar I, Memish ZA. Chikungunya virus: emergence of an arthritic arbovirus in Jeddah, Saudi Arabia. East Mediterr Heal J. 2013;19:506–8.
43. Humphrey JM, Cleton NB, Reusken CBEM, Glesby MJ, Koopmans MPG, Abu-Raddad LJ. Urban Chikungunya in the middle East and North Africa: a systematic review. PLoS Negl Trop Dis. 2017;11:e0005707. https://doi.org/10.1371/journal.pntd.0005707.

Rift Valley Fever in Travellers

11

Lucille Blumberg, Brett N. Archer, Peninah Munyua,
Osama Ahmed Hassan, David B. Wallace,
and Janusz Paweska

Abstract

Rift Valley fever (RVF) is a mosquito-borne viral zoonosis affecting humans,
livestock, and wildlife. The virus causes epizootics of abortions and deaths of
young livestock, resulting in substantial economic losses. A "One Health" (OH)

L. Blumberg (✉)
Division of Public Health Surveillance and Response, Centre for Emerging Zoonotic and
Parasitic Diseases, National Institute for Communicable Diseases a Division of the National
Health Laboratory Services, Sandringham, Johannesburg, South Africa
e-mail: lucilleb@nicd.ac.za

B. N. Archer
WHO Health Emergencies Programme, World Health Organization, Geneva, Switzerland
e-mail: archerb@who.int

P. Munyua
Global Disease Detection Center-Kenya, Division of Global Health Protection, Center for
Global Health, US Centers for Disease Control and Prevention, Nairobi, Kenya
e-mail: ikg2@cdc.gov

O. A. Hassan
Department of Community Medicine and Global Health, Institute of Health and Society,
Faculty of Medicine, University of Oslo, Oslo, Norway
e-mail: o.a.h.ahmed@medisin.uio.no

D. B. Wallace
Department Veterinary Tropical Diseases, Faculty of Veterinary Science, ARC-Onderstepoort
Veterinary Institute, University of Pretoria, Onderstepoort, Pretoria, South Africa
e-mail: WallaceD@arc.agric.za

J. Paweska
Centre for Emerging Zoonotic and Parasitic Diseases, National Institute for Communicable
Diseases a Division of the National Health Laboratory Services, Sandringham,
Johannesburg, South Africa
e-mail: januszp@nicd.ac.za

© The Author(s), under exclusive license to Springer Nature
Switzerland AG 2024
H. Leblebicioglu et al. (eds.), *Emerging and Re-emerging Infections in
Travellers*, https://doi.org/10.1007/978-3-031-49475-8_11

approach is critical for prevention and control strategies. The geographic range of RVF outbreaks has expanded to multiple African countries, with the first reports outside of the African continent in 2000 in Yemen and Saudi Arabia. The majority of human infections result from direct or indirect contact with blood or tissues from infected animals during handling, slaughter, assisting with animal births or through veterinary procedures rather than mosquito transmission. Occupational groups such as herders, farmers, slaughterhouse workers, and veterinarians are at higher risk of infection. To date, no human-to-human transmission of RVF has been documented. There is potential for the disease to expand to new, previously unaffected geographical locations through trade or transhumance and mosquitoes. RVF poses a very low risk to travellers outside of travel to areas affected by current epizootics and occupational risks. A detailed history of possible exposure to suspected or confirmed animals with RVF is key in performing a differential diagnosis in humans presenting with acute febrile illness. A low percentage of patients develop a much more severe form of the disease, but the overall mortality rate is <1%. Complications include ocular (retinal) disease (0.5–2% of patients), meningoencephalitis (<1%), hepatitis, or haemorrhagic fever (<1%). No specific treatment is available for RVF; management comprises general supportive therapy. Currently there is no approved RVF vaccine for humans.

11.1 Background

Rift Valley fever (RVF) is a mosquito-borne viral zoonosis affecting humans, livestock, and wildlife. The virus is in the family Phenuiviridae (genus *Phlebovirus*) and belongs to a group of viral haemorrhagic fever (VHF) agents due to the induction of severe clinical presentation with bleeding and multi-system disease in a small proportional group of infected humans, albeit with no human-to-human transmission [1]. The disease occurs predominantly in Africa and is mostly linked to exceptionally heavy rains, often after a period of relative drought, favouring the breeding of the mosquito vectors, with outbreaks documented in 12 African and two neighbouring countries from 2000 to 2019 [2, 3].

The virus causes epizootics of abortions and deaths of young livestock, predominantly sheep, goats and cattle, often resulting in substantial economic losses. Given the occurrence of the disease at the human/animal interface and climate and other environmental effects influencing transmission, a "One Health" (OH) approach [4–6] is critical for prevention and control strategies.

RVF is a World Organisation for Animal Health (WOAH)-listed disease. In 2015 was deemed a World Health Organization (WHO) priority disease for research and development of therapeutics, vaccines and rapid diagnostic tests. This is due to its potential to cause epizootics in livestock and consequently significant morbidity and mortality in humans and the lack of effective countermeasures [7]. RVFV is considered a potential bioterrorism weapon threat due to the ease of infection by inhalation.

11.2 Epidemiology

RVF virus was first characterized in 1931 in the Rift Valley region of Kenya. Between 1931 and 1950, outbreaks were reported in livestock in localized regions of Kenya and Tanzania. In the next four decades (1950–1996), the geographic range of RVF outbreaks expanded to multiple countries in the greater Horn of Africa area and southern and western Africa, with the first reports outside of the African continent in 2000 in Yemen and Saudi Arabia [2]. In the eastern Africa region, outbreaks normally occur every 5–15 years during periods of heavy and prolonged flooding, which increase habitat suitability for vector populations and influence the risk of disease emergence, transmission and spread [2, 8]. RVFV is likely maintained transovarially between outbreaks by *Aedes* mosquitoes and can survive in the eggs for many years during dry conditions. Breeding and generation of secondary vector mosquitoes of several genera, including *Culex, Anopheles* and *Mansonia*, and other biting flies (*Culicoides, Stomoxys* and tabanids) that feed on infected animals, result in rapid amplification of virus and mechanical transmission to other susceptible animal hosts and humans [9].

In contrast to the main vector in the Egyptian epidemic of 1977–1978, the principal mosquito vectors of RVFV in sub-Saharan Africa tend to be zoophilic and sylvatic. The majority of human infections result from direct or indirect contact with blood or tissues from infected animals during handling, slaughter, assisting with animal births, or through veterinary procedures. RVFV infects humans by either entry (parenteral route) through a wound or contact with broken skin or inhalation of aerosols produced during the slaughter or birthing of infected animals [10]. As such, occupational groups such as herders, farmers, slaughterhouse workers, veterinarians and animal health technologists are at higher risk of infection. Human infections have also resulted from the bites of infected mosquitoes, most commonly *Aedes* and *Culex* species, and the transmission of RVF virus by other haematophagous (blood-feeding) flies. There is limited evidence that humans may become infected by ingesting infected animals' unpasteurized or uncooked milk [11].

Accidental or intentional aerosolization of the virus may contribute to increased virus transmission by inhalational exposure. In 2009, RVFV was confirmed in six South African veterinary medicine students performing necropsies on cattle carcasses submitted to the Onderstepoort Veterinary Faculty for investigation. While direct contact with infected animal tissue was a possible source, given the level of contact precautions used, there is the real possibility that inhalation of infected aerosols generated by high-pressure hoses used to wash down the carcasses was the mode of transmission [12]. To date, no human-to-human transmission of RVF has been documented, and no transmission of RVF to healthcare workers has been reported when standard infection control precautions have been put in place [3].

A review of RVF in the eastern Africa region suggests an increase in the severity of human disease (morbidity and mortality) since the 1970s, with 478 deaths reported in 1998, 1107 reported cases with 350 deaths from 2006 to 2007, and 1174 cases with 241 deaths in 2008 [10, 13]. In 2018, simultaneous RVF outbreaks were reported in Kenya with 110 human cases and 8 deaths, 16 human cases and 7 deaths in Uganda and livestock cases in Rwanda.

A large nationwide outbreak of RVF occurred in South Africa during 2008–2011. During 2010 alone, at least 13,902 animal cases, including 8581 animal deaths, were laboratory-confirmed. During this period, cumulatively 302 human infections, including 25 human deaths, were reported. The vast majority (83%) of cases were farm-animal health workers or meat-industry workers with direct contact with animal tissues, blood or other body fluids (89%). Mosquito-borne transmission likely played a lesser role in the outbreak [14].

11.3 RVF as an Emerging Disease

In 2000, RVF spread outside of Africa to Yemen, probably as a result of the export of infected slaughtered animals. This highlights the potential for the disease to expand geographically to new unaffected areas through trade or transhumance [15] and mosquitoes. Importantly, the insect vectors that transmit RVFV are found in Europe, the Americas and in Asia, which opens the door to emergence in new locations and could cause considerable human morbidity and mortality, as well as economic damage. The international spread of West Nile, Chikungunya and Zika viruses is a good barometer for the potential impact of importation of another mosquito-borne virus such as RVFV. Climatic hazards (e.g., floods) occurring with increased frequency and intensity is expected to impact competent mosquito vector populations, increasing both frequency and distribution of RVF outbreaks.

11.4 Risks for Travellers

Outside of travel to areas affected by current epizootics, the risk RVF poses to travellers is generally considered low. Nonetheless, travellers should be encouraged to take precautions (clothing, suitable repellent and bednet use) to prevent mosquito bites, avoid direct contact with animal blood, body fluids or tissues, and avoid the unsafe consumption of fresh blood, raw milk or animal tissue. *Currently, there is no approved RVF vaccine for the general human population.*

Risks of infection increase greatly for travellers who may, for whatever reason, work with animals(livestock and wild animals) in RVF-endemic areas. In addition to the aforementioned precautions, such travellers should be encouraged to familiarize themselves with RVF and other zoonoses they may encounter, and take precautions such as wearing protective equipment to avoid direct contact with blood, tissue or other body fluids of potentially-infected animals.

Additional concern for female travellers, particularly pregnant women, is that RVF has been found for the first time to be associated with miscarriage [16]. This highlights the point that pregnant women may need to consider taking extra precautions when travelling to endemic regions of RVF, especially during an outbreak.

A small number of cases of RVF have been seen both in military and civilian travellers. For example, eight Swedish soldiers became positive for RVFV antibodies during their work with United Nation forces in Egypt in the Sinai desert in 1977 [17]. Similarly, French soldiers who worked in Chad in 2001 during the rainy season developed the disease [18]. A German woman who travelled to Kenya as a tourist returned home to Germany with severe hepatitis, suspected to be hepatitis A, but with RVF as an additional infection. She developed liver complications and died after being hospitalized for 11 days [19]. In 2018, the first imported case of RVF in China was confirmed. The patient was a man who was in Angola before returning to China [20, 21].

RVF may pose a potential risk to persons attending mass gatherings; this was highlighted when the RVF outbreak in South Africa coincided with the FIFA World Cup [22]. The concern was how to provide proper information on self-protection for hundreds of thousands of tourists expected to attend the event. RVFV was initially considered as the cause of an acute febrile illness in a German tourist who had visited a game farm in South Africa during the outbreak period and immediately before the World Cup event, prompting laboratory testing for RVF. An apparent positive serological test prompted a warning for RVF for tourists visiting South Africa for the event resulting in a large number of cancellations. On review, the traveller had in fact not had direct contact with animals in an area where RVF cases had been reported, and the clinical illness was more in keeping with African tick bite fever, which was subsequently confirmed. Repeat serology using IFA and ELISA on the acute and convalescent serum samples in two different laboratories was negative for RVFV [23]. This highlights the importance of collecting a careful epidemiological (including risk factors) and clinical history and ensuring accurate laboratory tests against a full differential diagnosis to definitively confirm the cause of infection before alerting travellers.

While it is an uncommon disease in 'leisure' travellers, RVF is important to consider in the differential diagnosis of persons with acute febrile illness, hepatitis and encephalitis who have travelled to endemic areas, especially where their occupations would place them at risk for infection.

Currently, there is no approved RVF vaccine for humans. Therefore, travellers to countries with endemic diseases should avoid contact with sick animals and their products and use personal protective measures against mosquito bites.

11.5 Pathogenesis

The liver is a major target, with histopathological examination showing moderate focal or midzonal coagulative necrosis. The pathophysiology of the retinitis is not well described. The mechanisms of the haemostatic derangements remain speculative [1].

11.6   Clinical Findings

RVF incubation period (interval from infection to onset of symptoms) varies from two to six days. In the vast majority of infected persons, the infection may be asymptomatic or manifest with very mild symptoms. Clinically it presents as a fever with "flu-like" symptoms (including myalgia, arthralgia and headache). Some patients may also develop neck stiffness, sensitivity to light (photophobia), pain behind the eyes, loss of appetite and vomiting; in such patients, the clinical presentation may be mistaken for meningitis. Symptoms of RVF usually last from four to seven days, after which the immune response becomes detectable with the appearance of antibodies, and the virus gradually disappears from the blood [24].

A small percentage of patients develop a much more severe form of the disease, but the overall mortality rate is <1%. Complications include *ocular (retinal)* disease (0.5–2% of patients), *meningoencephalitis* (<1%), *hepatitis*, or *haemorrhagic fever* (<1%). The mortality rate of patients developing the haemorrhagic form of the disease is high (50%) [24–29].

- **Ocular disease (retinitis):** The onset of retinitis is usually one to three weeks after the appearance of the first symptoms (which may be very mild or subclinical) and usually presents as blurred or decreased vision. It may resolve within 10–12 weeks with no sequelae. If lesions occur in the macula, about 50% of patients will experience permanent vision loss. Death in patients with only the ocular form of the disease is uncommon.
- **Meningoencephalitis:** The onset of meningoencephalitis usually occurs one to four weeks after the first symptoms (which may be very mild or subclinical) of RVF appear, and in some cases neurological complications can manifest >60 days after the initial symptoms. Clinical features may include intense headaches, loss of memory, hallucinations, confusion, disorientation, vertigo, convulsions, lethargy and coma. Although the mortality rate in patients who experience only this form of the disease is low, residual neurological deficit, which may be severe, is common.
- **Hepatitis:** This is characterized by markedly raised transaminase enzyme levels (ALT and AST), and may occur together with, or precede, other complications (e.g., haemorrhage or meningoencephalitis).
- **Haemorrhagic fever:** Manifestations appear two to four days after the initial onset of the illness. Usually, evidence of severe liver impairment (such as jaundice or elevated liver enzyme levels) is present, followed by haemorrhage. This may present as haematemesis (vomiting blood), melaena (passing blood in the faeces), a petechial /purpuric rash or ecchymoses, bleeding from the nose or gums, menorrhagia, and bleeding from venepuncture sites. There is often an associated hepatitis.

11.7 Laboratory Diagnosis

RVFV is classified as a Risk Group 3 agent, and biosafety level-3 (BSL-3) containment requirements are needed to work with the virus in the laboratory. The capacity for laboratory diagnosis of RVF is restricted to a limited number of reference laboratories worldwide [1, 30–32].

In the absence of haemorrhagic or specific organ manifestations, infections by VHF viruses are clinically difficult to recognize; consequently, definitive diagnosis depends largely on accurate laboratory tests. Serum specimens are commonly used for RVF diagnosis in humans. Although viraemia in infected individuals reaches high titres, it is of short duration, thus limiting the use of viral detection systems. In addition, most infected patients experience subclinical or mild infections; therefore, antigen and nucleic acid detection assays should be run in parallel with antibody-detecting techniques. Type-specific antibodies to RVFV are easily demonstrable shortly after exposure to the virus.

The virus is isolated in hamsters, infant or adult mice, and various cell cultures. Highly sensitive polymerase chain reaction (PCR) assays for the detection and quantification of RVFV have been reported, including reverse transcriptase PCR (RT-PCR) and real-time detection PCR (RTD-PCR) based on TaqMan probe technology. More recently, the real-time reverse-transcription loop-mediated isothermal amplification assay (RT-LAMP) was developed and evaluated to detect RVFV from a wide spectrum of isolates and clinical specimens. Apart from high analytical and diagnostic accuracy and speed of detection, another important practical advantage of the LAMP assay is that it utilizes simple and relatively inexpensive equipment, which renders it promising for use in resource-poor settings and as a portable device during RVF outbreaks in remote areas. The recent findings in Kenyan patients indicate that the quantitative real-time RT-PCR (qRT-PCR) can be used to rapidly identify patients with high viraemia associated with poor prognosis, thereby enabling them to be targeted for special or intensive clinical management. Diagnosis of recent infection is confirmed by demonstrating seroconversion or a four-fold or greater rise in antibody titre in paired serum samples or by detecting IgM antibodies. The classical methods for detecting antibodies to RVFV include haemagglutination inhibition, complement fixation, indirect immunofluorescence (IFA), and virus neutralization tests. Disadvantages of these techniques include health risks to laboratory personnel and restrictions for their use outside RVF endemic areas. Although regarded as a gold standard, the virus neutralization test is laborious, expensive, and requires 5–7 days for completion. It can be performed only when a standardized stock of live virus and tissue cultures is available. Consequently, it is rarely used and then only in highly specialized reference laboratories. Serology using IFA is widely used but is prone to false-positive results in inexperienced hands due to the presence of background non-specific fluorescence.

Following human infection, RVFV-specific IgM and IgG antibodies may remain detectable for prolonged periods. This should be considered when investigating persons with acute febrile illness living in endemic areas. Viral antigens can be detected in blood and other tissues using various immunological methods, including agar gel immunodiffusion and immunostaining assays. Histopathological examination of the liver reveals characteristic pathology. The development of rapid diagnostic tests would be particularly important for identifying outbreaks timeously.

11.8 Differential Diagnosis

RVF may be suspected when there is a sudden outbreak of febrile illness with headache and myalgia in humans, in association with the occurrence of abortions in domestic ruminants and deaths of young animals. Given the very non-specific presentation of usually low-grade fever and myalgia in humans, a key factor in the early recognition of RVF is close communication between veterinary and human health practitioners. When RVF is suspected or confirmed in animals, the epidemiological link in persons with direct animal contact or simply a resident in the area should prompt consideration of RVF in any person with an acute febrile illness or with one of the severe forms – hepatitis, disseminated intravascular coagulation or encephalitis. In persons with severe progressive illness, as for most VHFs, the non-specific presentation of RVF makes it difficult to diagnose clinically. Therefore, the differential diagnosis concerns a broad array of conditions, especially when first cases are encountered during a yet unrecognized outbreak. These include malaria, rickettsial infections, Q fever, typhoid fever, dysentery, plague, brucellosis, leptospirosis, meningitis, sepsis from other bacterial infections, viral hepatitis, other VHFs, including Lassa fever, Crimean-Congo haemorrhagic fever, Marburg virus disease, Ebola virus disease, and the haemorrhagic fever with renal syndrome associated with hantavirus infections. Disseminated intravascular coagulopathy and acute leukaemia should also be considered.

The availability of laboratory results and epidemiological information usually helps narrow the differential diagnosis spectrum. The tentative cause in endemic regions can be assumed based on recent travel and exposure history (e.g., mosquito bite, contact with animals or animal products). As for all VHFs, an RVF confirmatory diagnostic process has to consider all available laboratory results and clinical, pathological, and epidemiological data. Cases of RVF are sometimes only recognized late after infection from the occurrence of ocular complications. Late recognition of RVF infections is especially the case during inter-epizootic periods, when only very sporadic infections occur and are usually misdiagnosed. Haemorrhagic or encephalitic manifestations might also be indicative of RVF infection, and this is especially true in the rare instances when residents of RVF-free countries develop the illness following a visit to endemic areas.

When Should RVF Be Suspected?

Any person resident in or with recent travel (<21 days) to an area where RVF is known to occur, especially those with an epidemiological link* presenting with the following:

- Influenza-like illness (which may include fever, myalgia, arthralgia or headache), **OR.**
- Fever and features of encephalitis, haemorrhage, hepatitis and/or ocular pathology (retinitis) **OR.**
- Unexplained encephalitis or ocular pathology.

*High-risk categories/links include:

(i) Recent close contact with livestock/wild ruminants in or from RVF-affected areas, including.
   (a) Slaughtering and butchering (informal or commercial).
   (b) Disposal of carcasses/foetuses.
   (c) Assistance with birthing or other animal husbandry activities resulting in exposure to animal blood and body fluids.
   (d) veterinary procedures.
(ii) Residing in an RVF-affected area with a history of recent mosquito bites.
(iii) Consumption of unpasteurized/uncooked milk sourced from RVF-affected areas.

Note: other causes for these symptoms must be excluded where appropriate, including malaria, Crimean-Congo haemorrhagic fever (CCHF) and tick bite fever. Obtaining a thorough history, including other signs and symptoms, recent travel, arthropod (e.g., tick) exposures, contact with livestock etc., will assist clinicians in narrowing the differential diagnosis.

11.9 Management

No specific treatment is available for RVF; management comprises general supportive therapy. Early dialysis for patients with renal failure may improve outcomes. Ribavirin is not recommended for the treatment of RVF. Intravenous administration of ribavirin to patients during the 2000 outbreak in Saudi Arabia was quickly stopped due to the finding that it may increase the likelihood of neurological disease [28, 33]. Newer broad-spectrum antiviral drugs such as Favipiravir have shown some promise in rodent models [34, 35]. Identifying effective chemotherapeutic agents and/or human vaccine candidates is the focus of the WHO Blueprint for Research and Development, and a product profile and pathway is being developed [7].

Human-to-human transmission has not been demonstrated. Standard infection prevention and control precautions should be followed; patients do not require isolation or barrier nursing. However, should a patient present with a haemorrhagic fever or severe hepatitis where both RVF and other VHFs are part of the differential diagnoses, based on the clinical presentation, the epidemiological history, geographical area and possible exposures, the laboratory testing must include a panel of tests to cover the relevant VHFs. The laboratory results, particularly serology, must always be interpreted in conjunction with the clinical presentation and likelihood of exposure to that particular infection in the geographical setting. In the case of a patient presenting with fever and haemorrhage during an RVF outbreak, where there is geographical overlap with Crimean-Congo haemorrhagic fever, it is critically important to manage the patient in the interim as a possible VHF case until laboratory test results are available and to implement appropriate infection prevention and control measures (isolation, barrier nursing, etc.).

Follow-up of patients with RVF for at least 1 month after symptoms resolve is advised to monitor for possible development of ocular complications (retinitis in particular) or neurological complications.

Isolation of patients with RVF and follow-up of close contacts for disease is not required, given the absence of any evidence for person-to-person transmission.

11.10 Outbreak Prevention and Response

The most important first step in preventing significant human disease is early detection of animal cases through rigorous active surveillance and sentinel herd monitoring. Once infected animals and/or herds are located, further spread can be prevented by implementing mosquito control, animal movement control, a ban on livestock slaughtering, or at least the use of preventive measures (gloves, masks, and gowns) when handling carcasses or aborted foetuses. Public awareness and education about the signs, symptoms, and risk factors are critical to help limit further animal disease and spread to people. Targeted vaccination of animals may be beneficial as a control measure in high-risk areas. Still, animal vaccination may lead to disease spread due to the sharing of needles between livestock and may also be too late to halt further expansion [36].

Other ways to mitigate the spread of RVF involve control of the vector and protection against their bites. Larviciding measures at mosquito breeding sites are the most effective form of vector control if breeding sites can be clearly identified and are limited in size and extent. During flooding, however, the number and extent of breeding sites is usually too high for larviciding measures to be feasible.

11.11 Prevention and Advice for Travellers

Public health education and risk reduction play a vital role in preventing cases. Messages to the community, especially within affected areas, should focus on avoiding high-risk animal husbandry procedures and slaughtering practices through gloves, masks and other protective clothing, especially when handling sick animals. The unsafe consumption of fresh blood, raw milk or animal tissue should be avoided. All animal products (blood, meat, and milk) should be thoroughly cooked before consumption in epizootic regions. Slaughtering of animals for consumption should be discouraged during outbreaks. Personal and community protection against mosquito bites through insect repellents (containing 30–50% DEET), insecticide-treated bednets, and wearing light-coloured clothing should be encouraged [3, 37].

11.12 Vaccines

RVF presents a unique opportunity to merge facets of both veterinary and human vaccination strategies under the One Health concept. Livestock vaccination will not only help control epizootics but also prevent the chain of transmission to humans.

Since the 1960s, formalin-inactivated vaccines using pantropic strains of RVFV have been developed and tested in animals and humans for safety and immunogenicity [38, 39]. These have been available under special permission to protect lab workers at risk of exposure, requiring multiple priming events and regular follow-up boosters to maintain anti-RVFV antibody titre levels thought to be protective. To overcome these constraints, a mutagenized live attenuated vaccine (MP-12) was developed for human use and tested extensively in various animal and vector species [40]. More recently, Phase 1 trials in humans were followed by Phase 2 human clinical trials, including genetic stability studies of the vaccine (Pittman et al., 2016). Post-vaccinal reactions were mild, high neutralizing antibody titres were obtained, of long duration, and the vaccine did not revert to the virulent parental strain (ZH548). In addition, the Coalition for Epidemic Preparedness Innovations (CEPI) is busy supporting a number of technologies for a new human RVF vaccine [41] and a single dose vectored candidate vaccine utilizing the ChAdOx1 delivery platform is currently in phase 1 studies.

For livestock, a live attenuated vaccine was developed by neurotropic adaptation of the virus by Smithburn (Uganda) [41] and an inactivated vaccine was developed at the Onderstepoort Veterinary Institute (South Africa) [42, 43]. After further adaptation of the Smithburn vaccine in South Africa, it was found that a single dose was protective, although with a risk of causing abortion in pregnant animals. The inactivated vaccine was safer but requires a booster. Both vaccines are available commercially for use as preventative measures in endemic regions. Clone 13, a naturally occurring deletion mutant of RVFV, is a live attenuated RVF vaccine registered more recently for use in ruminants [43]. The vaccine is safe in pregnant animals, although overdose use is to be avoided, and proper storage is important. A more heat-stable version of the vaccine is now available from Morocco. In addition, MP-12 and a reverse-engineered variant have shown promise as candidate vaccines in livestock in Tanzania [44–46]. To address challenges experienced by developing farmers in Africa, multivalent virus-vectored vaccines are under development [47], and for countries non-endemic for RVF, a number of subunit vaccines have been developed and evaluated. However, none are yet available commercially [43].

- Veterinary authorities must communicate any suspicion/confirmation of Rift Valley fever (RVF) timeously with public health practitioners.
- The epidemiological link to animals with suspected RVF should prompt the consideration of RVF in a person with acute febrile non-specific illness.
- It is critically important to combine an accurate epidemiological history with the clinical picture, laboratory results and the diagnostic tests. All the different pieces of the "puzzle" must fit.
- Anything can occur anywhere, and RVF can emerge in new areas, so it must always be considered a cause of acute febrile illness when tests for other common conditions are negative.
- In a patient presenting with fever and bleeding, even in the presence of an RVF outbreak, other important diseases in that geographical area must be considered, for example, Crimean-Congo haemorrhagic fever and appropriate infection control precautions must be in place.

Acknowledgements Prof. Robert Swanepoel and Mr. Alan Kemp, thank you for your contributions to RVF knowledge over many years.

- Ms. Irma Latsky and Prof John Frean for collation and review of the manuscript.

Declaration of Interest We declare no conflict of interest.

References

1. Swanepoel B, Burt FJ. Principals and practice of clinical virology. John Wiley & Sons Ltd.; 2009.
2. Nanyingi MO, Munyua P, Kiama SG, Muchemi GM, Thumbi SM, Bitek AO, Bett B, Muriithi RM, Njenga MK. A systematic review of Rift Valley fever epidemiology 1931–2014. Infect Ecol Epidemiol. 2015;31(5):28024. https://doi.org/10.3402/iee.v5.28024.
3. Rift Valley fever. Fact sheet N°207. World Health Organization. Revised May 2010. Available from: http://www.who.int/mediacentre/factsheets/fs207/en/. Accessed 26 June 2019.
4. Coker R, Rushton J, Mounier-Jack S, Karimuribo E, Lutumba P, Kambarage D, Pfeiffer DU, Stärk K, Rweyemamu M. Towards a conceptual framework to support one-health research for policy on emerging zoonoses. Lancet Infect Dis. 2011;11(4):326–31.
5. Ahmed Hassan Ahmed, O. Rift Valley fever: challenges and new insights for prevention and control using the "One Health" approach. Umeå University, Faculty of Medicine, Department of

Clinical Microbiology, Virology. Umeå University, Faculty of Medicine, Department of Public Health and Clinical Medicine, Epidemiology and Global Health. (Magnus Evander). Doctoral thesis. http://umu.diva-portal.org/smash/record.jsf?pid=diva2%3A1040825&dswid=-8214

6. Hassan OA, Ahlm C, Evander M. A need for One Health approach—lessons learned from outbreaks of Rift Valley fever in Saudi Arabia and Sudan. Infect Ecol Epidemiol. 2014;4(1):20710. https://doi.org/10.3402/iee.v4.20710.

7. WHO Research and Development Blueprint. 2018 Annual review of diseases prioritized under the Research and Development Blueprint. https://www.who.int/emergencies/diseases/2018prioritization-report.pdf.

8. Anyamba A, Linthicum KJ, Small J, Britch SC, Pak E, de La Rocque S, Formenty P, Hightower AW, Breiman RF, Chretien JP, Tucker CJ. Prediction, assessment of the Rift Valley fever activity in East and Southern Africa 2006–2008 and possible vector control strategies. Am J Trop Med Hyg. 2010;83(Suppl. 2):43–51.

9. Gerdes GH. Rift Valley fever. Rev Sci Tech. 2004;23(2):613–23.

10. McMillen CM, Hartman AL. Rift Valley fever in animals and humans: current perspectives. Antivir Res. 2018;156:29–37.

11. Grossi-Soyster EN, Lee J, King CH, LaBeaud AD. The influence of raw milk exposures on Rift Valley fever virus transmission. PLoS Negl Trop Dis. 2019;13(3):e0007258. https://doi.org/10.1371/journal.pntd.0007258.

12. Archer BN, Weyer J, Paweska J, Nkosi D, Leman P, Tint KS, Blumberg L. 2011. Outbreak of Rift Valley fever affecting veterinarians and farmers in South Africa, 2008. S Afr Med J. 2011;101(4):263–6.

13. Baba M, Masiga DK, Sang R, Villinger J. Has Rift Valley fever virus evolved with increasing severity in human populations in East Africa? Emerg Microbes Infect. 2016;5:e58. https://doi.org/10.1038/emi.2016.57.

14. Archer BN, Thomas J, Weyer J, Cengimbo A, Landoh DE, Jacobs C, Ntuli S, Modise M, Mathonsi M, Mashishi MS, Leman PA, le Roux C, Jansen van Vuren P, Kemp A, Paweska JT, Blumberg L. Epidemiologic investigations into outbreaks of Rift Valley fever in humans, South Africa, 2008–2011. Emerg Infect Dis. 2013;19(12) https://doi.org/10.3201/eid1912.121527.

15. Soumare PL, Freire CC, Faye O, Diallo M, de Oliveira JVC, Zanotto PM. Phylogeography of Rift Valley fever virus in Africa reveals multiple introductions in Senegal and Mauritania. PLoS One. 2012;7(4):e35216.

16. Baudin M, Jumaa AM, Jomma HJ, Karsany MS, Bucht G, Näslund J, Ahlm C, Evander M, Mohamed N. Association of Rift Valley fever virus infection with miscarriage in Sudanese women: a cross-sectional study. Lancet Glob Health. 2016;4(11):e864–71.

17. Niklasson B, Meegan JM, Bengtsson E. Antibodies to Rift Valley fever virus in Swedish U.N. soldiers in Egypt and the Sinai. Scand J Infect Dis. 1979;11:313–4.

18. Ringot D, Durand JP, Tolou H, Boutin JP, Davoust B. Rift Valley Fever in Chad. Emerg Infect Dis. 2004;10(5):945–7.

19. Oltmann A, Kamper S, Staeck O, Chanasit JS, Gunther SG, Berg T, Frank C, Kruger DH. Fatal outcome of Hepatitis A Virus (HAV) infection in a Traveller with incomplete HAV vaccination and evidence of Rift Valley fever virus infection. J Clin Microbiol. 2008;46(11):3850–2.

20. Liu J, Sun Y, Shi W, Tan S, Pan Y, Cui S, Zhang Q, Dou X, Lv Y, Li X, Li X. The first imported case of Rift Valley fever in China reveals a genetic reassortment of different viral lineages. Emerg Microbes Infect. 2017;6(1):1–7.

21. Perez AM, Carrasco Medanic R, Thurmond MC. Rift Valley fever outbreaks in South Africa. Vet Record. 2010;166:798.

22. World Health Organization. Rift Valley fever, South Africa—update. Wkly Epidemiol Rec. 2010;85(21):185–6.

23. Hartman A. Rift Valley Fever. Clin Lab Med. 2017;37(2):285–301. https://doi.org/10.1016/j.cll.2017.01.004.

24. Laughlin LW, Meegan JM, Strausbaugh LJ, Morens DM, Watten RH. Epidemic Rift Valley fever in Egypt: observations of the spectrum of human illness. Trans R Soc Trop Med Hyg. 1979;73(6):630–3.

25. Freed I. Rift valley fever in man, complicated by retinal changes and loss of vision. S Afr Med J. 1951;25(50):930–2.
26. Al-Hazmi A, Al-Rajhi AA, Abboud EB, et al. Ocular complications of Rift Valley fever outbreak in Saudi Arabia. Ophthalmology. 2005;112(2):313–8.
27. Madani TA, Al-Mazrou YY, Al-Jeffri MH, et al. Rift Valley fever epidemic in Saudi Arabia: epidemiological, clinical, and laboratory characteristics. Clin Infect Dis. 2003;37(8):1084–92.
28. McIntosh BM, Russell D, dos Santos I, Gear JH. Rift Valley fever in humans in South Africa. S Afr Med J. 1980;58(20):803–6.
29. LaBeaud AD, Pfeil S, Muiruri S, et al. Factors associated with severe human Rift Valley fever in Sangailu, Garissa County, Kenya. PLoS Negl Trop Dis. 2015;9(3):e0003548.
30. Le Roux CA, Kubo T, Grobbelaar AA, van Vuren PJ, Weyer J, Nel LH, Swanepoel R, Morita K, Paweska JT. Development and evaluation of a real-time reverse transcription-loop-mediated isothermal amplification assay for rapid detection of Rift Valley fever virus in clinical specimens. J Clin Microbiol. 2009;47(3):645–51. https://doi.org/10.1128/JCM.01412-08.
31. Archer BN, Weyer J, Paweska J, Nkosi D, Leman P, Tint KS, Blumberg L. Outbreak of Rift Valley fever affecting veterinarians and farmers in South Africa, 2008. Afr Med J. 2011;101(4):263–6.
32. Pepin M, Bouloy M, Bird BH, Kemp A, Paweska J. Rift Valley fever virus (Bunyaviridae: Phlebovirus): an update on pathogenesis, molecular epidemiology, vectors, diagnostics and prevention. Vet Res. 2010;41(6):61.
33. Al-Hazmi M, Ayoola EA, Abdurahman M, Banzal S, Ashraf J, El-Bushra A, Hazmi A, Abdullah M, Abbo H, Elamin A, Al-Sammani E-T, Gadour M, Menon C, Hamza M, Rahim I, Hafez M, Jambavalikar M, Arishi H, Aqeel A. Epidemic Rift Valley fever in Saudi Arabia: a clinical study of severe illness in humans. Clin Infect Dis. 2003;36(3):245–52.
34. Scharton D, Bailey KW, Vest Z, Westover JB, Kumaki Y, Van Wettere A, Furuta Y, Gowen BB. Favipiravir (T-705) protects against peracute Rift Valley fever virus infection and reduces delayed-onset neurologic disease observed with ribavirin treatment. Antivir Res. 2014;104:84–92. https://doi.org/10.1016/j.antiviral.2014.01.016. Epub 2014 Jan 31
35. Caroline AL, Powell DS, Bethel LM, Oury TD, Reed DS, Hartman AL. Broad spectrum antiviral activity of favipiravir (T-705): protection from highly lethal inhalational Rift Valley fever. PLoS Negl Trop Dis. 2014;8(4):e2790.
36. Woods CW, Karpati AM, Grein T, McCarthy N, Gaturuku P, Muchiri E, Dunster L, Henderson A, Khan AS, Swanepoel R, Bonmarin I, Martin L, Mann P, Smoak BL, Ryan M, Ksiazek TG, Arthur RR, Ndikuyeze A, Agata NN. Peters CJ; World Health Organization Hemorrhagic Fever Task Force. An outbreak of Rift Valley fever in Northeastern Kenya, 1997-98. Emerg Infect Dis. 2002;8(2):138–44.
37. Boshra H, Lorenzo G, Busquets N, Brun A. Rift valley fever: recent insights into pathogenesis and prevention. J Virol. 2011;85(13):6098–105. https://doi.org/10.1128/JVI.02641-10.
38. Pittman PR, Liu CT, Cannon TL, Makuch RS, Mangiafico JA, Gibbs PH, Peters CJ. Immunogenicity of an inactivated Rift Valley fever vaccine in humans: a 12-year experience. Vaccine. 2000;18:181–9.
39. Rusnack JM, Gibbs P, Boudreau E, Clizbe DP, Pittman P. Immunogenicity and safety of an inactivated Rift Valley fever vaccine in a 19-year study. Vaccine. 2011;29:3222–9.
40. Pittman P, Norrisa SL, Brown ES, Ranadive MV, Schibly BA, Bettinger GE, Lokugamage N, Korman L, Morrill JC, Peters CJ. Rift Valley fever MP-12 vaccine Phase 2 clinical trial: safety, immunogenicity and genetic characterization of virus isolates. Vaccine. 2016;34(4):523–30.
41. Gerken KN, LaBeaud AD, Mandi H, L'Azou Jackson M, Breugelmans JG, King CH. Paving the way for human vaccination against Rift Valley fever virus: a systematic literature review of RVFV epidemiology from 1999 to 2021. PLoS Negl Trop Dis. 2022;16(1):e0009852. https://doi.org/10.1371/journal.pntd.0009852.
42. Smithburn KC. Rift Valley fever. The neurotropic adaptation of the virus and experimental use of the virus as a modified vaccine. Br J Exp Pathol. 1949;30(1):1–16.
43. Barnard BJH. Rift Valley fever vaccine—antibody and immune response in cattle to a live and an inactivated vaccine. J S Afr Vet Assoc. 1979;50(3):155–7.

44. Wallace DB, Ellis CE, Espach A, Smith SJ, Greyling RR, Viljoen GJ. Protective immune responses induced by different recombinant vaccine regimes to Rift Valley fever. Vaccine. 2006;24:7181–9.
45. Nyundo S, Adamson E, Rowland J, Palermo PM, Matiko M, Bettinger GE, et al. Safety and immunogenicity of Rift Valley fever MP-12 and arMP-12ΔNSm21/384 vaccine candidates in goats (*Capra aegagrus hircus*) from Tanzania. Onderstepoort J Vet Res. 2019;86(1):a1683. https://doi.org/10.4102/ojvr.v86i1.1683.
46. Adamson EK, Nyundo S, Rowland J, Palermo PM, Matiko MK, et al. Safety and immunogenicity of Rift Valley fever MP-12 and a Novel arMP-12ΔNSm21/384 recombinant vaccine candidate in native breed of Black Head Sheep (Ovis aries) from Tanzania. J Vaccines Vaccin. 2018;9(394):2. https://doi.org/10.4172/2157-7560.1000394.
47. Dungu B, Lubisi BA, Ikegami T. Rift Valley fever vaccines: current and future needs. Curr Opin Virol. 2018;29:8–15.

Yellow Fever in Travellers

12

Terezinha M. P. P. Castiñeiras and Luciana G. P. Brandão

Abstract

Yellow fever (YF) is an acute haemorrhagic flavivirus infection that is transmitted primarily by mosquitoes of the *Haemogogus*, *Sabethes* and *Aedes* genera, and affects humans and non-human primates (NHP). The disease is endemic and enzootic in several tropical regions in the Americas and Africa, with periodic upsurges and outbreaks. In its most severe form, it causes a haemorrhagic fever which has a high (20–50%) case-fatality rate. Besides the availability of safe and effective vaccines since 1937, the existence of a sylvatic cycle of transmission involving wild mosquitoes and NHPs makes eradication impractical. In the last years, explosive outbreaks have been documented in Africa and South America. The risk of major YF epidemics, especially in densely populated urban settings, has greatly increased due to reinvasion of urban settings by *Aedes aegypti*, rapid urbanization, intense population mobility, and waning immunization coverage. Importantly, people travelling to endemic regions represent a population at risk for YF virus exposure, and once infected, may contribute to disease spread to non-endemic areas. Vaccination is recommended for people aged ≥9 months

T. M. P. P. Castiñeiras (✉)
Departamento de Doenças Infecciosas e Parasitárias, Faculdade de Medicina, Universidade Federal do Rio de Janeiro, Rio de Janeiro, Brazil

Núcleo de Enfrentamento e Estudos de Doenças Infecciosas Emergentes e Reemergentes (NEEDIER), Universidade Federal do Rio de Janeiro, Rio de Janeiro, Brazil
e-mail: tmartapc@medicina.ufrj.br

L. G. P. Brandão
Laboratório de Pesquisa em Imunização e Vigilância em Saúde (LIVS), Instituto Nacional de Infectologia Evandro Chagas, Fundação Oswaldo Cruz, Rio de Janeiro, Brazil
e-mail: luciana.pedro@ini.fiocruz.br

H. Leblebicioglu et al. (eds.), *Emerging and Re-emerging Infections in Travellers*, https://doi.org/10.1007/978-3-031-49475-8_12

who live in or travel to endemic areas. The unusual resurgence events emphasize the relevance for considering YF as a serious threat to human health as well as the need for better understanding and monitoring the disease.

12.1 Background

Yellow fever (YF), the first-described haemorrhagic fever, is an acute viral disease, sometimes fatal, transmitted by infected mosquitoes. Yellow fever virus (YFV) originated in Africa and was brought to the western hemisphere during the slave trade era, with the first epidemic reported in 1648 in the Yucatan [1]. Over the centuries, the disease has been one of the great killers of mankind. YF epidemics decimated thousands of people in Europe, USA, Africa, and Central and South Americas, caused military forces failure and halted major engineering projects, as the first attempts to build the Panama Canal. Despite the availability of a highly effective and safe vaccine since 1930s, YF remains a disease of significant public health importance affecting 84,000–170,000 inhabitants annually in tropical regions of Africa and South America with an estimated 29,000–60,000 deaths, most in Africa [2]. Notably, it is a considerable hazard to unvaccinated travellers to endemic areas. Recent increases in the density and distribution of the urban mosquito vector, *Ae. aegypti*, as well as intense population mobility, increase the risk of introduction and spread of YF to areas of low vaccination coverage, that had never been affected (emergence) or had been free (re-emergence) from the disease for decades. Placing hundreds of millions of unvaccinated people at risk, the recent outbreaks have highlighted how the threat of YF beyond its classic endemic areas has been underestimated [3]. New research efforts are needed to better understand YFV and to develop effective tools in medical practice and public health policy against this arboviral disease.

12.2 Aetiology

Yellow fever virus (YFV) is an encapsulated single-stranded RNA virus, the prototype member of the genus *Flavivirus*, of the family *Flaviviridae* (Latin *flavus*, "yellow"), a group of viruses that are transmitted between vertebrates by arthropod vectors. At genomic level, seven major genotypes of YFV are distinguished [4], representing West Africa (02), Central-East Africa and Angola (03), and South America (02). Besides different genotypes, YFV is antigenically conserved, with a single serotype, which is critical to the effectiveness of virus strain (17D) vaccine.

12.3 Transmission

The primary mode of YFV transmission to humans is through the bite of an infected female mosquito and different vectors (*Aedes* spp., *Haemagogus* spp. or *Saebethes* spp.) are involved [5]. Occasionally, perinatal, breastfeeding, transfusion, and laboratory related transmission of YF were documented.

Infection of mosquitoes is initiated by ingestion of a blood meal from an infected human or non-human primate (NHP). After a median of 10 days at 25 °C (middle 95% = 2–37 days), that corresponds to extrinsic incubation time, virus is secreted in mosquito saliva, and the vector is capable of transmitting virus when it re-feeds on a susceptible host [6].

Human and NHP experience sufficient viraemia to infect naïve mosquitoes, and both are susceptible to infection and disease. The mosquito is the true reservoir of YF, persisting infected throughout its life, approximately 1–3 months [7]. Female mosquitoes can transmit the virus through transovarial route and infected eggs can resist the dry season. Also, venereal transmission in *Aedes* mosquitoes may have a role in the maintenance of arbovirus in interepidemic periods [5]. In nature, as virus is maintained in an enzootic cycle by these mosquitoes and NHPs, eradication of the disease is impractical.

Three types of transmission cycle are described [8]. In the *sylvatic (or jungle) cycle*, infected NHP are bitten by wild mosquito species found in forest canopy (*Haemagogus* spp. and *Sabethes* spp.), which pass the virus to other monkeys. Occasionally, humans working or travelling in the forest are bitten by infected mosquitoes and, if susceptible (unvaccinated), can develop yellow fever. In the *intermediate (or forest-savannah) cycle*, unique to Africa, semi-domestic tree hole-breeding mosquitoes (*Aedes* spp., such as *Ae. africanus*) infect both monkeys and humans in jungle border areas of savannah, leading to a constant transmission of YFV between mosquito, NHPs, and humans. This intermediate cycle provides an easy bridge for the viral disease to reach more densely populated areas, where an urban cycle can be initiated. Interesting, YFV-competent *Ae. albopictus* may play the role of "bridge vector" linking the forest cycle to the urban YFV cycle [3, 9]. In the *urban cycle*, a returning infected human from jungle or forest-savannah introduces the virus into heavily populated urban areas with high *Ae. aegypti* (Fig. 12.1) density and where many people are susceptible. In this scenario, infected mosquitoes transmit YFV from person to person and large epidemics may occur. The various cycles have different dynamics. This naturally leads to questions concerning the optimal routes for controlling the disease.

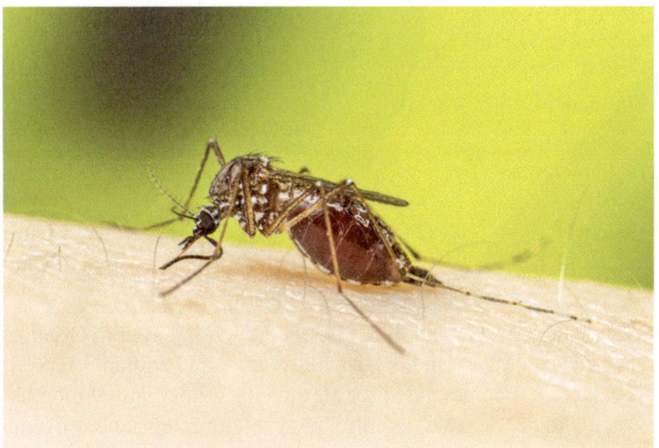

Fig. 12.1 *Aedes aegypti* adult female taking a blood meal. CDC library, 2022

12.3.1 Epidemiology

12.3.1.1 Geographic Distributions

Yellow fever is endemic and intermittently epidemic in sub-Saharan Africa and tropical South America, where 42 countries are considered endemic and at high-risk for YF re-emergence with explosive outbreaks (Table 12.1). While the principal vector of the YFV, *Ae. aegypti*, is largely present in Asia, there have been no documented cases of autochthonous transmission on this continent. In the continental area of Europe, *Ae. aegypti* is not established and therefore the risk of autochthonous transmission from travel-related cases is negligible. However, transmission of YF via the Asian tiger mosquito *Ae. albopictus*, which is present in large parts of Europe and in North America, cannot be entirely ruled out [10].

During the first half of the twentieth century, mosquito control associated with mass vaccination eliminated YFV transmission in urban areas. However, sporadic YF cases associated with sylvatic cycle continue to be registered and small outbreaks occur periodically in rural areas without a background of naturally acquired or vaccine-induced immunity [11]. Upsurges in YFV activity occurred in Africa in the 1960s and the late 1980s, and outbreaks affected Argentina, Paraguay, and Southern Brazil (2007–2009), Uganda (2010), Sudan and Ethiopia (2012–2013).

It has been estimated that in endemic regions of YF, 109,000 severe cases and 51,000 deaths occur annually [12]. These numbers are probably underestimated, as

Table 12.1 Countries with risk of yellow fever (YF) transmission[a]

Africa			
Holoendemic[b]	Part of the country[b]		
Angola	Gambia	Chad	Mauritania
Benin	Ghana	Ethiopia	Niger
Burkina Faso	Guinea	Kenya	Sudan
Burundi	Guinea-Bissau	Mali	
Cameroon	Liberia	Low risk of transmission[c]	
Central African Republic	Nigeria	Eritreia	Somália
Congo	Senegal	Ruanda	Tanzania
Cote d'Ivoire	Serra Leone	São Tomé	Zambia
DR of the Congo	South Sudan		
Equatorial Guinea	Togo		
Gabon	Uganda		
South and Central America			
Holoendemic[b]	Part of the country[b]		
French Guiana	Argentina	Panama	
Guyana	Bolivia	Peru	
Paraguay	Brazil[d]	Trinidad and Tobago	
Suriname	Colombia	Venezuela	
	Ecuador		

[a]Current as of December 2022. Defined by World Health Organization as areas where YF has been reported currently or in the past and vectors and animal reservoirs currently exist
[b]Vaccination recommended for all travellers older than 9 months
[c]Vaccination recommended only to special circumstances of high risk of exposures such as long permanence, no adherence for mosquito bite protection measures
[d]Brazil—substantial expansion of risk area in the last decade

most YF cases present with mild symptoms and are not detected or occur in remote areas without convenient access to care. In addition, limited laboratory diagnostic capacity and precarious surveillance systems contribute to underreporting in many poor-resourced endemic countries.

Recent and ongoing YF outbreaks have affected areas of YF endemicity in West Africa and extended into a region of southeastern Brazil that was previously labelled as low risk for transmission, dangerously approaching densely populated areas. Severe YF cases, including fatalities, have been reported among unvaccinated residents and travellers to these regions [13–15]. Consequently, YF has re-emerged as a major international public health threat [16].

12.3.1.2 Recent Outbreaks

In 2015–2016, an explosive outbreak occurred in Angola and expanded regionally to Democratic Republic of Congo. As of July 1, 2016, a total of 3552 suspected cases, including 875 laboratory-confirmed cases and 355 deaths, had been reported from all 18 provinces of Angola, with most cases occurring in Luanda Province [17]. The outbreak resulted in infection of expatriate workers, including at least 11 workers who returned to China, with one death [18]. The confirmed cases of yellow fever in China were the first-ever cases to be imported into Asia. Although no secondary case was described, due to the massive presence of *Ae. aegypti*, approximately two billion people in Asia were put at risk for yellow fever by international travellers. By September 2016, epidemic was controlled in Africa. Unfortunately, few months after, yellow fever upsurged in Brazil.

In late 2016, the largest outbreak of the last 80 years in the Americas took place in coastal areas of Brazil, where cases had not been reported since the 1940s, and vaccination was not routinely recommended. The outbreak, primarily associated with a sylvatic cycle of transmission, spread into forest areas contiguous to the country's largest megalopolises in the Southeast region, infested by *Ae. aegypti*, such as São Paulo and Rio de Janeiro, significantly increasing the risk of re-urbanization of the disease [19]. From December 2016 to June 2019, 2251 human cases and 772 deaths were confirmed in Brazil, an increase of 2.82 times the total of YF human cases in the previous 36 years [20]. A genetic investigation of the outbreak in Brazil demonstrated the origins and movement of YFV during the outbreak [21]. It was shown that the outbreak originated in northeastern Brazil and moved southward to areas where the virus had not been found previously. Surprisingly, YFV moved at a rate of 4.25 km/day, which probably explains the magnitude of the outbreak.

In these outbreaks in Angola and Brazil, the YF vaccine demands outstripped the available global vaccine supply and led to the unprecedented use of fractional doses of the vaccine to prevent further disease spread [22]. The WHO's recommendation for dose sparing was based on two clinical studies. The first, a Dutch study, is a non-inferiority, randomized controlled study that showed that the 0.1-ml fractional dose administered intradermally was non-inferior to the standard dose 0.5 ml administered subcutaneously [23]. The second, a dose-finding study of the 17DD substrain vaccine in healthy male army recruits in Brazil that showed seroconversion rates greater than 97% even with one-tenth fractions of the standard dose [24]. A recent study supports the use of one-fifth fractional doses of the four WHO-prequalified yellow fever vaccines for the general adult population when there are insufficient standard doses to protect the population at risk during an outbreak [25]. Studies are in progress to assess immunological non-inferiority and safety of fractional doses among children aged between 9 months and 5 years, and adults living with HIV. Despite the good performance of fractional doses in providing short-term protection, and first results showing that seroconverters to YF vaccine in reduced doses remained seropositive 8 years later [26], questions remain if they will provide the same long-term protective immunity as a full dose. Until definitive answers become available, fractional doses should only be considered in emergency scenarios with imminent threats of large-scale amplification.

YF outbreaks and resulting public health crises in Angola, the Democratic Republic of Congo, and Brazil underscored the need for a comprehensive, updated, and intensified strategy to eliminate YF epidemics. To that end, the multi-partner global Eliminate Yellow Fever Epidemics (EYE) Strategy was established in 2017 to improve detection, outbreak preparedness, and response [27]. The three objectives of the strategy include protecting at-risk populations through preventive mass vaccination campaigns and routine immunization, preventing international spread, and containing outbreaks rapidly. Developing strong surveillance with robust laboratory networks is key to these efforts.

As of 2021, yellow fever vaccine had been introduced in routine infant immunization programmes in 36 countries and territories at risk for yellow fever in Africa and the America. However, the current global coverage is estimated at 47% [28], not sufficient to provide herd immunity and prevent outbreaks. Of concern, there have been outbreaks detected in several high-risk countries in Africa since 2020, such as in Nigeria, Congo, Chad, Senegal, and Ghana [29].

12.3.1.3 Risks for International Travellers

More than nine million people from non-endemic countries in North America, Europe, and Asia travel to countries where YF is endemic, and these numbers are expected to progressively increase given the increasing travel globally.

It is difficult to estimate the exact risk of an individual traveller to acquire YF, as it may be influenced by many variables, such as destination, season, local YF rate of transmission at the time of travel, immunization status of endemic population and traveller, duration of stay, and travel occupational or recreational activities. As surveillance infrastructure is poor in many countries where yellow fever is endemic and difficulties are inherent in closely monitoring non-human hosts, it is difficult to precisely quantify YFV activity. Of note, a low level of transmission and a high level of immunity in the population of endemic areas may give a false perception of absence of risk.

The ecological determinants of YF transmission are variable. Depending on the season, the number of vectors may increase, facilitating YF transmission. In South America, the risk of infection by sylvatic vector is highest in rainy season (January–May). In rural West Africa, the risk is elevated during the transition of the rainy to dry season (July–October). However, *Ae. aegypti* may transmit YFV in rural and urban areas even in dry season.

The individual traveller variables may also impact risks. Therefore, unvaccinated profile, inadequate precautions against mosquito bites, long stay, and involvement in occupational or recreational activities which expose the traveller to the outdoors during prime mosquito biting hours can all facilitate YF acquisition.

All these risks should be taken into consideration by travel health practitioners during pre-travel appointments to accurately weigh risks and benefits for yellow fever vaccination on a case-by-case basis. As desirable for many aspects of travel medicine, a clinical decision requires up-to-date epidemiologic data to make informed choices. The careful assessment of risk is particularly important when dealing with those populations in which there is a higher risk of adverse events with attenuated vaccines.

Based on the risk of indigenous population, the risks for illness and for death due to YF for an unvaccinated traveller visiting an endemic area in South America are estimated as 5 per 100,000 and 1 per 100,000, respectively. For West Africa, corresponding estimated risks are 50 per 100,000 and 10 per 100,000 [30]. Nevertheless, as demonstrated in recent outbreaks in Angola and Brazil, the risk of infection for travellers is substantially higher during outbreaks. From 2016 through 2018, a record number of unvaccinated travellers associated with YF cases were reported (Fig. 12.2) including 11 Chinese workers returning from Angola [18] and 13 European travellers, most returning from Brazil [13].

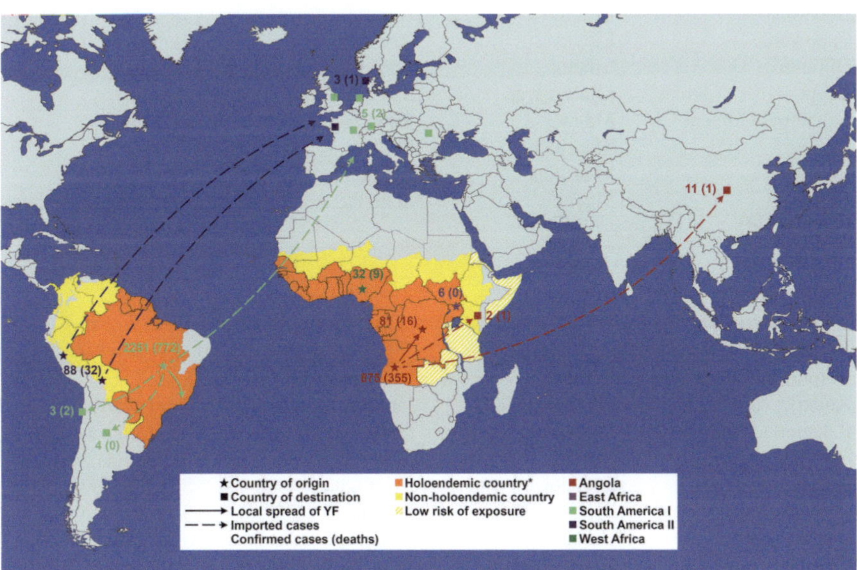

Fig. 12.2 Yellow fever transmission regions and outbreaks between 2016 and 2018. Countries and regions in orange represent high transmission risk zones, regions in yellow represent transmission risk zones in non-holoendemic countries. Full lines represent yellow fever spread regionally; dashed lines represent importation of cases. Stars represent the country of origin of the outbreak; squares represent the country where travellers returned to. Colours represent viral genotypes: South America I, light green; South America II, dark blue; Angola, red; West Africa, dark green; East Africa, purple

YF is unique amongst communicable diseases to be controlled by International Health Regulations (IHR, last updated in 2005). While some countries require travellers to be vaccinated for YF and proof of vaccination is necessary, others stipulate that proof of vaccination is necessary for travellers arriving from or through a country where yellow fever is endemic (Table 12.2). Of note, despite the risk of local YF transmission and the rationale of recommending YF vaccination, various endemic countries of South America and Africa do not systematically require vaccination for entrance.

Table 12.2 Countries that require yellow fever vaccination certificate for travellers

Africa			
For all travellers older than 9 months/1 year			
Angola	Cameroon	Ghana	Sierra Leone
Burkina Faso	Congo	Guinea-Bissau	South Sudan
Burundi	Côte d'Ivoire	Kenya	Sudan
Central African	DR of the Congo	Mali	Togo
Republic	Gabon	Niger	Uganda
Chad			
For travellers older than 9 months/1 year returning (or transiting) from countries with risk of YF			
Algeria	Guinea	Mozambique	South African
Benin	Kenya	Namibia	Swaziland
Botswana	Lesotho	Nigeria	Tanzania
Cape Verde	Libya	Réunion	Tunisia
Djibouti	Liberia	Rwanda	Uganda
Egypt	Madagascar	São Tomé and	Zambia
Equatorial Guinea	Malawi	Príncipe	Zimbabwe
Eritrea	Mauritania	Senegal	
Ethiopia	Mauritius	Seychelles	
Gambia	Mayotte	Somalia	
South and Central America			
For all travellers older than 9 months			
French Guyana			
For travellers older than 9 months/1 year returning (or transiting) from countries with risk of YF			
Antigua and Barbuda	Curaçao	Honduras	Saint Lucia
Aruba	Dominica	Jamaica	Saint Martin
Bahamas	Dominican	Martinique	Saint Vincent and
Barbados	Republic	Montserrat (UK)	the Grenadines
Belize	Ecuador	Nicaragua	Sint Eustatius
Bonaire	El Salvador	Panama	Sint Maarten
Bolivia	Grenada	Paraguay	Suriname
Colombia	Guadeloupe	Saint Barthelemy	Trinidad and Tobago
Costa Rica	Guatemala	Saint Eustatius	Uruguay
Cuba	Guyana	Saint Helena	Venezuela
	Haiti		

Table 12.2 (continued)

North America			
No requirement			
Europe			
For travellers older than 9 months/1 year returning (or transiting) from countries with risk of YF			
Albania	Malta		
Asia and Oceania			
For travellers older than 9 months/1 year returning (or transiting) from countries with risk of YF			
Afghanistan	India	Malaysia	Pitcairn Island (UK)
Australia	Indonesia	Maldives	Pakistan
Bahrain	Iran	Myanmar	Samoa
Bangladesh	Iraq	Nauru	Saudi Arabia
Brunei	Jordan	Nepal	Singapore
Cambodia	Kazakhstan	New Caledonia	Solomon Islands
China	Kiribati	Norfolk Island	Sri Lanka
Christmas Island	Kyrgyzstan	North Korea	Thailand
Fiji	Laos	Oman	Timor-Leste
French Polynesia	Malawi	Philippines	United Arab Emirates

12.4 Pathogenesis

YF pathogenesis is viscerotropic in humans and liver is the main target organ. After the intradermal inoculation by the infected mosquito, virus replication begins in dendritic cells in the epidermis, and then spreads through lymphatic channels to regional lymph nodes. In this tissue, YFV replicates in monocyte-macrophages and large histiocytes and primes the cellular immune response before spreading via bloodstream to reach the liver and other tissues and organs [31]. Large amounts of virus are produced in lymph nodes, liver and spleen and released into the blood.

In severe cases, YF is characterized by hepatic dysfunction, renal failure, bleeding diathesis, and shock. In the liver, YFV induces hepatocyte apoptosis and lytic necrosis, which, combined with steatosis, results in severe damage. Substantial lesions can also occur in the kidney, heart, thymus, spleen, and vascular endothelium. In addition to the virus-induced cytopathic effect, studies suggest that the immune response itself, via a systemic and unbalanced cytokine response (*"cytokine storm"*), is a major driver of hepatotoxicity [32]. Endothelium activation plays a role during severe YF triggering an intense cytokine-mediated inflammatory response in the liver parenchyma [33]. Haemorrhagic diathesis happens due to a combination of factors, including decreased synthesis of coagulation factors by the liver, platelet dysfunction and consumptive coagulopathy [34].

12.5 Clinical Findings

The clinical spectrum of YF varies from asymptomatic or very mild, nonspecific, febrile illness to a fulminating, sometimes fatal disease. It has been estimated that approximately 55% of infections are asymptomatic, 33% result in mild disease and 12% result in severe illness [35]. Frequently, people with minimal symptoms do not seek medical attention.

In symptomatic cases, the course of YF has been classically described in three phases, namely, infection, remission, and intoxication [11]. After an incubation period of in median 4.3 days (may vary from 2 to 9 days) [6], onset of *infection phase* is abrupt with fever, muscle pain, headache, weakness, loss of appetite, nausea, and vomiting. This initial unspecific *flu-like syndrome* usually lasts approximately 2–5 days, and most people recover completely within 1 week and become immune [30].

In approximately 10–15% of those infected, after a brief (2–48 h) *remission phase* of abatement of fever and symptoms, disease progress to the *intoxication phase*, characterized by the return of fever, abdominal pain, jaundice, bleeding diathesis, hepatic dysfunction, renal failure, coma, and shock. Bleeding can occur from the mouth, nose, eyes, or stomach. Recently, in severe YF cases, a critical metabolic acidosis, increased levels of serum lipase, and a high prevalence of pancreatitis are observed [14].

In this severe form, the case-fatality rate is 30–50%, or even higher. The main predictors of death are older age, elevated neutrophil count, elevated serum transaminases, jaundice, higher viral load, and changes in renal excretion [13–15, 36]. Death usually occurs 7–10 days after the onset of illness. For those that survive, there is a convalescent period, which is characterized by prolonged fatigue and weakness lasting several weeks.

12.6 Diagnosis

YF can be a challenge to diagnose because it mimics various acute febrile and febrile icteric diseases, especially tropical ones, such as leptospirosis, malaria, typhoid fever, rickettsia infections, acute viral hepatitis, dengue, Ebola, and other haemorrhagic fevers. Importantly, early detection of human YF infection in endemic or potential vulnerable regions is critical to control transmission and timely mitigate outbreaks.

A presumptive diagnosis of YF is typically made based on clinical symptoms, vaccination status and exposure risk, that is associated with epidemiological profile of the affected country or area and travel history. The definitive diagnosis of YF is performed through virological (detection of the viral genome, detection of viral antigens, or virus isolation) and/or serological methods [37]. Commercial diagnostic tests are not widely available, and testing is commonly performed at reference laboratories.

Virus isolations may be performed from different cell lines (Vero cell; C3/36; AP-61) but represent an extreme biohazard and should only be attempted in specialized laboratories. However, virus isolation capacity is important for the characterization of circulating strains, to produce diagnostic reagents and for research studies. More commonly used for diagnosis, reverse transcriptase polymerase chain reaction (RT-PCR) can detect the virus from blood, urine, or tissue samples from the first 3–4 days and up to 10 days of illness, although it may fail after the point when symptoms are more prominent [38].

Serodiagnosis is possible within 1 week of infection with IgM and IgG antibodies detectable using enzyme-linked immunosorbent assay (ELISA) or plaque reduction neutralization tests (PRNT). However, antibody testing comes with its own challenge, like cross-reactivity with other flavivirus (e.g. West Nile or dengue) and vaccine-induced antibodies [39]. Test results need to be accurately interpreted in the epidemiologic and clinical context.

In case of death, the diagnosis can be confirmed in various tissues by molecular tests and immunohistochemistry. Liver and kidney tissue should always be collected and additionally, spleen, heart, lung, and brain tissue can be collected [37].

12.7 Management

The management of YF remains primarily supportive and hospitalization in intensive care unit is recommended in severe cases [40]. Antiviral compounds have been evaluated to treat YF, such as ribavirin, and more recently sofosbuvir, but none has shown to be of value thus far [37]. Additionally, studies are being conducted to evaluate the potential use of an YFV monoclonal antibody (TY014) to interrupt the YF pathogenesis [41].

Care should include rest, adequate hydration, and nutrition. It is prudent to avoid sedatives and drugs dependent on hepatic metabolism or that increase the risk of bleeding. Gastric mucosal protection is also important, and other measures can be considered, such as fluid replacement, vasoactive drugs, treatment of bleeding with fresh-frozen plasma, antibiotics for secondary bacterial infections and administration of oxygen. Recently, Brazilian experience in treating critical patients showed that prophylactic anticonvulsant therapy, routine use of intravenous proton pump inhibitor, aggressive early haemodialysis, and high-volume plasma exchange may improve outcomes [14, 42].

Public health responses around management of an individual case, such as isolation measures, laboratory safety and protocols, contact precautions, advice and management for patient contacts, e.g. healthcare and household and other close contacts.

Case reporting is required nationally and by IHR. The infected patient needs to be isolated and follow adequate body fluids precautions. In some areas of the world, it may be necessary to protect the patient from mosquitoes to prevent transmission. Contacts should receive immunization promptly, wherever there is vector activity.

Health personnel providing care for infectious patients and laboratory personnel handling biological samples must be vaccinated against yellow fever and use appropriate personal protective equipment. All biological samples (whole blood, serum, or fresh tissue) should be considered as potentially infectious. Furthermore, for laboratories it is recommended to carry out all procedures in certified class II biosafety cabinets and to take all necessary precautions to avoid percutaneous exposure. Procedures for handling NHP samples should be carefully assessed according to national regulations [37].

12.8 Prevention and Advice for Travellers

All travellers to countries in which YF is endemic should be advised of the risks for the disease and available methods to prevent it, including vaccine and personal protective measures to avoid arthropod bites.

12.8.1 Vaccine

Vaccination is the most important means of preventing yellow fever. Live-attenuated YF vaccines derived from 17D strain have been widely available since 1937. The vaccine is safe, affordable, highly effective, and a single dose provides effective immunity within 10 days for 80–90% of people vaccinated, and robust and long-lived humoral and cellular immune responses within 30 days for more than 99% of people vaccinated [2]. Anti-YF neutralizing antibodies have been detected for as long as 30–35 years post-vaccination [43].

In 2014, the WHO Strategy Advisory Group of Experts on immunization concluded that a single primary dose of YF vaccine provides sustained immunity and lifelong protection. The current recommendation for YF vaccine is for a single lifetime dose [44] and the IHR were amended to specify this recommendation for travellers. Nevertheless, one-time booster administration can be considered for residents or travellers to endemic areas who last received YF vaccine more than 10 years prior if there are concerns with inadequate response to previous dose for long-term protection (e.g. vaccination during pregnancy, in a period of reduced immunocompetence, and maybe in early infancy). Additionally, it may be advisable in the context of higher risk settings, such as travelling to outbreaks areas or during peak transmission season, planning prolonged stays in endemic areas and for those working with the yellow fever virus in a laboratory setting [45, 46].

In general, YF vaccines are considered very safe. No substantial differences in immunogenicity or reactogenicity of the different YF-licensed vaccines have been reported. Reactions to YF vaccine are generally mild, occur in 10–30% of vaccinees, and include low-grade fever, myalgia, headache, that appears within days of vaccination and last 5–10 days [47, 48]. In the 1990s, despite 50 years of use and over 500 million doses distributed, new safety concerns about the live attenuated YF 17D vaccine have come to light, revealing that in rare circumstances the vaccine can cause a disease like wild-type virus. This fact has modified vaccine policy and regulations.

Although severe adverse events have been reported following vaccination, including yellow fever vaccine-associated viscerotropic disease (YEL-AVD) and acute neurotropic disease (YEL-AND), the incidence of these severe events remains very low, respectively, 0.4 and 0.8 case per 100,000 doses of YF vaccine administered [49].

YEL-AVD resembles wild-type YF with an even higher fatality rate (63%). Vaccine virus replicates intensively and causes injury to multiple organs and tissues and eventually death. Symptoms usually appear 4 days (range, 1–18 days) after vaccination. Risk factors include immunosuppression condition and thymus disease [50]. As the evidence for increased risk with old ages ($\geq$60) remains limited, decision to vaccinate should be made on a case-by-case basis after weighting the risk of contracting the disease [51].

YEL-AND include various neurological syndromes, such as Guillain-Barré syndrome, meningoencephalitis, encephalitis, and cranial nerve palsies. Although more commonly described among infants, people of all ages may be affected, and incidence is even higher in people older than 70 years [49, 52].

Immediate hypersensitivity reactions (rash, urticaria or bronchoespasm) to YFV are uncommon. Anaphylaxis is reported at a rate of 1.3 cases per 100,000 doses administered [48]. No evidence is available suggesting that the reporting rates of allergic reactions is higher than other egg-derived vaccine.

The medical practitioner administering live-attenuated YF vaccines should consider contraindications and precautions (Box 12.1). Live-attenuated YF vaccines is contraindicated in infants <6 months old, individuals with significant impaired immune function (symptomatic HIV infection or CD4+ T-lymphocytes <200/mm^3, primary immunodeficiencies, malignant neoplasm, solid organ transplantation, immunosuppressive and immunomodulatory therapies), and in cases of thymus disfunction or thymectomy. Precautions to receive YF vaccines include age 6–8 months, age $\geq$ 60 years, asymptomatic HIV infection with moderate immunosuppression, pregnancy and breastfeeding.

The yellow fever vaccine is indicated for individuals living in or travelling to an endemic area with 9 months of age or more. Yellow fever vaccine can be required for entrance in some non-endemic countries, and this requirement must be checked before travel [53]. To be considered valid, the primary vaccination must be administered at least 10 days before the trip, to give time for adequate protection.

Box 12.1 Contraindications and Precautions to Yellow Fever Vaccine

Contraindications

- Age < 6 months
- Symptomatic HIV infection or CD4+ T-lymphocytes <200/mm^3
  (or < 15% of total in children <6 years)
- Primary immunodeficiencies
- Thymus disorder associated with abnormal immune function or thymectomy
- Malignant neoplasms
- Solid organ transplantation
- Immunosuppressive and immunomodulatory therapies

Precautions

- Allergy to vaccine components*
- Age 6–8 months
- Age ≥60 years
- Pregnancy
- Breastfeeding

*Clinical experience in endemic areas suggests that the vaccine might be safe adopting systematic evaluation with allergy skin tests and desensitization protocols [53, 54]

12.8.2 Mosquito Protection Measures

As for many other arthropod-borne diseases, all travellers should take general measures to avoid mosquito and tick bites to prevent illness (Box 12.2). First, travellers should avoid known foci of epidemic yellow fever and other mosquito-borne diseases. Furthermore, to optimize protection, it is important to apply a repellent approved by regulatory agencies as both efficacious and safe for human use when applied according to the instructions on the label. Additionally, travellers may wear appropriate clothing to minimize areas of exposed skin by wearing long-sleeved shirts, long pants, socks, and closed shoes. Preferentially, clothing may be treated in advance of travel with permethrin, which retains repellent activity through multiple washes. Interestingly, besides mosquitoes, permethrin-treated clothing repels and kills ticks, chiggers and others biting arthropods. If permethrin is not available, repellents used on skin may be applied to clothing to provide shorter protection [48].

Repellents containing active ingredients such as DEET (N,N-diethyl-3-methyl-benzamide), Picaridin or Icaridin (2-(2-hydroxyethyl)-1-piperidinecarboxylic acid1-methylpropil ester), Oil of lemon eucalyptus (para-menthane-3,8-diol), IR3535 (3-[N-butyl-N-acetyl]-aminopropionic acid, ethyl ester) and 2-undercanona (methyl nonyl ketone) typically provide reasonably long-lasting protection when used in adequate concentrations. In general, higher concentrations of active ingredients (≥20%) provide longer protection time. Repellent should be used whenever outdoors (or indoors if mosquitoes can get inside) any time of day or night and must be applied and reapplied according to label instructions. Of note, combined sunscreen and repellent formulations are not recommended. Sunscreen may be applied first, followed by repellent.

Box 12.2 Protective Measures Against Diseases Transmitted by Mosquitoes and Ticks

- Yellow fever vaccination at least 10 days before travelling to an endemic area.
- Avoid travels during outbreaks and seasons with higher mosquito density.
- Minimize areas of exposed skin—wear long sleeves, pants, and socks.
- Stay in accommodations with air conditioning or adequate window screens. If not possible, sleep under a mosquito net. Treating bed nets with a pyrethroid insecticide helps maximize their efficacy.
- Use insect repellents with active ingredients and adequate concentrations.
- Reapply repellent if getting insect bites or according to the label instructions.
- Treat clothes with permethrin.
- Apply sunscreen first, then repellent.
- Use antimalarials when indicated.

12.8.3 General Advice Pre-travel and During Travel

Before travelling to a yellow fever endemic area, travellers should be strongly advised to have a pre-travel consultation. As these regions usually have other risks of infectious diseases that can be prevented, it is not only a matter of getting a yellow vaccine shot before travelling.

The absence of cases of yellow fever at the destination does not mean absence of risk, since in endemic areas people are generally protected by systematic vaccination. Epidemiologic silence can provide a false sense of security and lead to travel without the benefit of prophylactic measures [29]. It is also important to emphasize that some endemic countries do not require vaccination for entrance, but travellers should be vaccinated as a protective individual measure.

Travellers should be advised in advance that some items for individual protection against mosquito bites, such as repellents with adequate concentration of active ingredients and permethrin for impregnating clothes can be difficult to find in some regions, so it is important to plan to have them available.

A proof of yellow fever vaccination can be required (International Certificate of Yellow Fever or Prophylaxis—ICVP) for entering in many countries, including non-endemic ones. So as part of travel arrangements it is strongly recommended that yellow fever entry requirements be checked for all countries that the traveller intends to enter, including those for transit purposes [52].

For travellers with contraindication or precaution for vaccination, a medical waiver can be provided when going to non-endemic areas that require YF vaccination for entrance. If travelling to an endemic area with real risk of yellow fever, travellers with absolute contraindication to vaccination should be encouraged to cancel the trip or change the itinerary. Reasons other than medical contraindications are not acceptable for exemption from vaccination.

During travel and after the return, it is important for the traveller to be aware that fever can be a symptom of many different illnesses, including malaria that can be fatal if not diagnosed and treated early. Areas at risk for yellow fever can also be at risk for malaria and fever should be a warning to see a doctor. In some developing countries, the access to high-quality health service can be scarce and costly, so it is important to know in advance which health facilities to go to in case of emergency and consider health insurance with possibility of evacuation in some situations [55].

12.8.4　Specific Advice for Healthcare Workers

Healthcare workers should be aware that the risk of YF during travel is determined by multiple factors. Travellers to endemic areas should be vaccinated, independently of recent occurrences of cases since YFV can circulate silently between monkeys and mosquitoes, with few human cases in the local population, because of routine vaccination. Updated epidemiological information, even before official numbers are disclosed, is of paramount importance in the daily practice of travel medicine.

12.8.5　Specific Advice for Special People (e.g. Pregnant, Immunocompromised, Very Young, Elderly)

The vaccination of special groups in the context of outbreaks and travelling to high-risk areas can be challenging, and an individual risk-to-benefit assessment should be done based on the current epidemiological situation.

Age 6–8 months is a precaution for yellow fever vaccination, and infants at this age should be immunized only if there is a significant risk for natural infection. When possible, travel should be delayed until the age of 9 months. Precaution for vaccination of people with age beyond 60 years should also be considered, as the relative risk of serious adverse events increases in this age group, particularly beyond 70 years [49].

Live-attenuated YF vaccines should not be administered during pregnancy unless it is clearly required based on a high risk of natural infection, because of the hypothetical risk of transplacental infection and the recognition that young infants (and potentially the unborn foetus) are more susceptible to neuroinvasion by 17D virus. Nevertheless, inadvertent immunization of women (generally in the early stages of pregnancy) is not an indication for therapeutic abortion. If possible, women should wait until 4 weeks after vaccination before conceiving.

Breastfeeding is a precaution to yellow fever vaccination and a risk-to-benefit assessment must be conducted. YF vaccine virus can be transmitted into breastmilk.

Although the frequency of transmission is unclear, three cases of YEL-AND have been reported in exclusively breastfed infants whose mothers were vaccinated with yellow fever vaccine [56, 57].

Prior history of allergy to eggs or its products, chicken proteins, or egg-based vaccines or gelatin stabilizer in vaccines should not be considered an absolute contraindication to the use of 17D vaccine. Clinical experience in endemic areas suggests that the vaccine might be safe adopting systematic evaluation with allergy skin tests and desensitization protocols guided by an allergist [53, 54].

YF vaccine is contraindicated in primary or acquired immunosuppression conditions, because of the risk of serious adverse events. If feasible, individuals should be vaccinated at least 4 weeks before initiating immunosuppressive medications or the vaccination should be delayed if interruption of the medication is foreseen or can be planned.

12.9 Gaps in Knowledge that Need to Be Addressed

For an old disease preventable by an effective vaccine, recent re-emergence events demonstrate that YF is still a very real threat to human health and economies. Our knowledge of the YFV replication cycle, the YFV-induced mechanisms of disease and the molecular basis of attenuation remains limited. To answer these questions, research efforts should focus on the interplay between the virus and the immune system in the development of disease, the role of the cytokine storm in the disease process, the differential host-virus interactions and the genetic basis regulating YF disease susceptibility in humans [58]. Additionally, it is not definitively understood why upswings in enzootic transmission occur. Future work should include developing and comparing models for vector control methods incorporating the chemical, biological, and environmental tools and comparing interventions. Due to limited vaccine supply, efficient planning of interventions is vital to avoid large outbreaks. To facilitate this, robust estimates of disease burden and projections of future dynamics are key. Also, the 17D vaccine has been associated with severe adverse events, the pathogenesis of which are poorly known and improvements to the vaccine's safety will be required [60]. Finally, there are no specific drugs to treat the disease and studies must continue. While a significant amount has been learned in the last 100 years, clearly there is still much more to be discovered about yellow fever.

Acknowledgements The authors express their gratitude to Prof. Fernando Martins (1954–2022), for a life dedicated to the National Medical School and for the foundation of *Cives-UFRJ*, the first travel medicine centre in Brazil. We also thank the NEEDIER-UFRJ team for suggestions, and in particular the PhD student Guilherme Lira for contributions with tables and figures.

References

1. Staples JE, Monath TP. Yellow Fever: 100 Years of discovery. JAMA. 2008;300(8):960–2. https://doi.org/10.1001/jama.300.8.960.
2. World Health Organization (WHO). Yellow fever (Internet). 2019 (accessed on December 1, 2022). Available online: https://www.who.int/en/news-room/fact-sheets/detail/yellow-fever.
3. Douam F, Ploss A. Yellow Fever virus: knowledge gaps impeding the fight against an old foe. Trends Microbiol. 2018;26(11):913–28. https://doi.org/10.1016/j.tim.2018.05.012.
4. Beasley DW, McAuley AJ, Bente DA. Yellow fever virus: genetic and phenotypic diversity and implications for detection, prevention, and therapy. Antivir Res. 2015;115:48–70. https://doi.org/10.1016/j.antiviral.2014.12.010.
5. World Health Organization (WHO). Risk assessment on yellow fever virus circulation in endemic countries: working document from an informal consultation of experts: a protocol risk assessment at the field level. 2014. pp. 1–40. Available online: https://apps.who.int/iris/bitstream/handle/10665/112751/WHO_HSE_PED_CED_2014.2_eng.pdf?sequence=1 (accessed on October 12, 2022).
6. Johansson MA, Arana-Vizcarrondo N, Biggerstaff BJ, Staples JE. Incubation periods of Yellow fever virus. Am J Trop Med Hyg. 2010;83(1):183–8. https://doi.org/10.4269/ajtmh.2010.09-0782.
7. Vasconcelos PFC. Yellow fever. Rev Soc Bras Med Trop. 2003;36:275–93. https://doi.org/10.1590/S0037-86822003000200012.
8. Centers for Disease Control and Prevention (CDC). Transmission of Yellow fever virus. 2019. Available online: https://www.cdc.gov/yellowfever/transmission/index.html. (accessed on October 12, 2022).
9. Couto-Lima D, Madec Y, Bersot MI, et al. Potential risk of re-emergence of urban transmission of Yellow Fever virus in Brazil facilitated by competent Aedes populations. Sci Rep. 2017;7(1):4848. https://doi.org/10.1038/s41598-017-05186-3.
10. Benedict MQ, Levine RS, Hawley WA, Lounibos LP. Spread of the tiger: global risk of invasion by the mosquito Aedes albopictus. Vector Borne Zoonotic Dis. 2007;7(1):76–85. https://doi.org/10.1089/vbz.2006.0562.
11. Monath TP, Vasconcelos PF. Yellow fever. J Clin Virol. 2015;2015(64):160–73. https://doi.org/10.1016/j.jcv.2014.08.030.
12. Gaythorpe KAM, Jean K, Cibrelus L, Garske T. Quantifying model evidence for yellow fever transmission routes in Africa. PLoS Comput Biol. 2019;15(9):e1007355. https://doi.org/10.1371/journal.pcbi.1007355.
13. Hamer DH, Angelo K, Caumes E, et al. Fatal yellow fever in travellers to Brazil, 2018. MMWR Morb Mortal Wkly Rep. 2018;67:340–1. https://doi.org/10.15585/mmwr.mm6711e1.
14. Ho YL, Joelsons D, Leite GFC, et al. Severe yellow fever in Brazil: clinical characteristics and management. J Travel Med. 2019:26. https://doi.org/10.1093/jtm/taz040.
15. Kallas EG, D'Elia Zanella L, Moreira CHV, et al. Predictors of mortality in patients with yellow fever: an observational cohort study. Lancet Infect Dis. 2019;19(7):750–8. https://doi.org/10.1016/S1473-3099(19)30125-2.
16. Lindsey NP, Horton J, Barrett ADT, et al. Yellow fever resurgence: an avoidable crisis? NPJ Vaccines. 2022;7(1):137. https://doi.org/10.1038/s41541-022-00552-3.
17. Grobbelaar AA, Weyer J, Moolla N, Jansen van Vuren P, Moises F, Paweska JT. Resurgence of yellow fever in Angola, 2015–2016. Emerg Infect Dis. 2016;22(10):1854–5. https://doi.org/10.3201/eid2210.160818.
18. Barrett ADT. The reemergence of yellow fever. Science. 2018; https://doi.org/10.1126/science.aau8225.
19. Possas C, et al. Yellow fever outbreak in Brazil: the puzzle of rapid viral spread and challenges for immunisation. Mem Inst Oswaldo Cruz. 2018;113:e180278. https://doi.org/10.1590/0074-02760180278.

20. Silva NIO, Sacchetto L, de Rezende IM, et al. Recent sylvatic yellow fever virus transmission in Brazil: the news from an old disease. Virol J. 2020;17(1):9. https://doi.org/10.1186/s12985-019-1277-7.

21. Faria NR, Kraemer MUG, Hill SC, et al. Genomic and epidemiological monitoring of yellow fever virus transmission potential. Science. 2018;361(6405):894–9. https://doi.org/10.1126/science.aat7115.

22. World Health Organization (WHO). Fractional dose yellow fever vaccine as a dose-sparing option for outbreak response: WHO Secretariat information paper. World Health Organization; 2016. Available online: https://apps.who.int/iris/handle/10665/246236. (accessed on October 12, 2022)

23. Roukens AHE, Visser LG. Fractional-dose yellow fever vaccination: an expert review. J Travel Med. 2019;26(6):taz024. https://doi.org/10.1093/jtm/taz024.

24. Martins RM, de Maia MD, Farias RHG, et al. 17DD yellow fever vaccine: a double blind, randomized clinical trial of immunogenicity and safety on a dose-response study. Hum Vaccin Immunother. 2013;9:879–88. https://doi.org/10.4161/hv.22982.

25. Juan-Giner A, Kimathi D, Grantz KH, et al. Immunogenicity and safety of fractional doses of yellow fever vaccines: a randomised, double-blind, non-inferiority trial. Lancet. 2021;397(10269):119–27. https://doi.org/10.1016/S0140-6736(20)32520-4.

26. de Menezes Martins R, Maria de Lourdes SM, de Lima SM, et al. Duration of post-vaccination immunity to yellow fever in volunteers eight years after a dose-response study. Vaccine. 2018;36(28):4112–7. https://doi.org/10.1016/j.vaccine.2018.05.041.

27. World Health Organization (WHO). A global strategy to eliminate Yellow fever epidemics 2017–2026. Geneva: World Health Organization; 2018. Licence: CC BY-NCSA 3.0 IGO. Cataloguing-in-Pub

28. World Health Organization (WHO). Immunisation coverage. July 14, 2022. (Accessed on December 11, 2022); Available online https://www.who.int/news-room/fact-sheets/detail/immunization-coverage (accessed on October 12, 2023).

29. World Health Organization Africa. Yellow Fever in West and Central Africa. Weekly Bulletin on Outbreaks and Other Emergencies. Week 1: 27 December 2021–2 January 2022. Available online: https://iris.who.int/bitstream/handle/10665/350967/OEW01-271202012022.pdf?sequence=1&isAllowed=y (accessed on October 12, 2023).

30. Monath TP, Centron MS. Prevention of yellow fever in persons travelling to the tropics. Clin Infect Dis. 2002;34:1369–78. https://doi.org/10.1086/340104.

31. Monath TP, Barrett AD. Pathogenesis and pathophysiology of yellow fever. Adv Virus Res. 2003;60:343. https://doi.org/10.1016/s0065-3527(03)60009-6.

32. Quaresma JA, Pagliari C, Medeiros DB, Duarte MI, Vasconcelos PF. Immunity and immune response, pathology, and pathologic changes: Progress and challenges in the immunopathology of yellow fever. Rev Med Virol. 2013;23:305–18. https://doi.org/10.1002/rmv.1752.

33. Olímpio FA, Falcão LFM, Carvalho MLG, et al. Endothelium activation during severe yellow fever triggers an intense cytokine-mediated inflammatory response in the liver parenchyma. Pathogens. 2022;11(1):101. https://doi.org/10.3390/pathogens11010101.

34. Bailey AL, Kang LI, de Assis Barros D'Elia Zanella LGF, et al. Consumptive coagulopathy of severe yellow fever occurs independently of hepatocellular tropism and massive hepatic injury. Proc Natl Acad Sci U S A. 2020;117(51):32648–56. https://doi.org/10.1073/pnas.2014096117.

35. Johansson MA, Vasconcelos PFC, Staples JE. The whole iceberg: estimating the incidence of yellow fever virus infection from the number of severe cases. Trans R Soc Trop Med Hyg. 2014;108(8):482–7. https://doi.org/10.1093/trstmh/tru092.

36. Tuboi SH, Costa ZG, Costa Vasconcelos PF, Hatch D. Clinical and epidemiological characteristics of yellow fever in Brazil: analysis of reported cases 1998–2002. Trans R Soc Trop Med Hyg. 2007;101:169–75. https://doi.org/10.1016/j.trstmh.2006.04.001.

37. Pan American Health Organization (PAHO). Laboratory diagnosis of yellow fever virus infection. Washington, DC: Pan American Health Organization; 2018. Available online: https://www.paho.org/en/documents/laboratory-diagnosis-yellow-fever-virus-infection (accessed on October 12, 2023)

38. Waggoner JJ, Rojas A, Pinsky BA. Yellow fever virus: diagnostics for a persistent arboviral threat. J Clin Microbiol. 2018;56:e00827–18. https://doi.org/10.1128/JCM.00827-18.
39. Domingo C, Charrel RN, Schmidt-Chanasit J, Zeller H, Reusken C. Yellow fever in the diagnostics laboratory. Emerg Microbes Infect. 2018;7:129. https://doi.org/10.1038/s41426-018-0128-8.
40. Monath TP. Treatment of yellow fever. Antivir Res. 2008;78(1):116–24. https://doi.org/10.1016/j.antiviral.2007.10.009.
41. Low JG, Ng JHJ, Ong EZ, et al. Phase 1 Trial of a therapeutic anti-yellow fever virus human antibody. N Engl J Med. 2020;383(5):452–9. https://doi.org/10.1056/NEJMoa2000226.
42. Escosteguy CC, Pereira AG, Marques MRVE, Lima TRA, Galliez RM, Medronho RA. Yellow fever: profile of cases and factors associated with death in a hospital in the State of Rio de Janeiro, 2017–2018. Rev Saude Publica. 2019;53:89. https://doi.org/10.11606/s1518-8787.2019053001434.
43. Poland JD, Calisher CH, Monath TP, Downs WG, Murphy K. Persistence of neutralizing antibody 30–35 years after immunisation with 17D yellow fever vaccine. Bull World Health Organ. 1981;59:895–900.
44. World Health Organization (WHO). Vaccines and vaccination against yellow fever-WHO position paper. Weekly Epidemiol Rec. 2013;27(5):269–83. Available online: https://iris.who.int/bitstream/handle/10665/242089/WER8827_269-283.PDF?sequence=1 (accessed on October 12, 2023)
45. Staples JE, Bocchini JA Jr, Rubin L, Fischer M, Centers for Disease Control and Prevention (CDC). Yellow fever vaccine booster doses: recommendations of the Advisory Committee on Immunization Practices, 2015. MMWR Morb Mortal Wkly Rep. 2015;64(23):647–50.
46. Committee to Advise on Tropical Medicine and Travel (CATMAT). Statement on the use of booster doses of yellow fever vaccine. 2018. Available online: https://www.canada.ca/en/public-health/services/publications/diseases-conditions/use-booster-doses-yellow-fever-vaccine.html (accessed October 12, 2023).
47. Staples JE, Monath TP, Gershman MD, Barrett ADT. Yellow fever vaccine. In: Plotkin SA, Orenstein WA, Offit PA, editors. Vaccines. 8th ed. Philadelphia: Elsevier; 2022.
48. Gershman MD, Staples JE. Yellow fever - chapter 4 - travel-relates infectious disease. Yellow Fever. CDC Yellow Book 2024 | Travelers' Health | CDC (accessed October 12, 2023). Available online: https://wwwnc.cdc.gov/travel/yellowbook/2024/infections-diseases/yellow-fever (accessed October 12, 2023).
49. Lindsey NP, Rabe IB, Miller ER, Fischer M, Staples JE. Adverse event reports following yellow fever vaccination, 2007–13. J Travel Med. 2016;23(5) https://doi.org/10.1093/jtm/taw045.
50. Eidex RB. History of thymoma and yellow fever vaccination. Lancet. 2004;364:936. https://doi.org/10.1016/S0140-6736(04)17017-7.
51. Rafferty E, Duclos P, Yactayo S, Schuster M. Risk of yellow fever vaccine-associated viscerotropic disease among the elderly: a systematic review. Vaccine. 2013;31:5798–805. https://doi.org/10.1016/j.vaccine.2013.09.030.
52. Khromava AY, Eidex RB, Weld LH, Kohl KS, Bradshaw RD, Chen RT, et al. Yellow fever vaccine: an updated assessment of advanced age as a risk factor for serious adverse events. Vaccine. 2005;23:3256–63. https://doi.org/10.1016/j.vaccine.2005.01.089.
53. Cancado B, Aranda C, Mallozi M, Weckx L, Sole D. Yellow fever vaccine and egg allergy. Lancet Infect Dis. 2019;19:812.
54. Gerhardt CMB, Castro APBM, Pastorino AC, de Barros Dorna M, de Jesus Nunes-Santos C, Aquilante BP, et al. Safety of yellow fever vaccine administration in confirmed egg-allergic patients. Vaccine. 2020;38(42):6539–44. Available online: http://www.sciencedirect.com/science/article/pii/S0264410X20310513
55. Kácha O, Kovács BE, McCarthy C, Schuurmans AAT, Dobyns C, Haller E, et al. An approach to establishing international quality standards for medical travel. Front Public Health. 2016;4:29. https://doi.org/10.3389/fpubh.2016.00029.

56. Traiber C, Amaral PC, Ritter VRF, Winge A. Infant meningoencephalitis probably caused by yellow fever vaccine virus transmitted via breastmilk. J Pediatr. 2011; https://doi.org/10.2223/JPED.2067.
57. Kuhn S, Twele-Montecinos L, MacDonald J, Webster P, Law B. Case report: probable transmission of vaccine strain of yellow fever virus to an infant via breast milk. CMAJ. 2011;183:E243–5. https://doi.org/10.1503/cmaj.100619.
58. Staples JE, Barrett ADT, Wilder-Smith A, Hombach J. Review of data and knowledge gaps regarding yellow fever vaccine-induced immunity and duration of protection. NPJ Vaccines. 2020;5(1):54.
59. World Health Organization (WHO). International Travel and Health. Country vaccination requirements and WHO recommendations for vaccination against yellow fever, poliomyelitis, and malaria prophylaxis in international travellers. WHO, 18 November 2022 (Revised on 3 January 2023). Available online: https://cdn.who.int/media/docs/default-source/travel-and-health/vaccination-requirements-and-who-recommendations-ith-2022-country-list.pdf (accessed October 12, 2023).
60. Hansen CA, Barrett ADT. The Present and Future of Yellow Fever Vaccines. Pharmaceuticals (Basel). 2021;14(9):891. https://doi.org/10.3390/ph14090891.

Viral Hepatitis in Travellers

13

J. E. Arends, Maria C. Leoni, and Andrew Ustianowski

Abstract

Viral hepatitis poses a significant threat to global public health, with a myriad of causative agents, including hepatotropic viruses A through E. This chapter provides a comprehensive overview of the epidemiology, transmission, clinical course, diagnosis, and treatment of hepatitis A through E, focusing on travellers.

Hepatitis A, primarily transmitted through the faecal-oral route, exhibits varying endemicity levels across regions. Improved sanitation and vaccination programs have led to a decline in developed countries but continue to pose risks to travellers. The clinical course ranges from subclinical to acute hepatitis, with a well-defined diagnostic approach involving HAV-specific antibodies. Vaccination remains a key preventive measure.

J. E. Arends (✉)
Faculty of Health, Medicine and Life Sciences, Maastricht University, Maastricht, The Netherlands

Department of Internal Medicine and Infectious Diseases, University Medical Center Utrecht, Utrecht, The Netherlands
e-mail: j.e.arends@umcutrecht.nl

M. C. Leoni
Infectious Disease Unit, Spedali Riuniti, Livorno, Italy

A. Ustianowski
Regional Infectious Diseases Unit, North Manchester General Hospital, Manchester, UK

University of Manchester, Manchester, UK

H. Leblebicioglu et al. (eds.), *Emerging and Re-emerging Infections in Travellers*, https://doi.org/10.1007/978-3-031-49475-8_13

Hepatitis B and D, caused by DNA viruses, share transmission routes, including blood-blood contact and sexual interactions. Prevalence varies globally, influencing the risk for travellers. Chronic infections may lead to cirrhosis and hepatocellular carcinoma, emphasizing the importance of vaccination, especially in regions with moderate to high prevalence.

Hepatitis C, an RNA virus primarily transmitted through blood contact, exhibits diverse genotypes. Travel-related risks involve activities such as intravenous drug use and medical procedures. Screening and confirmation of HCV antibodies guide diagnosis, and recent advances in direct-acting antivirals revolutionize treatment.

Hepatitis E, caused by Hepeviridae, exhibits varied genotypes with different epidemiological patterns. While genotypes 1 and 2 cause epidemics in regions with poor sanitation, genotypes 3 and 4 pose risks in developed countries, often linked to consumption of contaminated meat. Diagnosis involves serology, and acute infections are typically self-limiting, while chronic cases in immunocompromised individuals may require antiviral therapy.

In conclusion, understanding the diverse characteristics of hepatitis A through E is crucial for travellers' health. Vaccination, hygiene practices, and awareness of transmission routes are pivotal for prevention and early intervention, ensuring the well-being of individuals in diverse global settings.

13.1 Introduction

Hepatitis is an inflammation of the liver which has many causes: toxic (alcohol, drugs, medication), autoimmunity, fatty liver, metabolic diseases and also infectious. Viral infections such as cytomegalovirus (CMV), Epstein-Barr virus (EBV) or Varicella zoster virus (VZV) can result in hepatitis accompanied by other manifestations. However, this chapter focuses on viruses that mainly infect hepatocytes (i.e. "hepatotropic")—hepatitis A through E.

Viral hepatitis infections are very prevalent worldwide, causing millions of infections every year. Depending on their mode of transmission, residents, as well as travellers are at risk of acquiring viral hepatitis. Hepatitis A and E cause acute hepatitis, although the latter can also become chronic in individuals with significant immunosuppression, such as transplant patients. Hepatitis B and C can both cause chronic infections and, over several decades, may cause liver cirrhosis and liver cancer in 20% of those infected.

This chapter explores the transmission, epidemiology, clinical course and treatment of viral hepatitis A through E (briefly summarized in Table 13.1).

Table 13.1 Overview of viral hepatitis characteristics

	A	B	C	D	E
Source of virus	Faeces	Blood/ blood-derived body fluids	Blood/ blood-derived body fluids	Blood/ blood-derived body fluids	Faeces
Route of transmission	Faeco-oral	Percutaneous/ permucosal	Percutaneous/ permucosal	Percutaneous/ permucosal	Faeco-oral
Chronic infection	No	Yes	Yes	Yes	No (GT 1/2/4) Yes (GT 3)
Prevention	Pre/post-exposure immunization	Pre/post-exposure immunization	Blood donor screening/risk behaviour modification	Pre/post-exposure immunization/ risk behaviour modification	Ensure safe drinking water/cook meat >70 °C
Genetics	RNA	DNA	RNA	RNA	RNA

13.2 Hepatitis A

13.2.1 Transmission and Epidemiology

Hepatitis A virus (HAV) is a single-stranded RNA virus belonging to the genus Hepatovirus in the Picornaviridae family. It is transmitted mainly through the faecal-oral transmission and can survive in water for months. Exposure to high temperatures (>85 °C) for longer than 1 min can kill HAV, though it can withstand temperatures below freezing. In the developed world, the risk of HAV infection has decreased drastically due to improved hygienic conditions over the past decades. Therefore, in general, all high-income global regions (Western Europe, Australia, New Zealand, Canada, the United States, Japan, the Republic of Korea, and Singapore) have low levels of HAV endemicity (< 50% of the population is exposed). This is in contrast to low-income regions with high endemicity levels (>90% of the population exposed) [1]. High-prevalence countries include those in Sub-Saharan Africa and India, where more than 90% of children get infected with HAV before the age of 10 years [1, 2]. In medium-prevalence regions like Northern Africa, parts of South America, China and some Eastern European countries, the reported rate of infections is relatively low, and outbreaks are not common.

Approximately 1.5 million new HAV clinical cases occur each year worldwide [3, 4]. It is estimated that travellers are exposed to HAV at a reported rate of 3–6 cases/1000 people/month. However, the risk varies with traveller age, duration of travel and local hygiene conditions. Cases of HAV imported into more developed countries are most common in adults and young immigrants who have recently visited families in regions with high HAV infection rates [5, 6]. Trips longer than 30 days were a strong predictor of acute HAV but were not associated with an increased incidence of HBV (probably because long-term travellers are less exposed to known risk factors (sexual contact, IV drugs or healthcare workers)).

Some recent studies indicate that the monthly incidence rate for HAV in non-immune travellers in non-industrialized countries has decreased due to improvements in sanitation, hygiene, food safety, and vaccination programs. However, vaccination against HAV continues to be encouraged for people travelling to or working in countries with high or intermediate risk of infection.

13.2.2 Clinical Course

The clinical picture can vary from being subclinical (mostly in children <6 years old) to an acute hepatitis with jaundice (which occurs in more than 70% of adults). Fulminant hepatitis, including hepatic failure, occurs in less than 1% of cases but is more often in older patients (1.8% mortality in those over the age of 50 years) and in those with existing liver disease, including chronic hepatitis C infection [7, 8]. This is of relevance as the "at risk" population for HAV infection has gradually aged (due to the reduced occurrence of naturally acquired immunity). For this group, the risk of a serious outcome is potentially greater. A group at particular risk recently are men having sex with men that acquire HAV through sexual contact [9]. International travel was demonstrated as a risk factor for acquisition through Epidemiological and laboratory investigations [10].

The incubation period of HAV varies between 2–7 weeks, with an average of 4 weeks. Symptoms can start abruptly and include fatigue, nausea, vomiting, anorexia and weight loss, fever, malaise and abdominal pain. After a few days to a week, jaundice, dark urine and decoloured stools occur (in >70% of adults), sometimes accompanied by itching due to cholestasis. Rash and arthralgias are the most common extra-hepatic symptoms (reported in 10–15% of patients).

Although the virus can remain detectable for a long time in the faeces (>80 days after symptom onset), patients appear to be the most contagious from 1 week before symptom onset to 1 week thereafter [11].

Elevated plasma transaminases, usually >1000 IU/L, which usually peak early in the icteric phase, can be detected. Complete clinical and biochemical recovery occurs in the majority of patients within 2–3 months; however, up to 10% of patients experience a biphasic course with relapse of symptoms in the first 6 months. Such relapses are generally milder than during the initial episode, but elevated transaminases may be present for months afterwards. In the recovery phase there is often a reported intolerance to fat, alcohol and tobacco. Chronic HAV has, however, never been described and after clinical recovery immunity is lifelong.

13.2.3 Diagnosis

The diagnosis of acute HAV can be made by detecting specific HAV IgM antibodies in the serum. The presence of HAV IgG antibodies indicates immunity from either natural infection or vaccination. After vaccination, immunity is deemed to be long-term and potentially lifelong.

Detection of the RNA virus by PCR is possible on faeces or in plasma (up to 6 weeks after the first day of illness). HAV-PCR is, however, not routinely performed and is used predominantly for surveillance purposes.

13.2.4 Therapy

HAV infection is self-limiting and only supportive care is possible. Several effective vaccines, requiring an initial shot and a booster vaccination, are available to prevent HAV for decades.

13.3 Hepatitis B and D

13.3.1 Transmission and Epidemiology

Hepatitis B virus (HBV) is a DNA virus that consists of an envelope (containing the hepatitis B surface antigen (HBsAg)) and a core (containing the hepatitis B core antigen (HBcAg) and the HBe antigen. (HBeAg)). It belongs to the hepadnaviridae family and is unrelated to the other human hepatotropic viruses. Hepatitis D virus (HDV) is an RNA virus that only enters the hepatocyte using HBsAg from concurrent HBV infection. The same HBsAg is then also necessary for its replication and subsequent distribution to other hepatocytes. HDV infection is, therefore, only possible in people who are living with actively replicating HBV.

Transmission of both HBV and HDV occurs largely via the same routes: through blood-blood contact, sexual contact, within-family contact or vertical/perinatally. The latter is probably rarer for HDV.

Worldwide, the prevalence of HBV is estimated at around 350 million people, of which 15 million people (5%) are probably also infected with HDV. The World Health Organisation (WHO) has set ambitious targets, including a 90% reduction in new chronic infections (with HBV and HCV) by 2030 [12].

The risk of a traveller acquiring HBV infection depends on the destination, since the prevalence of HBV varies widely. Areas of low prevalence (0.1%–2% HBsAg+) include Australia, the United States, Canada, and Western Europe; areas of intermediate prevalence (2%–7%) correspond to parts of central Asia, Central and South America, and Eastern Europe; China, Africa, and countries within the Middle East and Southeast Asia are areas where the prevalence is high ($\geq$8% HBsAg+ve). HDV is endemic in Central Africa, Eastern Turkey, Central Asia, some Eastern European countries and the Amazonian region of Brasil [13].

Other factors associated with the acquisition of HBV are specific risk activities, travel duration and the immune status of the traveller. Specific populations of travellers may be at greater risk, including expatriates, those visiting friends and relatives, and travellers engaging in casual sex, dental surgery, medical procedures, tattoos, piercings, and acupuncture. Organ transplantation and medical tourism have repeatedly been identified as risk factors for both HBV and HCV infection.

Prolonged duration of travel is associated with an increased likelihood of HBV infection. In susceptible expatriates residing in countries of high HBV endemicity, the estimated monthly incidence ranged from 25 per 100,000 for symptomatic infections to 80–420 per 100,000 for all HBV infections. However, volunteers, aid workers, and missionaries are recognized to be at further increased risk due to extended travel and close contact with the local population.

Apart from hepatitis A and influenza, HBV infection is the most common vaccine-preventable infection among travellers. The global prevalence of HBV infection (and of HDV as a consequence) and the risk to travellers are likely to decrease as universal vaccination of infants is progressively introduced and implemented [14]. Many national health authorities and the WHO recommend that HBV vaccination should be considered in non-immune travellers to countries with a moderate to high HBV prevalence (HBsAg $\geq$ 2%).

13.3.2 Diagnosis

Screening for HBV is strongly recommended in the following risk groups: injecting drug users, men who have sex with men (MSM), first-generation migrants from HBV endemic countries (i.e. an HBV prevalence $\geq$2% in the country of origin) and asylum seekers during the admission process.

The diagnosis of HBV is based on the detection of antigens (HBsAg and HBeAg) and antibodies (anti-HBs, anti-HBe, IgM anti-HBc and IgG anti-HBc) with serological tests. Approximately 4–8 weeks after infection with HBV HBsAg is detectable in the blood, followed by HBeAg. Subsequently antibody formation becomes detectable, initially IgM and subsequently IgG anti-HBc. Therefore, a high IgM anti-HBc titre fits in with an acute HBV infection; this antibody disappears after about 6 months. In those that control their infection and become HBsAg negative, antibodies against HBsAg appear as the abundance of HBsAg in the blood starts to disappear. Conversely, chronic HBV infection is associated with demonstrable HBsAg in blood for $\geq$6 months after infection, together with HBeAg or anti-HBe, but without anti-Hbs. According to the new international guideline definitions which depend on plasma transaminase levels, the various disease stages are now termed either chronic infection (normal transaminases) or chronic hepatitis (elevated transaminases) [15].

Viral replication can be demonstrated by HBV DNA PCR assay. Screening for total (combined IgM/IgG) antibodies against HDV is possible for HDV infection. Acute or persistent HDV infection can then be confirmed with an HDV RNA assay. Antibodies against HDV may disappear after clearing an HDV infection.

13.3.3 Clinical Course

For HBV we distinguish acute and chronic infections. It is not the HBV itself but the host's immune reaction that causes the majority of the (liver) damage and manifestations of the disease. An acute infection has an incubation period of about

6 weeks and can be asymptomatic (in approximately 90% of children but only 40% of adults) or symptomatic. Symptomatic infection classically has a prodromal phase with malaise and complaints such as nausea or vomiting, fever or joint symptoms. This can be followed by a phase with icterus, dark urine and putty-coloured stools that can last 2–6 weeks. In rare cases (approximately 0.1%), this can lead to fulminant hepatitis, resulting in death. However, those with a more symptomatic course also have a greater chance of recovery and subsequent viral clearance. Overall, after an acute infection, the risk of developing a chronic infection is highest for newborns (90%) and the lowest for adults (5–10%) [16].

Chronic HBV infection, in which HBsAg is detectable for more than 6 months, can vary from asymptomatic carriage to hepatitis with resulting cirrhosis. Chronic infection can be divided into HBeAg positive and negative infections, with seroconversion of HBeAg to anti-HBe being associated with a decrease in HBV replication and liver inflammation. However, HBeAg-negative disease is not benign, with the potential to still develop considerable liver damage.

The 5-year risk of developing cirrhosis and hepatocellular carcinoma in chronic untreated HBV infection ranges from 12–20% and 6–15%, respectively, with the risks being higher for patients from endemic areas such as Asia [17].

Either acute or chronic HBV infection may also be associated with extra-hepatic manifestations such as polyarteritis nodosa or glomerulopathy (membranous glomerulopathy and membranoproliferative glomerulonephritis).

HDV infection can be acquired as a co-infection (simultaneous infection with HBV) or a super-infection (in an individual with established HBV infection). Co-infection can result in severe hepatitis and liver failure but usually leads to clearance of both HBV and HDV (98%) [18]. Super-infection can temporarily cause hepatitis flares but often leads to chronic HDV infection. The prognosis varies per individual patient, but in general, the risk of progression to cirrhosis and hepatocellular carcinoma is estimated to be three times higher than for HBV mono-infections [19].

13.4 Hepatitis C

13.4.1 Transmission and Epidemiology

Hepatitis C virus (HCV) is a member of the Flaviviridae family and consists of a single RNA strand. There are at least seven genotypes described, differing by about 30% in their respective genomes. Transmission mainly takes place through blood-blood contact, such as associated with intravenous drug use or in procedures where improperly sterilized needles are used (including piercings/tattoos). In addition, high-risk sexual interaction in MSM populations and those infected with HIV is recognized as a transmission route. This is in contrast to discordant heterosexual couples in whom unprotected sex is much more rarely associated with transmission. Finally, HCV transmission is also possible vertically from mother to child during delivery (with rates dependent on viral load but thought to approximate 5%).

After transmission, acute HCV is cleared in up to 20–30% of individuals (potentially more commonly in those that have more severe symptoms at acquisition). If

HCV-RNA is detectable after 6 months, chronic HCV is deemed to have been established.

It is estimated that approximately 3% of the world's population is chronically infected by HCV [20]. The prevalence is high ($\geq$1.5%) in several countries in Latin America, Eastern Europe and the former Soviet Union, and certain countries in Africa, the Middle East, and Asia; the prevalence is reported to be highest (approximately 10%) in Egypt [21].

There is a lack of data on HCV acquisition in travellers, but the risk is thought to be low and will be related to the prevalence of HCV in the destination country. Activities that could expose travellers to a risk of acquiring HCV infection included tattooing or IDU. Travel has been associated with greater sharing of needles, syringes, and drug preparation equipment, as well as pooling money to buy drugs, heavy alcohol consumption, polysubstance use, and more sexual and injecting partners.

The latter has been demonstrated in studies among men having sex with men (MSM) that acquired acute HCV through sexual contact in a network of sexual contacts across Europe [22]. Acute HCV infection has been reported in travellers who received emergency medical care abroad, and there have been cases of HCV infection in travellers who received haemodialysis in Pakistan, Slovakia, Singapore, Bangladesh, India and more broadly in Asia [23–25].

Currently, no vaccine is available for HCV infection and immune globulin does not provide protection. Future travellers need to be advised about the modes of transmission and avoidance of activities associated with exposure to contaminated blood.

13.4.2 Diagnosis

The presence of HCV antibodies is evidence of exposure to HCV infection. A positive HCV antibody test must always be confirmed, for example, by an immunoblot or an HCV RNA determination. HCV antibodies may not be detectable at an early stage of the infection. Therefore, HCV RNA should also be determined in case of possible recent exposure.

If the HCV RNA is still positive after 6 months, the individual is defined as having chronic HCV infection. Until recently, HCV genotyping was performed because it was required for therapy choice and duration. However, this is no longer always necessary with the new generation pan-genotypic Direct Acting Antivirals (DAAs).

13.4.3 Clinical Course

The average incubation period of HCV is 7 weeks (range 2–26 weeks) and the clinical picture of acute HCV shows little difference from other acute viral hepatitis infections. The vast majority of chronic HCV patients either have no or only minimal symptoms - fatigue is a non-specific but common complaint and there may be extra-hepatic symptoms such as myalgia/arthralgia, cryoglobulinaemia or glomerulonephritis. HCV-related fulminant hepatitis is rare but occurs more frequently in the setting of HBV co-infection. Once chronic HCV is established, the risk of developing cirrhosis has been estimated as 14–19% after 20 years, and HCV patients with liver cirrhosis have an annual risk of 0–3% of hepatocellular carcinoma (HCC) development [26].

13.4.4 Treatment

Since the isolation of hepatitis C in 1989, strategies to eradicate the virus have evolved rapidly. Interferon was the first drug used to treat the infection, and with the addition of ribavirin, cure rates (known as sustained virological response (SVR) rates) of around 54–56% were achieved [27]. The real revolution came with the advent of directly acting antiviral drugs (DAAs): treatments of shorter duration achieve SVR rates above 95% for nearly all patient groups. Reinfection may occur as treatment does not result in any protective HCV-specific immunity [28]. Reinfection among PWID and MSM due to ongoing risk behaviour (sharing needles/syringes/other injecting equipment or unsafe sexual practices) could compromise both individual and population treatment benefits [29].

13.5   Hepatitis E

13.5.1 Transmission and Epidemiology

Hepatitis E virus (HEV) belongs to the Hepeviridae family and was first identified in 1983. Hepatitis E virus infections are prevalent worldwide, albeit geographical differences exist based on the different HEV genotypes. HEV genotypes 1 (Asia and Africa) and 2 (Mexico and Africa) cause epidemics in regions with poor sanitation, with large outbreaks reported, for example, from Uganda [30], China [31], India [32] and Mexico [33]. Furthermore, in these HEV-endemic countries, sporadic acute hepatitis E patients have been described. In Asia a fourth genotype has been found in 29 Chinese patients with an acute hepatitis E infection [34].

HEV genotypes 1 and 2 infections are also diagnosed in developed countries but almost exclusively among travellers from endemic countries [35]. During the past decade however, sporadic cases of HEV genotypes 3 and 4 infection have been reported in developed countries as autochthonous infections [36]. These infections have been linked to ingestion of raw or undercooked meat, especially from wild boar, swine or pig [37]. Reported seroprevalence for autochthonous genotype 3 infections in the general population in Europe is estimated to be around 2% in the Netherlands [38], 3–16% in France, depending on the region [39] and 1% in Spain [40]. However, studies from the United States show higher seroprevalence rates of 17–21% [41] whereas in Japan between 4.6 and 6.7% of the healthy populations was anti-HEV positive [42].

13.5.2 Diagnosis

The test of first choice in immunocompetent patients suspected of having an acute HEV infection is serology. In general, IgM and IgG are already positive early in the disease, but the sensitivity of the different assays varies (with Mikrogen and Wantei being the most sensitive). IgM generally disappears within 3 months, but IgG remains present for life (but probably does not protect against new infection). In immunocompromised patients, serology is unreliable and a negative IgM and/or IgG does not exclude acute or chronic HEV infection. Therefore, it is recommended to perform a HEV-RNA PCR on blood in these patients.

13.5.3 Clinical Course

The clinical picture of acute HEV infection varies from asymptomatic to fulminant hepatitis, with hepatic failure being described (especially in pregnant women with genotype 2). A mortality rate of 25% has been described. The clinical picture resembles that of hepatitis A with signs of nausea, jaundice and abdominal pain. Genotypes 3 and 4 are generally subclinical, but symptoms more often occur in elderly men and can even lead to liver failure. In addition to general and gastrointestinal symptoms, HEV GT 3 infection has been associated with neurological complaints such as Guillan-Barré, neuralgic amyotrophy and sensory neuropathy [43]. The clinical picture generally lasts for 1–4 weeks and recovers spontaneously. However, a chronic infection can develop in immunocompromised patients - defined by the detectable presence of HEV RNA for 6 months or longer. This has been described, among other things, in patients who have undergone haemopoietic stem cell or organ transplantation, HIV patients with a CD4 number < 200, oncology patients undergoing chemotherapy and patients using steroids or anti-TNF alpha therapy [44, 45]. In chronic infections the diagnosis is often only considered in case of unexplained persistent liver biochemistry disorders. However chronic HEV infection can result in rapidly progressive liver cirrhosis in the immunocompromised [46].

13.5.4 Treatment

Treatment of acute hepatitis E is usually based on supportive therapy and is often mild and self-limited in immunocompetent patients.

The role of antiviral therapy in immunocompromised patients is not well established, but retrospective studies have suggested the role of ribavirin in patients with chronic liver disease who are receiving immunosuppressive therapy [47]. Overall, treating chronic disease in immunocompromised patients involves reducing immunosuppression (if possible) and considering a 12-week course of ribavirin [48].

Declaration of Interest We declare no conflict of interest.

References

1. Jacobsen KH, Wiersma ST. Hepatitis A virus seroprevalence by age and world region, 1990 and 2005. Vaccine. 2010;28:6653–7.
2. Jefferies M, Rauff B, Rashid H, Lam T, Rafiq S. Update on global epidemiology of viral hepatitis and preventive strategies. World J Clin Cases. 2018;6:589–99.
3. Franco E, Meleleo C, Serino L, Sorbara D, Zaratti L. Hepatitis A: epidemiology and prevention in developing countries. World J Hepatol. 2012;4:68.
4. Henriquez-Camacho C, Serre N, Norman F, et al. Clinicoepidemiological characteristics of viral hepatitis in migrants and travellers of the +Redivi network. Travel Med Infect Dis. 2019. Published Online Feb 6; https://doi.org/10.1016/j.tmaid.2019.02.001.
5. Pham B, Duval B, De Serres G, et al. Seroprevalence of hepatitis A infection in a low endemicity country: a systematic review. BMC Infect Dis. 2005;5:56.
6. Faber MS, Stark K, Behnke SC, Schreier E, Frank C. Epidemiology of hepatitis A virus infections, Germany, 2007–2008. Emerg Infect Dis. 2009;15:1760–8.
7. Kemmer NM, Miskovsky EP. Hepatitis A. Infect Dis Clin N Am. 2000;14:605–15.
8. Bennett JE, John E, Dolin R, Mandell GL. Mandell, Douglas, and Bennett's principles and practice of infectious diseases, vol. 1. Churchill Livingstone Elsevier; 2010.
9. Alberts CJ, Boyd A, Bruisten SM, et al. Hepatitis A incidence, seroprevalence, and vaccination decision among MSM in Amsterdam, the Netherlands. Vaccine. 2019;37:2849–56.
10. Beebeejaun K, Degala S, Balogun K, et al. Outbreak of hepatitis A associated with men who have sex with men (MSM), England, July 2016 to January 2017. Eur Secur. 2017;22:30454.
11. Bower WA, Nainan OV, Han X, Margolis HS. Duration of viremia in Hepatitis A Virus infection. J Infect Dis. 2000;182:12–7.
12. Combating Hepatitis B and C to reach elimination by 2030 May 2016 Advocacy Brief. https://apps.who.int/iris/bitstream/handle/10665/206453/WHO_HIV_2016.04_eng.pdf?sequence=1 (accessed May 29, 2019).
13. Wedemeyer H, Manns MP. Epidemiology, pathogenesis and management of hepatitis D: update and challenges ahead. Nat Rev Gastroenterol Hepatol. 2010;7:31–40.
14. Johnson DF, Leder K, Torresi J. Hepatitis B and C infection in international travelers. J Travel Med. 2013;20:194–202.
15. EASL 2017 Clinical Practice Guidelines on the management of hepatitis B virus infection q. http://www.easl.eu/medias/cpg/management-of-hepatitis-B-virus-infection/English-report.pdf (accessed July 15, 2018).
16. Chen C-J, Yang H-I. Natural history of chronic hepatitis B REVEALed. J Gastroenterol Hepatol. 2011;26:628–38.
17. Iloeje UH, Yang H, Su J, et al. Predicting cirrhosis risk based on the level of circulating Hepatitis B viral load. Gastroenterology. 2006;130:678–86.
18. Farci P, Niro G. Clinical features of Hepatitis D. Semin Liver Dis. 2012;32:228–36.
19. Aberra H, Gordien E, Desalegn H, et al. Hepatitis delta virus infection in a large cohort of chronic hepatitis B patients in Ethiopia. Liver Int. 2018;38:1000–9.
20. Rosen HR. Chronic Hepatitis C Infection. N Engl J Med. 2011;364:2429–38.
21. Gower E, Estes C, Blach S, Razavi-Shearer K, Razavi H. Global epidemiology and genotype distribution of the hepatitis C virus infection. J Hepatol. 2014;61:S45–57. https://wwwnc.cdc.gov/travel/yellowbook/2018/infectious-diseases-related-to-travel/hepatitis-c
22. van de Laar T, Pybus O, Bruisten S, et al. Evidence of a large, international network of HCV transmission in HIV-positive men who have sex with men. Gastroenterology. 2009;136:1609–17.
23. Jauréguiberry S, Grandière-Pérez L, Ansart S, Laklache H, Métivier S, Caumes E. Acute hepatitis C virus infection after a travel in India. J Travel Med. 2006;12:55–6.
24. Bollepalli S, Wisinger D, Markov M, Patel P, Nadir A. Travel: a unique risk factor for acute hepatitis C virus. MedGenMed. 2006;8:17.

25. Ghafur A, Raza M, Labbett W, et al. Travel-associated acquisition of hepatitis C virus infection in patients receiving haemodialysis. Nephrol Dial Transplant. 2007;22:2640–4.
26. Thein H-H, Yi Q, Dore GJ, Krahn MD. Estimation of stage-specific fibrosis progression rates in chronic hepatitis C virus infection: a meta-analysis and meta-regression. Hepatology. 2008;48:418–31.
27. Strader DB, Seeff LB. A brief history of the treatment of viral hepatitis C. Clin Liver Dis. 2012;1:6–11.
28. Ingiliz P, Martin TC, Rodger A, et al. HCV reinfection incidence and spontaneous clearance rates in HIV-positive men who have sex with men in Western Europe. J Hepatol. 2017;66:282–7.
29. Midgard H, Weir A, Palmateer N, et al. HCV epidemiology in high-risk groups and the risk of reinfection. J Hepatol. 2016;65:S33–45.
30. Teshale EH, Howard CM, Grytdal SP, et al. Hepatitis E epidemic, Uganda. Emerg Infect Dis. 2010;16:126–9.
31. Bi SL, Purdy MA, McCaustland KA, Margolis HS, Bradley DW. The sequence of hepatitis E virus isolated directly from a single source during an outbreak in China. Virus Res. 1993;28:233–47.
32. Sailaja B, Murhekar MV, Hutin YJ, et al. Outbreak of waterborne hepatitis E in Hyderabad, India, 2005. Epidemiol Infect. 2009;137:234–40.
33. Velázquez O, Stetler HC, Avila C, et al. Epidemic transmission of enterically transmitted non-A, non-B hepatitis in Mexico, 1986–1987. JAMA. 1990;263:3281–5.
34. Harrison TJ, Erker JC, Wang Y, et al. A divergent genotype of hepatitis E virus in Chinese patients with acute hepatitis. J Gen Virol. 1999;80:169–77.
35. Bader TF, Krawczynski K, Polish LB, Favorov MO. Hepatitis E in a U.S. traveler to Mexico. N Engl J Med. 1991;325:1659.
36. Teshale EH, Hu DJ, Holmberg SD. The two faces of Hepatitis E virus. Clin Infect Dis. 2010;51:328–34.
37. Herremans M, Vennema H, Bakker J, et al. Swine-like hepatitis E viruses are a cause of unexplained hepatitis in the Netherlands. J Viral Hepat. 2007;14:140–6.
38. Verhoef L, Koopmans M, Duizer E, Bakker J, Reimerink J, Van Pelt W. Seroprevalence of hepatitis E antibodies and risk profile of HEV seropositivity in The Netherlands, 2006–2007. Epidemiol Infect. 2012;140:1838–47.
39. Boutrouille A, Bakkali-Kassimi L, Cruciere C, Pavio N. Prevalence of anti-hepatitis E Virus antibodies in French blood donors. J Clin Microbiol. 2007;45:2009–10.
40. Fogeda M, Avellón A, Echevarría JM. Prevalence of specific antibody to hepatitis E virus in the general population of the community of Madrid, Spain. J Med Virol. 2012;84:71–4.
41. Meng XJ, Wiseman B, Elvinger F, et al. Prevalence of antibodies to hepatitis E virus in veterinarians working with swine and in normal blood donors in the United States and other countries. J Clin Microbiol. 2002;40:117–22.
42. Tanaka E, Takeda N, Li T-C, et al. Seroepidemiological study of hepatitis E virus infection in Japan using a newly developed antibody assay. J Gastroenterol. 2001;36:317–21.
43. van den Berg B, van der Eijk AA, Pas SD, et al. Guillain-Barre syndrome associated with preceding hepatitis E virus infection. Neurology. 2014;82:491–7.
44. Carré M, Thiebaut-Bertrand A, Larrat S, et al. Fatal autochthonous fulminant hepatitis E early after allogeneic stem cell transplantation. Bone Marrow Transplant. 2017;52:643–5.
45. Kenfak-Foguena A, Schöni-Affolter F, Bürgisser P, et al. Hepatitis E virus seroprevalence and chronic infections in patients with HIV, Switzerland. Emerg Infect Dis. 2011;17:1074–8.
46. Maddukuri VC, Russo MW, Ahrens WA, et al. Chronic Hepatitis E with neurologic manifestations and rapid progression of liver fibrosis in a liver transplant recipient. Dig Dis Sci. 2013;58:2413–6.
47. Kamar N, Izopet J, Tripon S, et al. Ribavirin for chronic Hepatitis E Virus infection in transplant recipients. N Engl J Med. 2014;370:1111–20.
48. Dalton HR, Kamar N, Baylis SA, Moradpour D, Wedemeyer H, Negro F. EASL Clinical Practice Guidelines on hepatitis E virus infection. J Hepatol. 2018;68:1256–71.

Chikungunya Virus Infection in Travellers

14

Alfonso J. Rodriguez-Morales, Natalia Millan-Benavides, and Jaime A. Cardona-Ospina

Abstract

Over the last decades, especially in the previous 10 years, the epidemiological importance of the chikungunya virus (CHIKV) has significantly increased. After 2014, epidemics in multiple countries in the Americas and with imported cases abroad, especially in Europe and North America, called attention to the relevance

A. J. Rodriguez-Morales (✉)
Grupo de Investigación Biomedicina, Faculty of Medicine, Fundacion Universitaria Autónoma de las Américas-Institucion Universitaria Vision de las Americas, Pereira, Risaralda, Colombia

Universidad Cientifica del Sur, Lima, Peru

Gilbert and Rose-Marie Chagoury School of Medicine, Lebanese American University, Beirut, Lebanon

School of Medicine, Universidad Privada Franz Tamayo, Cochabamba, Bolivia
e-mail: alfonso.rodriguez@uam.edu.co; arodriguezmo@cientifica.edu.pe; alphonso.morales@lau.edu.lb

N. Millan-Benavides
Grupo de Investigación Biomedicina, Faculty of Medicine, Fundacion Universitaria Autónoma de las Américas-Institucion Universitaria Vision de las Americas, Pereira, Risaralda, Colombia

J. A. Cardona-Ospina
Grupo de Investigación Biomedicina, Faculty of Medicine, Fundacion Universitaria Autónoma de las Américas-Institucion Universitaria Vision de las Americas, Pereira, Risaralda, Colombia

Division of Infectious Diseases and Vaccinology, School of Public Health, University of California, Berkeley, CA, USA

Emerging Infectious Diseases and Tropical Medicine Research Group, Instituto para la Investigación en Ciencias Biomédicas - Sci-Help, Pereira, Colombia
e-mail: jaime.cardona@uam.edu.co

© The Author(s), under exclusive license to Springer Nature Switzerland AG 2024
H. Leblebicioglu et al. (eds.), *Emerging and Re-emerging Infections in Travellers*, https://doi.org/10.1007/978-3-031-49475-8_14

of arboviral diseases in travel and migration. Introduction and autochthonous transmission in the Caribbean, Colombia, Brazil and the rest of the countries of the region of Latin America was the consequence of travelers from endemic and epidemic areas arriving at places with suitable conditions for transmission. The last has been highlighted, especially in climate change and variability, global warming, travel, and migration, for Europe, where autochthonous transmission has also occurred during summer seasons in the south of the continent. In the current chapter, we reviewed the epidemiological and clinical aspects related to CHIKV, especially in the context of travel medicine, but also considered the importance of long-term consequences for the affected patients, such as the case of the potential development of chronic rheumatological and non-rheumatological sequelae.

14.1 Background

14.1.1 Brief History

The chikungunya virus infection (CHIKV) was first reported in Tanzania, Africa, in 1952 [1]. Several other epidemics followed that in the Central African Republic, Guinea, Burundi, Angola, Uganda, Malawi, Nigeria, Democratic Republic of the Congo, and several other states, which unfortunately were poorly recognized and few clinical researches were derived from. Almost half a million cases were reported in June 2004 in an outbreak in Kenya, with a seroprevalence rate of 75% [2]. Several other epidemics occurred in subsequent years on the southwestern Indian Ocean islands, except Madagascar, from 2005 to 2007, particularly in La Reunión island, France [3]. Although previously considered a self-limited arthritogenic febrile illness, by 2006, significant increases in the numbers of CHIKV-associated neurological complications, mortality rate, and foetal infections were observed [4–6].

In Asia, CHIKV was first reported in Bangkok, Thailand, in 1958. The virus spread to other surrounding regions in 1964 and then reemerged in 1975 and 1976. About 20 Indian states experienced several disastrous epidemics. Significant outbreaks that increased concerns about CHIKV occurred in India in 2005, affecting 1.4 million people [7].

In Europe, the first CHIKV outbreak was reported in Emilia-Romagna, Italy, in 2007, mainly favoured by the presence of the vector of CHIKV, *Aedes albopictus*, which was present in almost 20 European countries [8]. In 2014, an outbreak of autochthonous CHIKV cases occurred in France, Puerto Rico, Miami (Florida, USA), and Haiti. Since then, CHIKV has spread to almost half of the Pacific Island countries, including Australia, New Zealand, Papua New Guinea, the Cook Islands, and the Marshall Islands. The epidemiological findings indicate that the global distribution of *A. albopictus* and *A. aegypti* and travelers are involved in the ongoing transmission of the disease in localities previously free of this infection [9]. In fact, after this, it has been recognized that the risk of CHIKV is an emerging condition with the potential for autochthonous transmission in the continent, especially in the south Mediterranean coastal areas, due to climate change and migration [9–11]. Over the last years, multiple imported cases of CHIKV have been investigated in Europe [12–14]. Although between 2018 and 2023, no autochthonous cases have been reported in Europe, especially in 2017, outbreaks with local cases were reported in France [9, 10] and Italy [10].

In the Americas, CHIKV emerged in 2013 in the tourist Saint Martin islands, and the virus spread to 17 countries in South America [15]. By 2014, the US Centres for Disease Control and Prevention (CDC) had reported 55,992 travel-related and locally acquired cases of CHIKV from 14 islands of French Guiana and the Caribbean. That outbreak caused more than 2.9 million confirmed and suspected cases and 296 deaths in late 2016, which was an important burden and cost in Latin America [16–20]. The first case of local transmission of CHIKV in Colombia was notified in August 2014 by the Department of Bolivar [21]. According to reports, the cost and burden of this outbreak during 2014 represented a total Disability-Adjusted Life Years (DALYs) loss of 40.44 to 45.14 lost/100,000 population and at least US\$73.6 million [19]. After intensive circulation of Chikungunya, Zika and dengue during 2015–2016, the years 2017 and 2018 showed a significant decrease in all the arboviral disease burdens [22], but remain endemic [23] with its potential implications in public health as well as for travel medicine in the region.

14.1.2 Importance of the Disease

Chikungunya is a clinically and economically significant arbovirus, spread worldwide in the twenty-first century [1, 24]. While rarely fatal [25], its derived chronic sequelae can significantly impact the quality of life of patients [3], mental health [26] and their productivity [3, 20, 24] (Fig. 14.1). At least half of the patients with CHIK could develop chronic rheumatologic sequelae, especially in women and older patients, which can persist for months or years [16, 27, 28].

Unfortunately, little information is available on the real economic costs of CHIKV infection. Healthcare costs during the La Reunion in 2005–2006 epidemic were estimated: the medical management of CHIKV was associated with a significant economic burden, with 60% of the CHIKV-related expenditure attributable to direct medical costs, such as medical consultation, hospitalization, and drug consumption [29]. Loss of productivity, measured as absenteeism costs, is also high

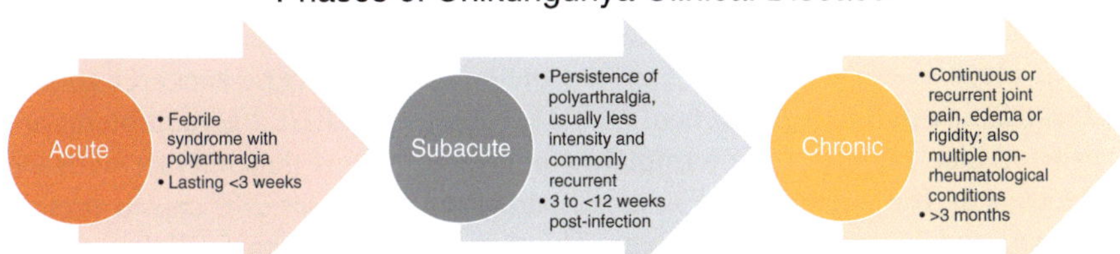

Fig. 14.1 Clinical evolution of CHIKV-associated disease

[30]. In Colombia, a total DALYs loss of 40.44–45.14 lost/100,000 population was estimated. The 2014 outbreak estimated costs were at least US$73.6 million [19]. Reported costs associated with CHIKV diseases are substantial and vary by region, age group, and public/private delivery of healthcare services. Its burden includes chronicity, severe infections, increased hospitalization risks, and related mortality. The disease can impact the economy in several spheres, significantly affecting the health system and national economies. Understanding and measuring the full impact of this reemerging disease is essential [31].

14.1.3 Why Is It Classified as Emerging and/or Reemerging?

CHIKV virus infectious disease is considered both emerging and reemerging. In the first place, it is occurring as a recently identified and previously unknown infectious agent, which causes public health problems at local, regional or global levels [32], especially in the Americas during 2014–2016. Then, gradually, it expanded to other parts of the world; since 2004, it has caused sustained epidemics of unprecedented magnitude in Asia and Africa. It was extended later to other regions, such as Europe and the Americas [33, 34].

In the second instance, it is a reemerging disease, mainly due to the cyclical presentation of epidemics, with inter-epidemic periods ranging between 4 and 30 years [35]. CHIKV has spread since 1953 in many Southeast Asian countries. In 1990, it resurfaced in the Indian Ocean, South Pacific and America after the weakening of the active control of the transmitting mosquito and its proliferation in urban areas [36]. In Asia, CHIKV is endemic and causes recurrent and sometimes large epidemics [37], especially in the Indian subcontinent and in Southeast Asia [30].

14.2 Aetiology

Chikungunya is an RNA virus of the genus Alphavirus, Togaviridae family. The name chikungunya originated in the Kimakonde dialect of a word whose meaning is "one who bends or bows" or "to be contorted", which describes the inclined appearance of people suffering from the characteristic and painful arthralgia [38, 39].

Structurally, the virus has a simple RNA chain of positive polarity, which codes for four non-structural (nsP1-4) and three structural (C, E1–2) proteins. It consists of a small spherical particle, approximately 60–70 nm in diameter, with a phospholipid envelope where the E1 and E2 glycoproteins form 80 trimeric anchored spikes, each consisting of 3 heterodimers of E1/E2 glycoproteins. E1/E2 glycoproteins are transmembrane proteins with terminal cytoplasmic regions that interact with the nucleocapsid. The nucleocapsid is icosahedral and comprises 240 capsid protein monomers and the genomic RNA chain. The virion binds to the host cell through the E2 glycoprotein, which includes a fusion peptide that mediates the entry of the nucleocapsid into the cytoplasm from the endosome [36, 40].

14.3 Transmission

For the transmission of the disease, they must be present simultaneously: the virus, the vector and the susceptible host [41]. The CHIKV virus is transmitted from one person to another by the bite of infected female mosquitoes. To transmit the disease, the mosquito must have bitten a person infected with the virus during the period of viremia and then bites another human being [39].

The mosquito species involved are *Aedes aegypti* and *Aedes albopictus*, which can transmit other viruses such as dengue and Zika. These vectors are typically present in temperate latitudes (less than 2000 metres above sea level) [42] and usually bite throughout the day. However, their activity may be at its maximum at the beginning of the morning and the end of the afternoon. Both species bite outdoors, but *A. aegypti* can also do it indoors. The female of the *A. aegypti* mosquito is a transmitter after an average period of extrinsic incubation of 10 days; the disease usually appears between 4 and 8 days after the infected mosquito's bite, although the interval can range between 2 and 12 days [39].

Within the reservoirs are the human beings in the epidemic period and monkeys, rodents and birds (jungle cycle) in the interepidemic period. *Aedes aegypti* is an efficient vector given the high susceptibility to the virus, preferential feeding with human blood, diurnal feeding, almost imperceptible sting and ability to sting several people quickly [42].

In addition to *A. aegypti* and *A. albopictus*, now in the region of the Americas, *A. vitattus* represents a risk for transmission. It has been reported sporadically in some Caribbean islands in 2020 and after [43–46], then may be detected in other places, as well as in continental countries, already endemic for CHIKV.

Host susceptibility occurs in anyone who has not previously become ill with the virus and moves to endemic areas. It is believed that once exposed to CHIKV, individuals develop prolonged immunity that protects them against reinfection [41].

Evidence also suggests that the infective virus is excreted in the saliva and could be a source of infection [47, 48]. Vertical transmission has been reported, too [6, 49]. Despite some studies failing to show CHKV infection's effect during pregnancy on significant obstetrical outcomes or congenital anomalies, long-term follow-up studies have reported poor neurocognitive outcomes of newborns and even more unsatisfactory results in patients with neonatal CHIKV encephalopathy [50, 51].

14.4 Epidemiology

14.4.1 Geographic Distributions

Chikungunya has been identified in nearly 40 countries.

Countries having documented endemic or epidemic Chikungunya are [52]:

Asia: Human chikungunya virus infection has been reported in Cambodia, East Timor, India, Indonesia, Laos, Malaysia, Maldives, Myanmar, Pakistan, Philippines, Réunion, Seychelles, Singapore, Taiwan, Thailand and Vietnam.

Africa: Chikungunya occurs in Benin, Burundi, Cameroon, Central African Republic, Comoros, Congo (DRC), Equatorial Guinea, Guinea, Kenya, Madagascar, Malawi, Mauritius, Mayotte, Nigeria, Senegal, South Africa, Sudan, Tanzania, Uganda and Zimbabwe.

Europe and the Americas: Aside from minor incidence rates caused by imported cases from travelers, Italy and France are the only European countries with outbreaks (Table 14.1). The Americas have not had any significant outbreaks between 2017 and 2021, but the disease is endemic in most places where CHIKV caused epidemics in 2014-2016. After 2021, specifically in late 2022, CHIKV increased in multiple countries of South America, especially in Argentina, Paraguay, Brazil, Bolivia and Uruguay, with outbreaks declared particularly in early 2023.

Table 14.1 Outbreaks of CHIKV reported in Europe, 2007–2017 (from ECDC.europa.eu)

Year	Country, region, municipalities	Number of autochthonous cases	Period of circulation (probable)	Origin of the primary travel-related case (probable)	Virus
2007	Italy, region of Emilia Romagna (main transmission areas in Castiglione di Cervia and Castiglione di Ravenna)	≈ 330 suspected, probable and confirmed	July–September	India	CHIKV ECSA
2010	France, Var department, Fréjus	2	September	India	CHIKV ECSA
2014	France, Hérault department, Montpellier	12	September–October	Cameroon	CHIKV ECSA
2017	France, Var department, Le Cannet-les-Maures and Taradeau	17 (11 in Cannet-des-Maures and 6 in Taradeau)	July–September	Central Africa	CHIKV ECSA
2017	Italy, Lazio region (Anzio, Latina and Roma) and Calabria region (Guardavalle marina)	270 confirmed and 219 probable	August–November	Asia (India/Pakistan)	CHIKV ECSA, belonging to a branch of Indian Ocean Lineage (IOL), reported from the Indian subcontinent (India, Pakistan)

14.4.2 Recent Epidemics/Outbreaks

Chikungunya was first identified in Tanzania in early 1952 and has caused periodic outbreaks in Asia and Africa since the 1960s [4, 5].

Outbreaks are often separated by periods of more than ten years. Between 2001 and 2011, several countries reported chikungunya outbreaks.

2005–2006: More than 272.000 people were infected during an outbreak of Chikungunya in the Indian Ocean islands of Réunion and Mauritius, where Ae. albopictus was the presumed vector.

2006: Outbreak in India, more than 1.500.000 chikungunya cases were reported with *A. aegypti* implicated as the vector.

2007: The migration of infected people introduced the infection in a coastal village in Italy. This outbreak (197 cases) confirmed that mosquito-borne outbreaks by *A. albopictus* are plausible in Europe.

2013: France reported two laboratory-confirmed autochthonous cases on the Caribbean island of St Martin [39].

2014: France confirmed 4 cases of locally acquired chikungunya infection in Montpellier, France. In late 2014, outbreaks were reported in the Pacific islands [39].

2015: 693.489 suspected cases and 37.480 confirmed cases of Chikungunya were reported to the PAHO, of which Colombia bore the most significant burden with 356.079 suspected cases [39].

2016: 349.936 suspected and 146.914 laboratory-confirmed cases were reported to the PAHO. Countries reporting the most cases were Brazil (265.000 suspected cases), Bolivia and Colombia (19.000 suspected cases) [39].

2017–2022: Outbreaks reported in the Americas, with 273,685 cases. CHIKV cases were reported in 14 of the 52 countries and territories in the Americas, of which 138,438 were confirmed (50.6%). The regional cumulative incidence in 2022 was 27.55 cases per 100,000 population. The rate of growth of the curve for 2021 was 48.7% from the epidemiological week (EW) 1 until the peak on EW22, while the rate of growth for the curve in 2022 was 81.3% from EW 1 until the peak on EW 18. Peak transmission was in EW 22 for 2021 and EW 18 for 2022. A total of 87 deaths were reported associated with chikungunya infection. The highest number of cases in the region has been reported by Brazil, with 265,289 cases, which represents (96.9%) of total regional cases. Belize follows in case counts with 2509 cases (0.9%), followed by Paraguay with 2443 cases (0.9%), Guatemala with 2086 cases (0.8%), and Peru with 595 cases (0.2%).

2023: Outbreaks reported in South American countries, especially in Argentina. As of 7 June 2023, 214,317 cases and 281 deaths have been reported. The majority of cases have been reported from Brazil (124,270), Paraguay (85,889), Argentina (1336), and Bolivia (1233). Deaths have been reported in Brazil (25) and Paraguay (256).

14.4.3 Risk Factors

Mainly, unprotected exposure to mosquito bites in endemic areas is key for CHIKV transmission.

14.4.4 Risks for International Travelers

In most places, the risk for travelers is low, especially compared with dengue, probably the arbovirus with the highest incidence in most countries in the Americas, Africa and Asia [22]. But during outbreaks, as described before, there is an increased risk for travelers to those areas.

14.4.5 Considerations in Migrants

In migrants from CHIK-endemic countries, this should be considered a differential diagnosis during acute febrile and rheumatological syndromes, but also in patients with chronic arthralgia without other apparent etiological causes.

14.5 Pathogenesis

After it enters the human host, the CHIKV replicates in primary targets like the skin fibroblasts, mononuclear cells and macrophages [53–56], which help in virus replication and dissemination. Its replicative cycle is swift, about 4 h [57, 58]. After the infection of these cells, CHIKV triggers an early type I interferon response [59], enters the circulatory system, and disseminates to immune-privileged niches where it can persist and replicate. This persistence is associated with extensive inflammatory cell recruitment, especially in joints and skeletal muscles [53, 59–63].

Viral persistence in immune-privileged niches is associated with the expression of IFN-α, IL-10, and monocyte chemotactic protein 1 (MCP-1 or CCL2) [59]. And apparently, they are associated with bone reabsorption and bone loss, and CHIKV seems to favour a pro-osteoclastic microenvironment disrupting the receptor activator of nuclear factor-kB ligand/osteoprotegerin (RANKL/OPG) ratio [61, 64].

Regarding adaptive immune response, IgM titers are detectable early during the infection, and higher and early increase of IgG3 titers has been correlated with efficient viral clearance and long-term viral protection [65]. During sub-acute and chronic disease, activated and effector CD4+ and CD8+ T cells play an essential role [66, 67], and chronic arthritis has been correlated with higher levels of effector T cells and levels of IL-10 [68].

14.6 Clinical Findings

The clinical picture of CHIKV infection is divided into three phases: Acute (<3 weeks), subacute (between 3–12 weeks) and chronic (>12 weeks) (Fig. 14.1). The acute disease is characterized by a self-limited, undifferentiated febrile illness that can course with polyarthralgia or polyarthritis affecting limbs. Atypical and lethal cases have been reported. Atypical cases comprise neurological, ophthalmologic, respiratory, cardiovascular and cutaneous involvement, among others, that could evolve to death [17, 69–75] with mortality rates that range between 0.082–0.738 [17]. Older age, gender, and comorbidities are associated with the appearance of severe cases, death and evolution to chronic forms of the disease. However, baseline risk factors related to disease progression require further characterization [69, 76]. Notwithstanding, febrile illness usually lasts less than 7 days, and according to retrospective analysis, nearly 80% of the patients progress to subacute disease [77].

Patients continue experiencing polyarticular involvement during subacute disease, and apparently, the progression to subacute illness is a good indicator of progression to chronic disease (RR = 5.208; 95%CI 2.51–10.797) [77]. The chronic disease is characterized by articular manifestations like joint pain, stiffness, or swelling that persist continuously or recurrently after 3 months of acute phase onset [78]. However, other causes of chronic articular pain like inflammatory rheumatic diseases (rheumatoid arthritis, ankylosing spondyloarthritis, psoriatic rheumatism), gout or osteoarthritis should be ruled out [78].

Although most studies have centred on the characterization of rheumatologic involvement, evidence suggests that the spectrum of chronic disease is broader than expected. Evidence from different locations shows that the patient can develop mental health impairment with anxiety, depression and detriment to their quality of life—other plausible chronic derived sequelae with implications for the long-term.

14.7 Laboratory Diagnosis

Specific etiological diagnosis of CHIKV, during acute and non-acute phases, is mainly rendered in serological tests, such as ELISA, looking for IgG and IgM against CHIKV. During the acute phase, in the first week, molecular tools, including PCR, can be performed to detect the RNA of the virus. Molecular assays previously described for CHIKV and other alphaviruses require further evaluation, standardized protocols and the availability of international standards representing the genetic diversity of the viruses [79]. Detection of specific IgM would benefit from further investigations to clarify the extent of cross-reactivity of CHIKV with

O'nyong-nyong (ONNV) and Mayaro virus (MAYV) [79, 80], the sensitivity of the assays, and the possible interfering role of cryoglobulinemia. Implementation of reference panels and external quality assessments for both molecular and serological assays is necessary.

Regarding seroepidemiological studies, no reported high-throughput assay can distinguish among these different viruses in areas of potential co-circulation. New specific tools and improved standardized protocols are needed to enable large-scale epidemiological studies of public health relevance to be performed. Considering the high risk of future CHIKV, MAYV and ONNV outbreaks, the GloPID-R (Global Research Collaboration for Infectious Disease Preparedness) Chikungunya (CHIKV), O'nyong-nyong (ONNV) and Mayaro virus (MAYV) Working Group recommend that a major investigation should be initiated to fill the existing diagnostic gaps [79, 81–83].

14.8 Differential Diagnosis

The initial differential diagnosis includes other arboviruses, such as dengue, Zika and Mayaro [84–86]. These four arboviruses clinically overlap (ChikDenMaZika) and should be considered between them in the differential diagnosis [84], but also co-infections between them occur, even with triple coinfections (CHIKV-DENV-ZIKV), as has been especially reported in Colombia [87–91]. Coinfections with other tropical agents should also be considered, as well as in the differential diagnosis, e.g. leptospirosis [92]. Other viruses, depending on the geographic place [93, 94], should be considered and include West Nile fever (e.g. the United States and Europe), Adenovirus infection, O'nyong-nyong fever, Ross River fever (e.g. Australia), Sindbis fever (e.g. Europe, Africa), Crimean-Congo fever, Bussuquara fever, Ebola fever, Hantavirus infection, Kyasanur Forest disease (e.g. India), Lassa fever (e.g. Africa), Rubella (e.g. Venezuela), Parvovirus B19 infection, Hepatitis B, Mumps, Infection with herpes viruses. Other differential diagnoses include malaria, Rickettsial infections, gonococcemia, postinfectious reactive arthritis, and group A streptococcal infection. During the COVID-19 pandemic, infection due to SARS-CoV-2 in endemic areas was also a differential diagnosis.

14.9 Treatment

Management of CHIKV is directly depending on the phase of the disease as well as the degree of severity. In recent years, the expert group in France have developed guidelines for CHIKV in the acute and non-acute phases [95]. Also, in Brazil, the Brazilian Society of Rheumatology has recently developed recommendations for diagnosing and treating chikungunya fever [96].

14.10 Prevention

As the CDC recommends, travelers to endemic areas should select accommodations with well-screened windows and doors or air conditioning when possible. *Aedes* mosquitoes typically live indoors and often are found in dark, cool places (e.g. in closets, under beds, behind curtains, in bathrooms, and on porches). Wear clothing that covers the arms and legs, especially during the early morning and late afternoon, when the risk of being bitten by *Aedes* species mosquitoes is most remarkable. The use of insect repellent is also relevant. For longer-term travelers, empty and clean or cover any standing water that can be a mosquito-breeding site in the local residence (e.g. water storage tanks, flowerpots) (https://wwwnc.cdc.gov/travel/yellowbook/2024/).

14.11 Advice for Travellers

14.11.1 General Advice

As with other endemic diseases, especially vector-borne diseases, it is critical to pre-travel advice and plan according to all the travel conditions (e.g. places to be visited, time, specific risk, individual condition and travellers' health, among others) and appropriate preventive measures. When available, vaccines against CHIKV would probably be helpful for infection and other associated outcomes prevention. In 2023 a candidate at phase 3 (VLA1553) showed promising results with a robust immune response and the generation of seroprotective titers in almost all vaccinated participants, suggesting that the vaccine is an excellent candidate for disease prevention [97]. VLA1553 is a live-attenuated vaccine [98].

14.11.2 Specific Advice for Healthcare Workers

Healthcare workers should consider CHIKV in all febrile patients and those presenting CHIKV-related symptoms from endemic areas. Searching reports and epidemiology at updated sites like ProMEDmail.org is highly recommended. Consider appropriate diagnostic tests, including PCR and serology, according to the time of disease.

14.11.3 Specific Advice for Special People (e.g. Pregnant, Immunocompromised)

CHIKV is relevant for pregnant women, as it impacts the evolution and outcome across the gestational period, especially perinatal [6, 91, 99]. CHIKV may cause congenital infection [6, 99]. Then pregnant women should avoid exposure. There is little information regarding immunosuppression's impact on CHIKV infection [100]. However, some data suggest that CHIKV may induce cellular immunosuppression and an increased risk for secondary infections, especially respiratory [100, 101]. A recent study indicates that among HIV-treated populations, CHIKV had no significant impact on associated disease [102]. Among patients with diabetes, CHIKV infection has a significant negative effect on glycemic control and, compared with non-diabetic patients, results in more considerable morbidity. Close clinical and glycemic observation is recommended in patients with diabetes concurrently with CHIKV infection [103].

Box 14.1: Key Websites for Travellers and Healthcare Workers About CHIKV
ProMEDmail: http://www.promedmail.org/
    CDC Yellow Book 2024: https://wwwnc.cdc.gov/travel/yellowbook/2024/
    International Society for Travel Medicine: https://www.istm.org/
    Latin American Society for Travel Medicine: https://www.slamvi.org/

Box 14.2: Things Commonly Forgotten About CHIKV
- Patients exposed to the risk for CHIKV are simultaneously at risk for other arboviral diseases, such as DENV, ZIKV, if in urban areas, but even to yellow fever, Mayaro and arboviral encephalitis, if in rural areas in Latin America, Africa and/or Asia. But also for other non-viral vector-borne diseases and in general tropical diseases, many ecoepidemiological conditions are shared with CHIKV.
- In non-less than 25%, but even in 50%, of patients exposed to infection, there is a risk of chronic disease associated with CHIKV, which mainly affects joints, and in general with rheumatological consequences, but also with non-rheumatological consequences, that should be considered, and approached in a multidisciplinary way.
- Also, in connection to that, in travellers to endemic areas, returning to non-endemic areas, this exposure would lead to chronic disease. Then, in travellers without fever but with continuous or recurrent joint pain, edema and rigidity lasting more than 3 months, CHIKV should be considered a differential diagnosis and serological tests should be performed (IgG). PCR is recommended to confirm acute infection during the first 7–10 days of disease.

Declarations of Conflict of Interest AJRM has been a speaker/consultant for Sanofi, MSD, and Valneva in connection with emerging diseases and CHIKV. The rest of the authors have no conflict of interest.

References

1. Musso D, Rodriguez-Morales AJ, Levi JE, Cao-Lormeau VM, Gubler DJ. Unexpected outbreaks of arbovirus infections: lessons learned from the Pacific and tropical America. Lancet Infect Dis. 2018;18:e355–e61.
2. Renault P, Balleydier E, D'Ortenzio E, Baville M, Filleul L. Epidemiology of Chikungunya infection on Reunion Island, Mayotte, and neighboring countries. Med Mal Infect. 2012;42:93–101.
3. Rodríguez-Morales AJ, Simon F. Chronic Chikungunya, still to be fully understood. Int J Infect Dis. 2019;86:133–4.
4. Borgherini G, Poubeau P, Staikowsky F, Lory M, Le Moullec N, Becquart JP, et al. Outbreak of Chikungunya on Reunion Island: early clinical and laboratory features in 157 adult patients. Clin Infect Dis. 2007;44:1401–7.
5. Sergon K, Njuguna C, Kalani R, Ofula V, et al. Seroprevalence of Chikungunya Virus (CHIKV) infection on Lamu Island, Kenya, October 2004. Am Soc Trop Med Hyg. 2008;78:333–7.
6. Villamil-Gómez W, Alba-Silvera L, Menco-Ramos A, Gonzalez-Vergara A, Molinares-Palacios T, Barrios-Corrales M, et al. Congenital Chikungunya virus infection in Sincelejo, Colombia: a case series. J Trop Pediatr. 2015;61:386–92.
7. Yang CF, Su CL, Hsu TC, Chang SF, Lin CC, Huang JC, et al. Imported Chikungunya virus strains, Taiwan, 2006–2014. Emerg Infect Dis. 2016;22:1981–4.
8. Liumbruno GMCD, Petropulacos K, Mattivi A, Po C, Macini P, Tomasini I, Zucchelli P, Silvestri AR, Sambri V, Pupella S, Catalano L, Piccinini V, Calizzani G, Grazzini G, Liumbruno GM, Calteri D, Petropulacos K, Mattivi A, Po C, Macini P, Tomasini I, Zucchelli P, Silvestri AR, Sambri V, Pupella S, Catalano L, Piccinini V, Calizzani G, Grazzini G. Blood Transfus. 2008;6:199–210.
9. Delisle E, Rousseau C, Broche B, Leparc-Goffart I, L'Ambert G, Cochet A, et al. Chikungunya outbreak in Montpellier, France, September to October 2014. Euro Surveill. 2015;20(17):21108.
10. Calba C, Guerbois-Galla M, Franke F, Jeannin C, Auzet-Caillaud M, Grard G, et al. Preliminary report of an autochthonous chikungunya outbreak in France, July to September 2017. Euro Surveill. 2017;22:17-00647.
11. Roiz D, Bousses P, Simard F, Paupy C, Fontenille D. Autochthonous Chikungunya transmission and extreme climate events in southern France. PLoS Negl Trop Dis. 2015;9:e0003854.
12. Rossi B, Barreca F, Benvenuto D, Braccialarghe N, Campogiani L, Lodi A, et al. Human arboviral infections in Italy: past, current, and future challenges. Viruses. 2023:15.
13. Gossner CM, Hallmaier-Wacker L, Briet O, Haussig JM, de Valk H, Wijermans A, et al. Arthropod-borne diseases among travellers arriving in Europe from Africa, 2015–2019. Euro Surveill. 2023;28:2200270.
14. Trojánek M, Grebenyuk V, Manďáková Z, Sojková N, Zelená H, Roháčová H, et al. Epidemiology of dengue, chikungunya and Zika virus infections in travellers: a 16-year retrospective descriptive study at a tertiary care centre in Prague, Czech Republic. PLoS One. 2023;18:e0281612.
15. Yactayo S, Staples JE, Millot V, Cibrelus L, Ramon-Pardo P. Epidemiology of Chikungunya in the Americas. J Infect Dis. 2016;214:S441–S45.
16. Cardona-Ospina JA, Diaz-Quijano FA, Rodriguez-Morales AJ. Burden of Chikungunya in Latin American countries: estimates of disability-adjusted life-years (DALY) lost in the 2014 epidemic. Int J Infect Dis. 2015;38:60–1.
17. Cardona-Ospina JA, Henao-SanMartin V, Paniz-Mondolfi AE, Rodriguez-Morales AJ. Mortality and fatality due to Chikungunya virus infection in Colombia. J Clin Virol. 2015;70:14–5.
18. Cardona-Ospina JA, Rodriguez-Morales AJ, Villamil-Gomez WE. The burden of Chikungunya in one coastal department of Colombia (Sucre): estimates of the disability adjusted life years (DALY) lost in the 2014 epidemic. J Infect Public Health. 2015;8:644–6.

19. Cardona-Ospina JA, Villamil-Gomez WE, Jimenez-Canizales CE, Castaneda-Hernandez DM, Rodriguez-Morales AJ. Estimating the burden of disease and the economic cost attributable to Chikungunya, Colombia, 2014. Trans R Soc Trop Med Hyg. 2015;109:793–802.

20. Rodriguez-Morales AJ, Cardona-Ospina JA, Villamil-Gomez W, Paniz-Mondolfi AE. How many patients with post-chikungunya chronic inflammatory rheumatism can we expect in the new endemic areas of Latin America? Rheumatol Int. 2015;35:2091–4.

21. Villero-Wolf Y, Mattar S, Puerta-Gonzalez A, Arrieta G, Muskus C, Hoyos R, et al. Genomic epidemiology of Chikungunya virus in Colombia reveals genetic variability of strains and multiple geographic introductions in outbreak, 2014. Sci Rep. 2019;9:9970.

22. Zambrano LI, Rodriguez E, Espinoza-Salvado IA, Rodriguez-Morales AJ. Dengue in Honduras and the Americas: the epidemics are back! Travel Med Infect Dis. 2019;31:101456.

23. Cardona-Ospina JA, Trujillo AM, Jiménez-Posada EV, Sepúlveda-Arias JC, Tabares-Villa FA, Altieri-Rivera JS, et al. Susceptibility to endemic Aedes-borne viruses among pregnant women in Risaralda, Colombia. Int J Infect Dis. 2022;122:832–40.

24. Rodriguez-Morales AJ, Gil-Restrepo AF, Ramirez-Jaramillo V, Montoya-Arias CP, Acevedo-Mendoza WF, Bedoya-Arias JE, et al. Post-chikungunya chronic inflammatory rheumatism: results from a retrospective follow-up study of 283 adult and child cases in La Virginia, Risaralda, Colombia. F1000Res. 2016;5:360.

25. Cardona-Ospina JA, Jiménez-Canizales CE, Vásquez-Serna H, Garzón-Ramírez JA, Alarcón-Robayo JF, Cerón-Pineda JA, et al. Fatal dengue, chikungunya and leptospirosis: the importance of assessing coinfections in febrile patients in tropical areas. Trop Med Infect Dis. 2018;3(4):123.

26. Rodriguez-Morales AJ, Hernandez-Moncada AM, Hoyos-Guapacha KL, Vargas-Zapata SL, Sanchez-Zapata JF, Mejia-Bernal YV, et al. Potential relationships between Chikungunya and depression: solving the puzzle with key cytokines. Cytokine. 2018;102:161–2.

27. Delgado de la Mora J, Licona-Enriquez JD, Alvarez-Hernandez G. Brote de Chikungunya en el estado de Sonora. El problema de las enfermedades febriles exantemáticas en regiones de clima seco. Salud Publica Mex. 2017;59:127.

28. Rodriguez-Morales AJ, Restrepo-Posada VM, Acevedo-Escalante N, Rodriguez-Munoz ED, Valencia-Marin M, Castrillon-Spitia JD, et al. Impaired quality of life after chikungunya virus infection: a 12-month follow-up study of its chronic inflammatory rheumatism in La Virginia, Risaralda, Colombia. Rheumatol Int. 2017;37:1757–8.

29. Soumahoro MK, Boelle PY, Gauzere BA, Atsou K, Pelat C, Lambert B, et al. The Chikungunya epidemic on La Reunion Island in 2005-2006: a cost-of-illness study. PLoS Negl Trop Dis. 2011;5:e1197.

30. Rezza G, Weaver SC. Chikungunya as a paradigm for emerging viral diseases: evaluating disease impact and hurdles to vaccine development. PLoS Negl Trop Dis. 2019;13:e0006919.

31. Costa LB, Barreto FKA, Barreto MCA, Santos T, Andrade MMO, Farias L, et al. Epidemiology and economic Burden of Chikungunya: a systematic literature review. Trop Med Infect Dis. 2023;8(6):301.

32. Durich JO. Enfermedades emergentes y reemergentes: algunas causas y ejemplos. Med Int. 2000;36:79–82.

33. Maguiña-Vargas C. Fiebre de Chikungunya: Una nueva enfermedad emergente de gran impacto en la salud pública. Rev Méd Herediana. 2015;26:55–9.

34. Saydam FN, Erdem H, Ankarali H, El-Arab Ramadan ME, El-Sayed NM, Civljak R, et al. Vector-borne and zoonotic infections and their relationships with regional and socioeconomic statuses: an ID-IRI survey in 24 countries of Europe, Africa and Asia. Travel Med Infect Dis. 2021;44:102174.

35. Mohan A, Kiran DH, Manohar IC, Kumar DP. Epidemiology, clinical manifestations, and diagnosis of Chikungunya fever: lessons learned from the reemerging epidemic. Indian J Dermatol. 2010;55:54–63.

36. Morrison CR, Plante KS, Heise MT. Chikungunya virus: current perspectives on a reemerging virus. Microbiol Spectr. 2016;10:143–61.

37. Begum MM, Ulvi O, Karamehic-Muratovic A, Walsh MR, Tarek H, Lubinda J, et al. Quantifying media effects, its content, and role in promoting community awareness of Chikungunya epidemic in Bangladesh. Epidemiologia (Basel, Switzerland). 2021;2:84–94.

38. Organización Panamericana de la Salud CfDCaP. Preparación y respuesta ante la eventual introducción del virus chikungunya en las Américas, Washington DC; 2011.

39. Organización Mundial de la Salud (OMS) OPdlSO. Chikungunya; 2017.

40. Wahid B, Ali A, Rafique S, Idrees M. Global expansion of chikungunya virus: mapping the 64-year history. Int J Infect Dis. 2017;58:69–76.

41. Colombiana MS. Curso virtual en enfermedades transmitidas por vectores. Iladiba ed; 2015.

42. Sharp TM, Lorenzi O, Torres-Velasquez B, Acevedo V, Perez-Padilla J, Rivera A, et al. Autocidal gravid ovitraps protect humans from chikungunya virus infection by reducing Aedes aegypti mosquito populations. PLoS Negl Trop Dis. 2019;13:e0007538.

43. Outammassine A, Zouhair S, Loqman S. Global potential distribution of three underappreciated arboviruses vectors (Aedes japonicus, Aedes vexans and Aedes vittatus) under current and future climate conditions. Transbound Emerg Dis. 2022;69:e1160–e71.

44. Yee DA, Reyes-Torres LJ, Dean C, Scavo NA, Zavortink TJ. Mosquitoes (Diptera: Culicidae) on the islands of Puerto Rico and Vieques, U.S.A. Acta Trop. 2021;220:105959.

45. Pagac BB, Spring AR, Stawicki JR, Dinh TL, Lura T, Kavanaugh MD, et al. Incursion and establishment of the Old World arbovirus vector Aedes (Fredwardsius) vittatus (Bigot, 1861) in the Americas. Acta Trop. 2021;213:105739.

46. Alarcón-Elbal PM, Rodríguez-Sosa MA, Newman BC, Sutton WB. The First Record of Aedes vittatus (Diptera: Culicidae) in the Dominican Republic: Public Health Implications of a Potential Invasive Mosquito Species in the Americas. J Med Entomol. 2020;57:2016–21.

47. Gardner J, Rudd PA, Prow NA, Belarbi E, Roques P, Larcher T, et al. Infectious Chikungunya virus in the saliva of mice, monkeys and humans. PLoS One. 2015;10:e0139481.

48. Rolph MS, Zaid A, Mahalingam S. Salivary Transmission of the Chikungunya Arbovirus. Trends Microbiol. 2016;24:86–7.

49. Vasani R, Kanhere S, Chaudhari K, Phadke V, Mukherjee P, Gupta S, et al. Congenital Chikungunya—a cause of neonatal hyperpigmentation. Pediatr Dermatol. 2016;33(2):209–12.

50. Fritel X, Rollot O, Gerardin P, Gauzere BA, Bideault J, Lagarde L, et al. Chikungunya virus infection during pregnancy, reunion, France, 2006. Emerg Infect Dis. 2010;16:418–25.

51. Gerardin P, Samperiz S, Ramful D, Boumahni B, Bintner M, Alessandri JL, et al. Neurocognitive outcome of children exposed to perinatal mother-to-child Chikungunya virus infection: the CHIMERE cohort study on Reunion Island. PLoS Negl Trop Dis. 2014;8:e2996.

52. (WHO) WHO. 2019.

53. Ekchariyawat P, Hamel R, Bernard E, Wichit S, Surasombatpattana P, Talignani L, et al. Inflammasome signaling pathways exert antiviral effect against Chikungunya virus in human dermal fibroblasts. Infect Genet Evol. 2015;32:401–8.

54. Schilte C, Buckwalter MR, Laird ME, Diamond MS, Schwartz O, Albert ML. Cutting edge: independent roles for IRF-3 and IRF-7 in hematopoietic and nonhematopoietic cells during host response to Chikungunya infection. J Immunol. 2012;188:2967–71.

55. Gardner J, Anraku I, Le TT, Larcher T, Major L, Roques P, et al. Chikungunya virus arthritis in adult wild-type mice. J Virol. 2010;84:8021–32.

56. Poo YS, Nakaya H, Gardner J, Larcher T, Schroder WA, Le TT, et al. CCR2 deficiency promotes exacerbated chronic erosive neutrophil-dominated chikungunya virus arthritis. J Virol. 2014;88:6862–72.

57. Restrepo Jaramillo BN. Infección por el virus del Chikungunya. Rev CES Med. 2014;28:313–23.

58. Martínez Fernández L, Torrado Navarro YP. Fiebre Chikungunya. Rev Cubana Med. 2015;54:74–96.

59. Hoarau JJ, Jaffar Bandjee MC, Krejbich Trotot P, Das T, Li-Pat-Yuen G, Dassa B, et al. Persistent chronic inflammation and infection by Chikungunya arthritogenic alphavirus in spite of a robust host immune response. J Immunol. 2010;184:5914–27.

60. Ozden S, Huerre M, Riviere JP, Coffey LL, Afonso PV, Mouly V, et al. Human muscle satellite cells as targets of Chikungunya virus infection. PLoS One. 2007;2:e527.
61. Herrero LJ, Taylor A, Wolf S, Mahalingam S. Arthropod-borne arthritides. Best Pract Res Clin Rheumatol. 2015;29(2):259–74.
62. Labadie K, Larcher T, Joubert C, Mannioui A, Delache B, Brochard P, et al. Chikungunya disease in nonhuman primates involves long-term viral persistence in macrophages. J Clin Invest. 2010;120:894–906.
63. Her Z, Malleret B, Chan M, Ong EK, Wong SC, Kwek DJ, et al. Active infection of human blood monocytes by Chikungunya virus triggers an innate immune response. J Immunol. 2010;184:5903–13.
64. Chen W, Foo SS, Taylor A, Lulla A, Merits A, Hueston L, et al. Bindarit, an inhibitor of monocyte chemotactic protein synthesis, protects against bone loss induced by chikungunya virus infection. J Virol. 2015;89:581–93.
65. Kam YW, Simarmata D, Chow A, Her Z, Teng TS, Ong EK, et al. Early appearance of neutralizing immunoglobulin G3 antibodies is associated with chikungunya virus clearance and long-term clinical protection. J Infect Dis. 2012;205:1147–54.
66. Miner JJ, Aw-Yeang HX, Fox JM, Taffner S, Malkova ON, Oh ST, et al. Chikungunya viral arthritis in the United States: a mimic of seronegative rheumatoid arthritis. Arthritis Rheumatol. 2015;67:1214–20.
67. Dias CNS, Gois BM, Lima VS, Guerra-Gomes IC, Araujo JMG, Gomes JAS, et al. Human CD8 T-cell activation in acute and chronic chikungunya infection. Immunology. 2018;155:499–504.
68. Kulkarni SP, Ganu M, Jayawant P, Thanapati S, Ganu A, Tripathy AS. Regulatory T cells and IL-10 as modulators of chikungunya disease outcome: a preliminary study. Eur J Clin Microbiol Infect Dis. 2017;36:2475–81.
69. Economopoulou A, Dominguez M, Helynck B, Sissoko D, Wichmann O, Quenel P, et al. Atypical Chikungunya virus infections: clinical manifestations, mortality and risk factors for severe disease during the 2005-2006 outbreak on Reunion. Epidemiol Infect. 2009;137:534–41.
70. de la Hoz JM, Bayona B, Viloria S, Accini JL, Juan-Vergara HS, Viasus D. Fatal cases of Chikungunya virus infection in Colombia: diagnostic and treatment challenges. J Clin Virol. 2015;69:27–9.
71. Torres JR, Cordova LG, Saravia V, Arvelaez J, Castro JS. Nasal skin necrosis: an unexpected new finding in severe Chikungunya fever. Clin Infect Dis. 2016;62(1):78–81.
72. Lebrun G, Chadda K, Reboux AH, Martinet O, Gauzere BA. Guillain-Barre syndrome after chikungunya infection. Emerg Infect Dis. 2009;15:495–6.
73. Villamil-Gomez W, Silvera LA, Paez-Castellanos J, Rodriguez-Morales AJ. Guillain-Barre syndrome after Chikungunya infection: a case in Colombia. Enfermedades Infecciosas Microbiol Clin. 2016;34:140–1.
74. Oehler E, Fournier E, Leparc-Goffart I, Larre P, Cubizolle S, Sookhareea C, et al. Increase in cases of Guillain-Barre syndrome during a Chikungunya outbreak, French Polynesia, 2014–2015. Euro Surveill. 2015:20.
75. Mahendradas P, Avadhani K, Shetty R. Chikungunya and the eye: a review. J Ophthal Inflam Infect. 2013;3:35.
76. Rodriguez-Morales AJ, Hoyos-Guapacha KL, Botero-Castano G, Aroca-Gomez KD, Imbacuan-Unigarro JL, Guinchin D, et al. Baseline risk factors associated with the development of one and two years post-Chikungunya chronic inflammatory rheumatism, La Virginia, Risaralda, Colombia, 2015–2017. Int J Infect Dis. 2018;73:194–5.
77. Rodriguez-Morales AJ, Ochoa-Orozco SA, Ocampo-Serna S, Meneses-Quintero OM, Sanchez-Castano DM, Hoyos-Guapacha KL, et al. Subacute disease (3-to-11 weeks) predicts post-Chikungunya chronic inflammatory rheumatism (>12 weeks): findings of an ambispective cohort in La Virginia, Risaralda, Colombia. Int J Infect Dis. 2018;73:168–9.

78. Cardona-Ospina JA, Rodriguez-Morales AJ, Teixeira MG, Gerardin P. Need for accurate and consistent definition of chronic Chikungunya arthritis: comment on the article by Chang et al. Arthritis Rheumatol. 2018;70:1891.

79. Pezzi L, Reusken CB, Weaver SC, Drexler JF, Busch M, LaBeaud AD, et al. GloPID-R report on Chikungunya, O'nyong-nyong and Mayaro virus, part I: Biological diagnostics. Antivir Res. 2019;166:66–81.

80. Arenivar C, Rodriguez Y, Rodriguez-Morales AJ, Anaya JM. Osteoarticular manifestations of Mayaro virus infection. Curr Opin Rheumatol. 2019;31:512–6.

81. Pezzi L, LaBeaud AD, Reusken CB, Drexler JF, Vasilakis N, Diallo M, et al. GloPID-R report on chikungunya, o'nyong-nyong and Mayaro virus, Part 2: Epidemiological distribution of o'nyong-nyong virus. Antivir Res. 2019;172:104611.

82. Pezzi L, Rodriguez-Morales AJ, Reusken CB, Ribeiro GS, LaBeaud AD, Lourenço-de-Oliveira R, et al. GloPID-R report on chikungunya, o'nyong-nyong and Mayaro virus, Part 3: Epidemiological distribution of Mayaro virus. Antivir Res. 2019;172:104610.

83. Pezzi L, Diallo M, Rosa-Freitas MG, Vega-Rua A, Ng LFP, Boyer S, et al. GloPID-R report on chikungunya, o'nyong-nyong and Mayaro virus, Part 5: Entomological aspects. Antivir Res. 2020;174:104670.

84. Paniz-Mondolfi AE, Rodriguez-Morales AJ, Blohm G, Marquez M, Villamil-Gomez WE. ChikDenMaZika Syndrome: the challenge of diagnosing arboviral infections in the midst of concurrent epidemics. Ann Clin Microbiol Antimicrob. 2016;15:42.

85. Zambrano LI, Rodriguez E, Espinoza-Salvado IA, Fuentes-Barahona IC, Lyra de Oliveira T, Luciano da Veiga G, et al. Spatial distribution of dengue in Honduras during 2016–2019 using a geographic information systems (GIS)-Dengue epidemic implications for public health and travel medicine. Travel Med Infect Dis. 2019;32:101517.

86. Bonilla-Aldana DK, Bonilla-Aldana JL, García-Bustos JJ, Lozada CO, Rodríguez-Morales AJ. Geographical trends of Chikungunya and Zika in the Colombian Amazonian gateway department, Caqueta, 2015–2018—implications for public health and travel medicine. Travel Med Infect Dis. 2020;35:101481.

87. Carrillo-Hernandez MY, Ruiz-Saenz J, Villamizar LJ, Gomez-Rangel SY, Martinez-Gutierrez M. Co-circulation and simultaneous coinfection of dengue, Chikungunya, and zika viruses in patients with febrile syndrome at the Colombian-Venezuelan border. BMC Infect Dis. 2018;18:61.

88. Mercado-Reyes M, Acosta-Reyes J, Navarro-Lechuga E, Corchuelo S, Rico A, Parra E, et al. Dengue, chikungunya and zika virus coinfection: results of the national surveillance during the zika epidemic in Colombia. Epidemiol Infect. 2019;147:e77.

89. Rodriguez-Morales AJ, Villamil-Gomez WE, Franco-Paredes C. The arboviral burden of disease caused by co-circulation and coinfection of dengue, Chikungunya and Zika in the Americas. Travel Med Infect Dis. 2016;14:177–9.

90. Villamil-Gomez WE, Gonzalez-Camargo O, Rodriguez-Ayubi J, Zapata-Serpa D, Rodriguez-Morales AJ. Dengue, Chikungunya and Zika co-infection in a patient from Colombia. J Infect Public Health. 2016;9:684–6.

91. Villamil-Gómez WE, Rodríguez-Morales AJ, Uribe-García AM, González-Arismendy E, Castellanos JE, Calvo EP, et al. Zika, dengue, and chikungunya co-infection in a pregnant woman from Colombia. Int J Infect Dis. 2016;51:135–8.

92. Cardona-Ospina JA, Jimenez-Canizales CE, Vasquez-Serna H, Garzon-Ramirez JA, Alarcon-Robayo JF, Ceron-Pineda JA, et al. Fatal dengue, Chikungunya and leptospirosis: the importance of assessing coinfections in febrile patients in tropical areas. Trop Med Infect Dis. 2018;3:123.

93. Lutwick LI, Rodriguez-Morales AJ. Central America. Infect Dis. 2017:317–34.

94. Nogueira Angerami R, Jacintho da Silva L, Rodriguez-Morales AJ. South America. Infect Dis. 2017:335–55.

95. Simon F, Javelle E, Cabie A, Bouquillard E, Troisgros O, Gentile G, et al. French guidelines for the management of Chikungunya (acute and persistent presentations). November 2014. Med Mal Infect. 2015;45:243–63.

96. Marques CDL, Duarte A, Ranzolin A, Dantas AT, Cavalcanti NG, Goncalves RSG, et al. Recommendations of the Brazilian Society of Rheumatology for the diagnosis and treatment of chikungunya fever. Part 2—Treatment. Rev Bras Reumatol Engl Ed. 2017;57(Suppl. 2):438–51.

97. Schneider M, Narciso-Abraham M, Hadl S, McMahon R, Toepfer S, Fuchs U, et al. Safety and immunogenicity of a single-shot live-attenuated chikungunya vaccine: a double-blind, multicentre, randomised, placebo-controlled, phase 3 trial. Lancet (London, England). 2023;401:2138–47.

98. Stephenson KE. Live-attenuated Chikungunya vaccine: a possible new era. Lancet (London, England). 2023;401:2090–1.

99. Alvarado-Socarras JL, Ocampo-González M, Vargas-Soler JA, Rodriguez-Morales AJ, Franco-Paredes C. Congenital and neonatal Chikungunya in Colombia. J Pediatr Infect Dis Soc. 2016;5:e17–20.

100. Ríos L, Rodriguez-Morales AJ, Castrillón-Spitia JD, Henao-SanMartin V, Londoño JJ, Bedoya-Rendón HD, et al. Chikungunya virus infection, immunosuppression and respiratory tract infections: are they associated? Int Marit Health. 2018;69:149–50.

101. Jaller Raad J, Segura Rosero A, Vidal Martínez J, Parody A, Jaller Raad R, Caballero Tovar D, et al. Respuesta inmunitaria de una población del Caribe colombiano infectada con el virus chikungunya. Rev Colomb Reumatol. 2016;23:85–91.

102. Pircher M, Pitono E, Pierre-François S, Molcard S, Brunier-Agot L, Fagour L, et al. The effects of chikungunya virus infection on people living with HIV during the 2014 Martinique outbreak. PLoS One. 2020;15:e0234267.

103. Jean-Baptiste E, von Oettingen J, Larco P, Raphaël F, Larco NC, Cauvin MM, et al. Chikungunya virus infection and diabetes mellitus: a double negative impact. Am J Trop Med Hyg. 2016;95:1345–50.

Dengue in Travellers

15

Huynh Trung Trieu, Angela McBride, and Sophie Yacoub

Abstract

Dengue is the most common arboviral infection in humans. It is transmitted by infected Aedes mosquitos. Dengue transmission occurs in over 100 countries, and around 400 million people are infected annually. It is spreading rapidly to new regions due to global warming and urbanization. There are four different dengue serotypes, and there is no lasting cross-serotype immunity after infection. Approximately 80% of infections are asymptomatic, but symptoms include fever, muscle pain, abdominal pain, nausea, vomiting, and bleeding. Severe complications include shock, respiratory distress, severe bleeding, and multi-organ failure due to plasma leakage and impaired coagulation. Severe complications typically occur between days 3 and 7 of the illness and are often preceded by warning signs; mortality is about 5% of those with severe dengue. Children and adults infected with dengue have some phenotypic differences in clinical manifestations and complications. Risk factors for severe illness include secondary infection with a different dengue serotype, younger age/elderly, obesity, diabetes, and other chronic comorbidities. Dengue can be diagnosed early using the NS1 antigen rapid test, or PCR tests; after

H. T. Trieu (✉)
Paediatric Intensive Care Unit, Hospital for Tropical Diseases, Ho Chi Minh City, Vietnam
e-mail: trieuht@oucru.org

A. McBride
Oxford University Clinical Research Unit, Ho Chi Minh City, Vietnam

Department of Global Health and Infection, Brighton and Sussex Medical School, Brighton, UK
e-mail: amcbride@oucru.org

S. Yacoub
Oxford University Clinical Research Unit, Ho Chi Minh City, Vietnam
e-mail: syacoub@oucru.org

H. Leblebicioglu et al. (eds.), *Emerging and Re-emerging Infections in Travellers*, https://doi.org/10.1007/978-3-031-49475-8_15

day 5 of illness, these tests may be falsely negative and paired serology can be used to confirm diagnosis. There is no specific treatment for dengue, the main management is supportive care. Intravenous fluids should be administered judiciously during plasma leak and stopped promptly once no longer necessary. Recently, TAK-003 has become the first vaccine to be approved by the European Commission for individuals above 4 years of age, regardless of previous dengue exposure.

15.1 Background

15.1.1 Brief History

When Was the First Dengue Case Reported?

There are many different theories on the origins of dengue. A dengue-like illness was first recorded in a Chinese medical encyclopaedia from the Jin Dynasty (265-420 AD), and later in the Tang Dynasty (610 AD), and the Northern Sung Dynasty (992 AD) [1]. The disease was described as a "water poison" and was said to be associated with flying insects. Probable dengue outbreaks were later described in the West Indies in 1635 and in Panama in 1699. A dengue-like illness was given the name "breakbone fever" in 1789 by Benjamin Rush, describing an outbreak in Philadelphia in the 1780s, and soon afterward similar epidemics were reported across Asia, Africa, and North America [1].

Why Is the Disease Named Dengue?

The name dengue is thought to derive from the Swahili phrase "Ka-dinga pepo" which means "cramp-like seizure caused by an evil spirit"—the word "dinga" describes the gait of a person with bone pain. Later the disease was known as "Dandy Fever", taken from a description of slaves in the West Indies who contracted dengue and had the posture of a dandy during the St Thomas epidemic in 1827 [2]. The first use of the name "dengue" was in Spain in 1802. Subsequently, during an 1828 epidemic of dunga in Cuba, the Spanish recognized the similarity to dengue in Spain, and changed the name dunga to dengue [1].

15.1.2 Importance of the Disease

Why Is Dengue an Important Infectious Disease?

Estimation of the global burden of dengue is difficult because around 80% of those infected are thought to be asymptomatic; amongst the remainder of patients the range of clinical manifestations is broad and differentiation from other febrile illnesses is challenging, especially where rapid diagnostic tests are not widely available. Despite this, it has been estimated that 3.9 billion people across 129 countries are at risk of dengue infection [3]. One modelling study estimated that 390 million dengue infections occur annually, of which 96 million manifest clinical symptoms [4] and about 4% of symptomatic cases require hospital admission [5].

In addition to the massive burden on public health services, the economic impact of dengue is substantial. A study merging healthcare cost data from 108 countries with information on 95 million symptomatic cases found that 60% of dengue cases occurred in countries with GDP per capita below 6000 USD. The global cost for reduced productivity, premature death and healthcare utilization related to dengue was 39.3 billion USD or about 414 USD per case (18.5 billion USD for productivity loss, 11.1 billion USD for premature death and 9.8 billion USD for healthcare utilization). About 40% of the total costs were incurred in South East Asia, 24.7% in the Americas, 21.6% in the Western Pacific Region, 5.9% in Africa and 6.1% in the Eastern Mediterranean Region [6].

15.1.3 Why It Is Classified as Emerging and/or Re-emerging

According to recent WHO figures, the number of reported dengue cases increased more than eightfold over two decades, from 505,430 in 2010 to 4.2 million in 2019. The number of fatal cases also increased, from 960 reported deaths in 2000–4032 in 2015. Among the WHO's six geographical regions it is estimated that more than 70% of the world's at-risk population for dengue live in the Western Pacific and South-East Asia Regions. India alone accounts for 34% of the total, while the Americas and Africa contribute 14% and 16% of the total respectively [4].

Not only is the incidence of dengue infection high in these regions, dengue is also spreading rapidly to new regions. Before 1970, dengue epidemics were only reported in nine countries in South-East Asia and the Western Pacific. Dengue is now reported from more than 100 countries worldwide, including several European nations. Imported cases and local transmission have been described in France, Croatia, Portugal and 10 other European countries [7]. In 2019, alongside the highest reported number of dengue infections ever from a global perspective, dengue cases were reported from Afghanistan for the first time [7]. Thus the geographical reach of dengue continues to expand globally, with the overall footprint now encompassing much of the tropics and subtropics. Further expansion of the mosquito vector, and thus disease occurrence, is predicted [8], especially in light of changing climate/environmental factors.

15.2 Aetiology

15.2.1 Transmission

How Does Dengue Transmit Rapidly?

Dengue is transmitted by infected female Aedes mosquitos. Aedes mosquitoes like warm humid environments and preferentially feed on humans when breeding. A week after taking a blood meal from a person infected with dengue virus, the mosquito can transmit dengue virus to another person through saliva inoculated with her bites. A female mosquito can live for 2–4 weeks and breeds about 300 eggs during her lifespan in small collections of standing water, such as in flower pots, plastic jars, bottles, cans and discarded tires. The rise in uncontrolled urban development, often combined with poor sanitation and inadequate waste disposal services, resulted in the expansion of these mosquito populations and facilitated major disease outbreaks from the 1950s onwards, especially in huge Asian megacities such as Bangkok, Manila, Jakarta, and Ho Chi Minh City.

Global warming may be another factor contributing to the spread of dengue. Higher environmental temperatures serve to lengthen the dengue season in endemic regions and also promote dengue infection in new areas such as southern Europe. In addition, the effects of flooding in rural areas can result in significant migration into urban areas, increasing overcrowding and exerting pressure on the often-limited public health resources [9]. Finally, air travel has been associated with the rapid spread of many diseases in the modern era, and recent data has shown that the spread of dengue is associated with air transportation [10, 11].

Can Dengue Transmit from Mother to Her Child?

In-utero and peri-partum maternal-foetal transmission of dengue have been reported [12]. Regardless of whether the child is infected, maternal dengue infection during pregnancy results in a higher risk of premature birth, low birth weight, or even death for both mother and the child [13, 14].

15.2.2 Epidemiology

15.2.2.1 Geographic Distributions

Dengue is prevalent in more than 100 countries in the Americas, Africa, the Middle East, Asia, and the Pacific Islands. The list of these countries can be found here:
https://www.cdc.gov/dengue/areaswithrisk/around-the-world.html.

15.2.2.2 Recent Epidemics/Outbreaks

The recent outbreaks of dengue have been updated on this website:
https://www.healthmap.org/dengue/en/

15.2.2.3 Risk Factors

Any person living in or travelling to a dengue endemic-country, who is bitten by mosquitos is at risk for dengue infection. Risk of infection is often higher in urban environments.

Risk factors for severe illness include secondary infection with a different dengue serotype [15], younger age [16], female, obesity, diabetes, renal failure and other chronic comorbidities [17].

15.2.2.4 Risks for International Travellers

International travellers are at risk of infection with dengue if they travel to endemic regions. Risk of severe infection is highest with secondary infection; this is much less likely to occur in a short-term traveller compared to someone resident in a high-burden area, but theoretically those who travel between regions where different dengue serotypes are endemic are at risk for severe disease.

15.2.2.5 Differing Issues for Migrants and Those "visiting Friends and Relations" (VFR)

Migrants and VFR are less likely to have access to bite reduction measures such as mosquito repellent and air-conditioning. They may also have a primed immune response from prior dengue virus infection while resident in the endemic region, which could increase risk for severe disease if subsequently infected with a different serotype.

Updated information about dengue epidemiology can be found on some websites (Box 15.1).

15.2.3 Pathogenesis

What Is Special Feature of Dengue Virus?

Dengue virus is an RNA virus belonging to the family Flaviviridae and includes four serotypes DENV-1 to DENV-4. All four viral serotypes co-circulate at the same time to varying degrees, and all can cause both symptomatic infection and severe disease. The immune response following infection with one serotype does not offer long-term protection against infection with different serotypes; this means a person may be infected with dengue up to four times.

Would Secondary Dengue Infection Have Milder Symptoms?

No. The innate and adaptive immune response after the first infection does not offer better protection; conversely, it can induce more severe disease in subsequent infections with a different serotype. In one study, the risk of progressing to severe dengue for children with pre-existing dengue antibodies was eightfold higher than for those without pre-existing antibodies [18]. In particular, this phenomenon presents difficulties for tetravalent dengue vaccine development.

How Long Does the Immunity Protect the Body from Subsequent Dengue Infection?

During the first (primary) infection with any dengue serotype, long-lived immunity develops against that particular serotype, but protection against other serotypes is short-lived, estimated at 2–3 months by Sabin in the 1950s [19]. More recent evidence suggests the length of cross-protection can be up to 2.6 years [20]. Thereafter, waning cross-immunity predisposes to more severe disease.

What Are Important Features in the Pathogenesis of Dengue Infection?

There are two major features:

1. Vascular leakage—if severe, this may result in dengue shock or respiratory distress.
2. Bleeding–varies from mild to severe, accompanied by low platelets and impaired coagulation.

15.2.4 Clinical Findings

The dengue manifestations can be divided into three phases: febrile, critical, and recovery phase.

1. The febrile phase occurs from day 1 to 3 of the onset of illness. Dengue patients develop a sudden high-grade fever which usually lasts 2–7 days accompanied by generalized body aches, muscle pain, joint pain, facial flushing, skin erythema, retro-orbital eye pain, and headache. Other non-specific symptoms are sore throat, anorexia, nausea, and vomiting. Symptoms may be difficult to differentiate from other common viral infections.
2. The critical phase is from day 4 to 7 of illness and is marked by an abrupt cessation of fever. A minority of patients with vascular leak may develop warning signs (abdominal pain or tenderness, persistent vomiting, mucosal bleeding, restlessness, hepatomegaly); these may or may not progress to severe complications including shock, bleeding and/or multi-organ impairment. Dengue shock syndrome (DSS) is more common in children than in adults. Bleeding and multi-organ impairment are seen more often in adults than children [21, 22]. More unusual presentations of severe dengue may include severe liver and/or renal injury, cardiac arrhythmias and dysfunction, or central nervous system involvement.
3. Patients usually enter the recovery phase after day 6 of illness. Among those who have not developed severe disease, clinical symptoms improve with stable status, appetite, and increased urine volume. A recovery rash often appears on the extremities, often accompanied by pruritus. Bradycardia is commonly seen during this phase.

15.2.5 Laboratory Diagnosis

During the febrile or early critical phases of illness, an NS1 antigen or PCR test is often positive. Thereafter, a negative NS1 or PCR test does not reliably exclude infection; paired serology may be used to make a diagnosis. Dengue IgM can often be detected after day 5 of illness. Dengue IgG will be negative during the acute phase of illness in primary infection, but positive in secondary dengue.

There are changes in haematological tests including decreases in white blood cell count, low platelets, and high haematocrit. The platelet level is often lowest on day 6 of illness then recovers gradually afterward. Prolonged coagulation, and decreased fibrinogen levels often occur during the critical phase without severe bleeding. Liver enzymes increase during the illness and recover gradually during convalescence.

Different courses with changes in clinical manifestations and laboratory tests are described in Fig. 15.1.

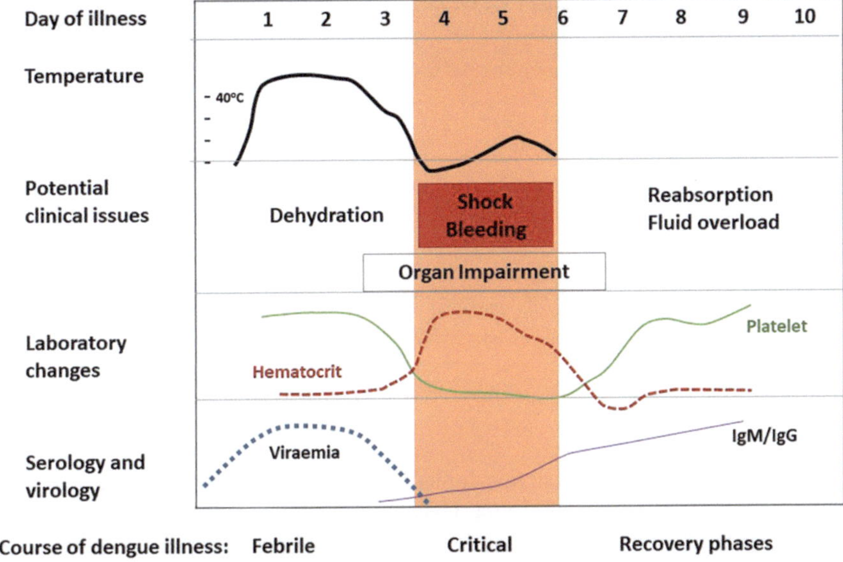

Fig. 15.1 The course of dengue illness retrieved from the WHO handbook of dengue management [22]. Source: Yip WCL, 198025

15.2.6 Differential Diagnosis

Dengue can present with similar clinical manifestations and haematological changes to other infections caused by viruses, bacteria, or parasites and non-infective illnesses (such as autoimmune diseases or drug reactions, leukaemia, idiopathic thrombocytopenic purpura). It can be helpful to combine clinical examination, epidemiological risk and virological diagnostics to confirm the diagnosis. Rarely, co-infection with dengue and other viral infections, malaria, or bacterial sepsis have been reported.

– Viral infection:
   Hanta
   Zika
   Chikungunya
   Yellow fever, Lassa fever, Ebola, Marburg
   Rubella
   Measles
   Infectious mononucleosis
   Human immunodeficiency virus

Acute viral hepatitis A, B, C, D, E
Adenoviruses
Influenza
SARS, COVID-19
Parvovirus B19
Herpes virus type 6
Enterovirus
- Bacterial infection:
  Typhoid
  Typhus
  Scarlet fever
  Staphylococcal infection
  Leptospirosis
  Rickettsiae
- Parasite: Malaria
- Autoimmune disease: Systemic lupus erythematosus, Kawasaki disease, idiopathic thrombocytopenic purpura, Henoch-Schonlein purpura
- Cancer: Leukaemia, lymphoma
- Drug reaction
- Acute cholecystitis

15.2.6.1 Diagnostic Hints

A traveller presenting with fever, myalgia, headache +/− rash, who has returned from an area with active dengue transmission within the past 7 days, and whose initial blood tests show leucopenia, low platelet count and moderately elevated liver enzymes should arouse suspicion for dengue; the appropriate confirmatory virological tests should be conducted, depending on the illness phase at presentation.

15.3 Management

There are currently no specific treatments for dengue, therefore the management relies on supportive care. Depending on the clinical presentation, a dengue patient will be classified as having dengue with or without warning signs or severe dengue (see Fig. 15.2). Dengue management varies by severity.

- Fever can be managed with paracetamol. Aspirin, ibuprofen and other non-steroidal anti-inflammatory medications should not be used as they may increase the risk of bleeding.
- Dengue patients without warning signs can stay at home for self-care. After 3 days of illness, patients managed at home should have daily contact with clinicians or revisit clinicians during the critical phase to monitor for development of warning signs or severe disease until the recovery phase.

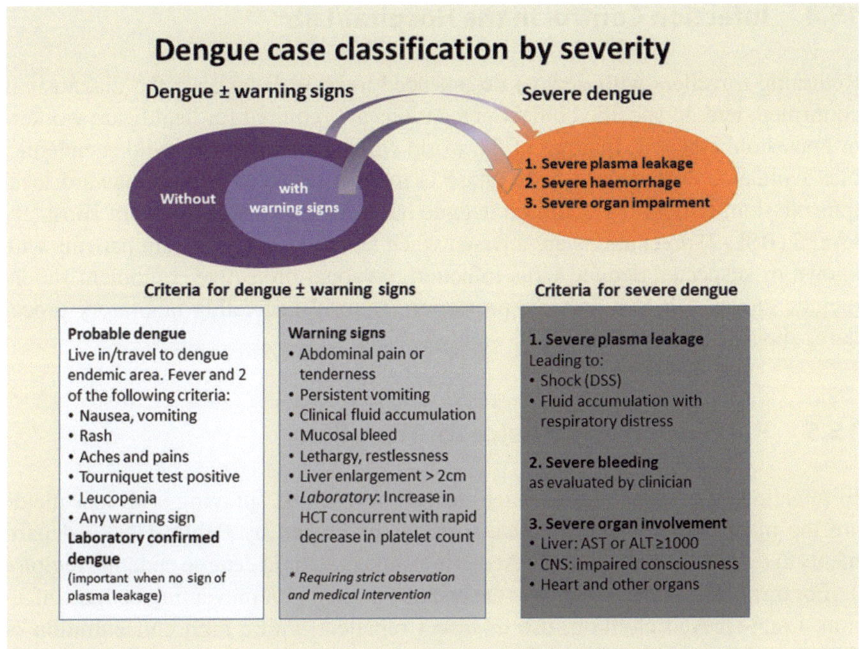

Fig. 15.2 Clinical presentations and laboratory tests at different levels of severity, retrieved from WHO handbook of dengue management [22] (Fig. 15.1, page 7)

– Dengue patients with warning signs or those with comorbidities (pregnancy, infancy, old age, obesity, diabetes, renal failure, liver failure, haematological abnormalities, cardiac abnormalities) or those with social problems (living alone, living far from healthcare centres) should be admitted to hospital for close monitoring. Oral fluid intake is recommended for all patients with warning signs. The use of parenteral fluid is only indicated for those who have persistent vomiting or diarrhoea.

– Severe dengue should be managed in high dependency units or intensive care units. Patients with dengue shock require fluid infusion for 24–48 h until plasma leak ceases; it should be discontinued promptly thereafter [23]. Those with severe bleeding often need support with multiple blood products, and may need nasal packing/management of gastrointestinal bleeding. Patients with respiratory distress or multiple organ failure may need organ support including non-invasive/invasive ventilation, vasopressors and/or haemodialysis.

The dengue illness specifically follows its clinical courses which is different from other viral infections. Box 15.2 lists some common thoughts that are inappropriate for dengue and need to be noticed. Information resources for dengue patients are shown in Box 15.3.

15.4 Infection Control in the Hospital/Lab

Returning travellers with dengue do not need to be isolated once the diagnosis is confirmed, and no specific contact precautions are required for healthcare workers or household contacts. In areas of the world where the Aedes mosquito is endemic, bite avoidance during the febrile phase is recommended to prevent onward local transmission. Laboratory acquired dengue has been reported; laboratory Biosafety level 2 (BSL-2) precautions are advised when handling samples from patients with known or suspected dengue virus infection. Personal protective equipment should include gloves, lab coat and eye protection. Aerosol-generating laboratory procedures should be performed in a biosafety cabinet.

15.5 Prevention and Advice for Travellers

Elimination of breeding habitats by clearing refuse and spraying with insecticide are the most common preventative methods employed by Public Health departments to reduce the burden of the Aedes mosquito vector in dengue endemic regions.

For travellers, bite avoidance is the primary strategy for preventing dengue infection. Long-sleeved clothing, use of insect repellent with a high concentration of DEET, residing in high-floor accommodation and the use of air conditioning will reduce the likelihood of contact with biting Aedes mosquitoes. Those at highest risk of severe dengue (pregnant, very young and elderly, obese, co-morbid) should take particular care to avoid being bitten. Since Aedes mosquitoes typically bite by day, insecticide-treated bed nets are of limited utility in reducing transmission.

In 2022, the tetravalent dengue vaccine QDENGA (TAK-003) was licensed in the European Union for prevention of dengue in populations aged ≥ 4 years. This is the first dengue vaccine licensed for use in dengue-naïve travellers. Whether the vaccine will be included in routine pre-travel vaccination schedules, or its efficacy in preventing infection in travellers with short−/medium-term risk-exposure are yet to be seen.

15.6 Gaps in Knowledge that Need to Be Addressed

- There have been no effective antiviral drugs for dengue.
- There have been no clinical studies investigating efficacy of host-directed therapies, including immune modulators for dengue.

- There is a lack of evidence to support or against the use of synthetic colloid solutions for patients with dengue shock syndrome.
- The long-term safety and efficacy of the new TAK003 dengue vaccine need further investigation in endemic regions, particularly in dengue naïve persons.

Box 15.1 Key Websites for Travellers and Healthcare Workers

https://www.cdc.gov/dengue/
https://www.who.int/news-room/fact-sheets/detail/dengue-and-severe-dengue
https://apps.who.int/iris/handle/10665/76887
https://www.who.int/publications/i/item/9789241547871
https://www.ecdc.europa.eu/en/dengue-monthly
https://www.healthmap.org/dengue/en/

Box 15.2 Things Commonly Forgotten

Common thoughts	Truth
When the fever ceases, the patient is recovering	The critical phase coincides with abrupt cessation of the fever; it is the host-immune response that may trigger development of severe/complicated dengue
Previous dengue infection is protective against subsequent dengue infection	There are four different dengue serotypes and an infection with one serotype does not protect against infection with another serotype
The second infection with dengue is associated with milder disease	Secondary infection with a different serotype increases the risk of severe dengue
The vascular system is leakier during dengue infection resulting in intravascular volume depletion; therefore, prophylactic fluid infusion may prevent shock	The more volume of fluid given to a dengue patient, the higher risk of developing respiratory distress due to pulmonary vascular leakage and interstitial oedema. There is no evidence that dengue shock syndrome can be prevented by prophylactic fluid infusion
Dengue results low platelets which increases the risk of bleeding; therefore, prophylactic platelet infusion is helpful to improve outcomes	Prophylactic platelet infusion may result more adverse events and it was not superior than supportive care in preventing bleeding [24]

Box 15.3 Information Resources for Patients
https://www.cdc.gov/dengue/resources/Caring-for-a-Family_Dengue-P.pdf

https://www.cdc.gov/zika/pdfs/sick-with-chikv-denv-zika.pdf

Declarations of Conflict of Interest None.

References

1. Gubler DJ. Dengue/dengue haemorrhagic fever: history and current status. Novartis Found Symp. 2006;277:3–16. discussion -22, 71-3, 251-3
2. Christie J. On epidemics of dengue fever: their diffusion and etiology. Glasgow Med J. 1881;16(3):161–76.
3. Brady OJ, Gething PW, Bhatt S, Messina JP, Brownstein JS, Hoen AG, et al. Refining the global spatial limits of dengue virus transmission by evidence-based consensus. PLoS Negl Trop Dis. 2012;6(8):e1760.
4. Bhatt S, Gething PW, Brady OJ, Messina JP, Farlow AW, Moyes CL, et al. The global distribution and burden of dengue. Nature. 2013;496(7446):504–7.
5. Cattarino L, Rodriguez-Barraquer I, Imai N, Cummings DAT, Ferguson NM. Mapping global variation in dengue transmission intensity. Sci Transl Med. 2020;12(528)
6. Castro MC, Wilson ME, Bloom DE. Disease and economic burdens of dengue. Lancet Infect Dis. 2017;17(3):e70–e8.
7. WHO. Dengue and severe dengue; 2022. (Available from: https://www.who.int/news-room/fact-sheets/detail/dengue-and-severe-dengue).
8. Messina JP, Brady OJ, Golding N, Kraemer MUG, Wint GRW, Ray SE, et al. The current and future global distribution and population at risk of dengue. Nat Microbiol. 2019;4(9):1508–15.
9. Whitehorn J, Yacoub S. Global warming and arboviral infections. Clin Med (Lond). 2019;19(2):149–52.
10. Quam MB, Khan K, Sears J, Hu W, Rocklov J, Wilder-Smith A. Estimating air travel-associated importations of dengue virus into Italy. J Travel Med. 2015;22(3):186–93.
11. Tian H, Sun Z, Faria NR, Yang J, Cazelles B, Huang S, et al. Increasing airline travel may facilitate co-circulation of multiple dengue virus serotypes in Asia. PLoS Negl Trop Dis. 2017;11(8):e0005694.
12. Basurko C, Matheus S, Hilderal H, Everhard S, Restrepo M, Cuadro-Alvarez E, et al. Estimating the risk of vertical transmission of dengue: a prospective study. Am J Trop Med Hyg. 2018;98(6):1826–32.
13. Pouliot SH, Xiong X, Harville E, Paz-Soldan V, Tomashek KM, Breart G, et al. Maternal dengue and pregnancy outcomes: a systematic review. Obstet Gynecol Surv. 2010;65(2):107–18.
14. Basurko C, Carles G, Youssef M, Guindi WE. Maternal and fetal consequences of dengue fever during pregnancy. Eur J Obstet Gynecol Reprod Biol. 2009;147(1):29–32.
15. Vaughn DW, Green S, Kalayanarooj S, Innis BL, Nimmannitya S, Suntayakorn S, et al. Dengue viremia titer, antibody response pattern, and virus serotype correlate with disease severity. J Infect Dis. 2000;181(1):2–9.
16. Lam PK, Tam DT, Dung NM, Tien NT, Kieu NT, Simmons C, et al. A prognostic model for development of profound shock among children presenting with dengue shock syndrome. PLoS One. 2015;10(5):e0126134.
17. Sangkaew S, Ming D, Boonyasiri A, Honeyford K, Kalayanarooj S, Yacoub S, et al. Risk predictors of progression to severe disease during the febrile phase of dengue: a systematic review and meta-analysis. Lancet Infect Dis. 2021;
18. Katzelnick LC, Gresh L, Halloran ME, Mercado JC, Kuan G, Gordon A, et al. Antibody-dependent enhancement of severe dengue disease in humans. Science. 2017;358(6365):929–32.

19. Sabin AB. Research on dengue during World War II. Am J Trop Med Hyg. 1952;1(1):30–50.
20. Montoya M, Gresh L, Mercado JC, Williams KL, Vargas MJ, Gutierrez G, et al. Symptomatic versus inapparent outcome in repeat dengue virus infections is influenced by the time interval between infections and study year. PLoS Negl Trop Dis. 2013;7(8):e2357.
21. Trung DT, Thao le TT, Dung NM, Ngoc TV, Hien TT, Chau NV, et al. Clinical features of dengue in a large Vietnamese cohort: intrinsically lower platelet counts and greater risk for bleeding in adults than children. PLoS Negl Trop Dis. 2012;6(6):e1679.
22. World Health Organization. Handbook for clinical management of dengue. WHO; 2012.
23. WHO. Dengue: Guidelines for diagnosis, treatment, prevention and control: new edition. Geneva: WHO Guidelines Approved by the Guidelines Review Committee; 2009.
24. Lye DC, Archuleta S, Syed-Omar SF, Low JG, Oh HM, Wei Y, et al. Prophylactic platelet transfusion plus supportive care versus supportive care alone in adults with dengue and thrombocytopenia: a multicentre, open-label, randomised, superiority trial. Lancet. 2017;389(10079):1611–8.

Zika Virus Infection in Travellers

Chantal B. E. M. Reusken, Barry Rockx, and Isabella Eckerle

Abstract

Zika virus (ZIKV) was first isolated in 1947 from a rhesus macaque held captive in the Zika forest in Uganda as a sentinel for yellow fever virus circulation. The first suggestion of its potential to cause sporadic human disease dates from the early sixties in the same country, but it was not until 2007 with the outbreak in Yap state (Micronesia) that ZIKV was recognized as a cause of outbreaks of mild febrile human disease. The general perception of ZIKV as a cause of benign infections transformed with the first indications of association with Guillain-Barré Syndrome (GBS) during the 2013/14 outbreak in French Polynesia. Following its rapid emergence across the Americas in 2015/16, the declaration of "clusters of microcephaly cases and other neurological disorders in areas affected by Zika virus" as a Public Health Emergency of International Concern by WHO in February 2016 further substantiated concerns about the potential severity of ZIKV infections. By 2017, it was established that although ZIKV generally

Chantal B. E. M. Reusken (✉)
Centre for Infectious Disease Control, National Institute for Public Health and the Environment, Bilthoven, The Netherlands
e-mail: chantal.reusken@rivm.nl

B. Rockx
Department of Viroscience, Erasmus University Medical Center, Rotterdam, The Netherlands

Department of Virology & Molecular Biology, Wageningen Bioveterinary Research, Lelystad, The Netherlands
e-mail: barry.rockx@wur.nl

I. Eckerle
Centre for Emerging Viral Diseases, University Hospitals of Geneva and University of Geneva, Geneva, Switzerland
e-mail: Isabella.Eckerle@hcuge.ch

H. Leblebicioglu et al. (eds.), *Emerging and Re-emerging Infections in Travellers*, https://doi.org/10.1007/978-3-031-49475-8_16

causes mild or asymptomatic infections, it is a cause of GBS in adults, and congenital ZIKV infection may result in microcephaly and other congenital central nervous system (CNS) malformations, pre-term birth and miscarriage.

Since the outbreak in Micronesia ZIKV has rapidly expanded its geographic distribution, and it is currently known to affect > 85 countries in Africa, Asia, the Pacific, the Americas and the Caribbean. An estimated 2 billion people live in areas of the world with environmental suitability for ZIKV circulation. Although most countries in the Americas and the Caribbean see a decline in the number of ZIKV cases, the situation in Africa remains obscure, while for Asia, increasing evidence from retro- and prospective studies points to a wide geographical circulation. The affected countries include many popular travel destinations for European citizens, and indeed many import cases of ZIKV infections in returning travellers have been reported and continue to be reported.

Given the profile of ZIKV as a (re-)emerging pathogen and as aetiology of severe disease, clinicians and public health officials should remain vigilant about the risk of ZIKV infection in (returning) travellers and for ongoing local transmission. Pre-travel advice to prevent infection, especially in case of pregnancy or pregnancy wish, is necessary. To maintain this awareness to prevent, identify, manage and investigate ZIKV cases, this chapter reviews ZIKV epidemiology, pathogenesis, diagnostics and treatment.

16.1 Background

Zika virus (ZIKV) was first isolated in 1947 from a rhesus macaque held captive in the Ziika forest in Uganda as a sentinel for yellow fever virus circulation [1, 2]. The first suggestion of its potential to cause sporadic human disease dates from the early sixties in the same country [3] but it was not until 2007 with the outbreak in Yap state (Micronesia) that ZIKV was recognized as a cause of outbreaks of mild febrile human disease [4]. The general perception of ZIKV as a cause of benign infections transformed with the first indications of association with Guillain-Barré Syndrome (GBS) during the 2013/14 outbreak in French Polynesia [5, 6]. Following its rapid emergence across the Americas in 2015/16, the declaration of 'clusters of microcephaly cases and other neurological disorders in areas affected by Zika virus' as a Public Health emergency of International Concern by WHO in February 2016 further substantiated concerns about the potential severity of ZIKV infections [7]. By 2017, it was established that although ZIKV generally causes mild or asymptomatic infections, it is a cause of GBS in adults, and congenital ZIKV infection may result in microcephaly and other congenital central nervous system (CNS) malformations, pre-term birth and miscarriage [8].

Since the outbreak in Micronesia, ZIKV has rapidly expanded its geographic distribution, and it is currently known to affect almost 90 countries in Africa, Asia, the Pacific, the Americas and the Caribbean [9, 10]. An estimated 2 billion people live in areas of the world with environmental suitability for ZIKV circulation [11].

Although most countries in the Americas and the Caribbean have seen a decline in the number of ZIKV cases, the situation in Africa remains obscure, while for Asia, increasing evidence from retro- and prospective studies points to a wide geographical circulation [12, 13]. The affected countries include many popular travel destinations for European citizens, and indeed many import cases of ZIKV infections in returning travellers have been reported and continue to be reported [14, 15].

Given the profile of ZIKV as a (re-)emerging pathogen and as aetiology of severe disease, clinicians and public health officials should remain vigilant about the risk of ZIKV infection in (returning) travellers and for ongoing local transmission [16]. Pre-travel advice to prevent infection, especially in case of pregnancy or pregnancy wish, is necessary. To maintain this awareness to prevent, identify, manage and investigate ZIKV cases, this chapter reviews ZIKV epidemiology, pathogenesis, diagnostics and treatment.

16.2 Aetiology

ZIKV is a virus that belongs to the genus *Orthoflavivirus* in the family *Flaviviridae*. This genus comprises >50 virus species, including clinically important viruses like dengue virus (DENV), West Nile virus (WNV), tick-borne encephalitis virus (TBEV), Japanese encephalitis virus (JEV) and yellow fever virus (YFV). YFV is the type species of the genus with 'flavivirus' derived from the Latin word 'flavus', meaning yellow, which refers to jaundice, which is common in yellow fever cases.

Species demarcation within the genus *Orthoflavivirus* is based on seven criteria, including nucleotide and deduced amino acid sequence data, antigenic characteristics, and geographic and vector association [17]. ZIKV is classified by the ICTV within the Ntaya group of mosquito-borne orthoflaviviruses together with a.o. Ilheus virus, Tembusus virus and Bagaza virus. Although all orthoflaviviruses are serologically related (see also section diagnostics), more closely related serogroups have been identified within the genus based on levels of cross-reactivity in neutralization assays. ZIKV belongs with Spondweni virus (SPOV) to the Spondweni virus serogroup [17, 18].

ZIKV is a positive-stranded RNA virus with a single genome segment of approximately 10.8 kb that is packaged in an enveloped, 50 nm icosahedral virion. Two virus forms can be distinguished in host cells: immature virions with viral proteins pre-membrane (prM) and envelope (E) proteins associated with the membrane and mature virions in which prM has been proteolytically cleaved into M. The genome comprises a single open reading frame flanked by a type 1 cap-5′-and 3′-untranslated region and encoding a large polyprotein that is cleaved by viral and host proteases into three structural proteins (Capsid, [pr]M, E) and seven non-structural proteins (NS1, NS2A, NS2B, NS3, NS4A, NS4B, NS5) [17, 19, 20].

Phylogenetic analysis based on whole coding region sequences shows the existence of two ZIKV lineages, an Africa lineage that includes two sublineages (West Africa and East Africa), and an Asia lineage that includes three sublineages

(American, Southeast Asian and Pacific) [21, 22]. ZIKV is thought to originate from east Africa and the two lineages were estimated to have diverged in ~1834 [23, 24]. The Asian lineage was responsible for the outbreaks in the Americas and Caribbean.

16.3 Transmission

Since its initial discovery, ZIKV has been recognized as a mosquito-borne virus [25]. Since then, several other secondary, non-mosquito-borne transmission modes have been identified, including sexual transmission, transmission through substances of human origin (SOHO) and maternofoetal transmission. Limited studies have suggested intrapartum transmission and, transmisison via breastfeeding, laboratory exposure, or animal bites and need further investigations [26–30].

Mosquito-borne transmission. Mosquito-borne transmission is considered the primary transmission mode for ZIKV for which both a sylvatic and urban transmission cycle are known (Fig. 16.1) [31, 32]. ZIKV has been found in 26 mosquito

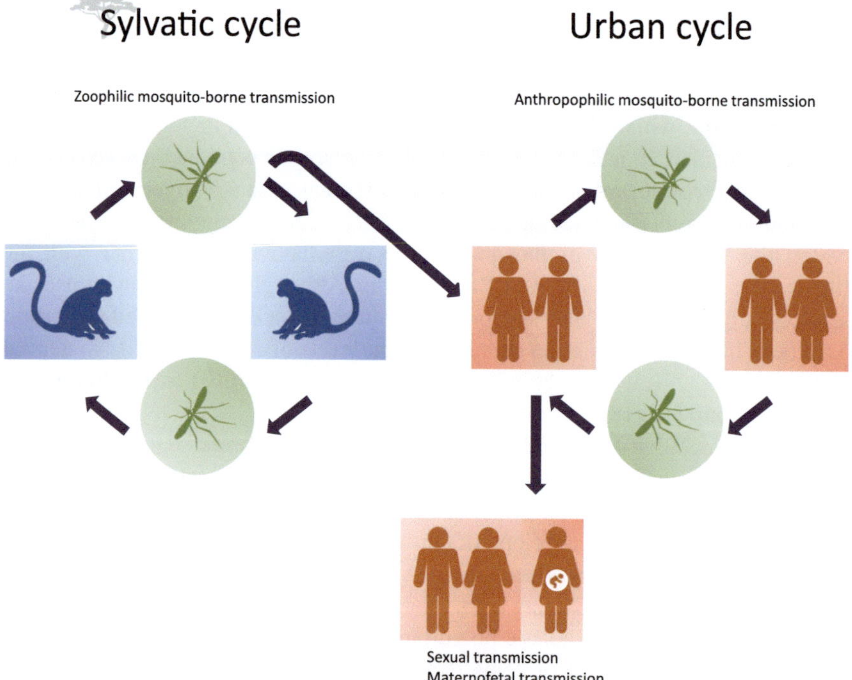

Fig. 16.1 Mosquito-borne and non-mosquito-borne transmission of ZIKV
Mosquito-borne circulation of ZIKV can occur in two parallel cycles. A sylvatic cycle involving non-human primates and zoophilic (bush) mosquitoes and an urban cycle involving humans and anthropophilic mosquitoes. Non-mosquito-borne transmission can occur through sexual intercourse and intra-uterine

species in the field, primarily *Aedes* spp. [33]. ZIKV originates from Africa, where it circulates in a sylvatic cycle between non-human primates and forest-dwelling zoophilic mosquitoes. Human exposure to sylvatic ZIKV might occur through these arboreal mosquito species. To date it is unknown whether ZIKV has established sylvatic circulation in Asia and the New World [31, 34]. However, modelling has suggested a high likelihood of the establishment of a sylvatic cycle in a wide range of settings, including the forests of South America [35, 36]. Studies are needed to determine the existence (Asia and the Americas) and the impact of the sylvatic cycle on the incidence of human ZIKV infections [31, 34, 37]. Similar to DENV, YFV and chikungunya virus (CHIKV), ZIKV has adapted to maintenance in an urban cycle between humans and anthropophilic mosquitoes, primarily *Ae. aegypti*. The ZIKV outbreaks in Micronesia, French Polynesia, the Americas, and the Caribbean were all outbreaks resulting from an urban ZIKV cycle. Besides transmission to vertebrates, there is evidence for the maintenance of ZIKV in mosquito populations through vertical and venereal transmission, which has been demonstrated for *Ae. aegypti* [32, 38–41].

Sexual transmission. ZIKV was the first arthropod-borne (arbo) virus for which sexual intercourse was implicated as a mode of transmission [42, 43]. The initial report dates from 2008 when an American scientist who developed ZIKV disease (including prostatitis and haematospermia) 6 days upon return from mosquito fieldwork in Senegal transmitted the virus to his wife who had no recent travel history to destinations outside the United States. Ten days after the scientist's return, the wife developed symptoms compatible with ZIKV disease. ZIKV infection was confirmed in both patients based on serology on paired serum samples. The couple had sexual intercourse the day after the scientist returned to the United States while competent mosquito species were absent in the region where the couple lived. Since early 2016, accumulating reports involving local transmission in Europe and the United States through travellers returning from areas with ZIKV circulation confirmed sexual intercourse as a transmission mode for ZIKV [31, 44–46]. Reported sexual transmission of ZIKV involves predominantly transmission from symptomatic men-to-women, while some cases of asymptomatic men-to-women transmission have been published [47–49]. Sporadic reports on transmission from women-to-men and men–to men exist [44, 50]. Modes of sexual transmission include unprotected vaginal, oral and anal intercourse. The sexual transmission events can occur before, during and after the index's symptom development [51]. The longest period reported between the onset of symptoms of two sexual partners is 44 days [52] with a median of 12 days (based on 15 couples, [47]). Infectious virus in human semen was detected for a median duration of 9.5 days (95% CI: 1.2–20.3 days) based on 22 cases [47] and for a maximum of 69 days upon onset of symptoms [53]. Two cohort studies, including 184 and 55 subjects, showed the presence of ZIKV RNA in semen with a median of 35 and 34 days (95% CI:53-28-41) post-onset symptoms [54, 55], respectively. The longest detection of ZIKV RNA shedding in semen described in the literature is 370 days post-onset illness [56]. Based on data from 15 women, the presence of ZIKV RNA in women vaginal excretions was determined to be a median of 13.9 days (95% CI: 7.2–19.6) [47], while a recent case description reported the presence of ZIKV RNA in vaginal secretions and endocervical samples up to 31 days after onset of symptoms [57]. For these cases of extended ZIKV RNA detection in male and female genital tracts, it is unknown whether the presence of ZIKV RNA represents a viable virus.

Per definition, the estimated proportion of ZIKV cases due to sexual transmission is underestimated as it is nearly impossible to ascertain this mode of transmission in regions with active ZIKV circulation. Nevertheless, upon correction for systematic testing of pregnant women, a 90% higher incidence of infection was found in sexually active women (15–65 years old) when compared to men in the same age group in a study in Rio de Janeiro. This difference was not observed in other age groups and was attributed to sexual transmission [58]. Multiple modelling studies have attempted to estimate the impact of sexual transmission on the incidence of human infections, resulting in a wide range of estimated proportions of cases or contributions to the R_0 [59–63].

Maternofoetal transmission. Upon its emergence in the Americas, it became rapidly clear that ZIKV is transmitted transplacental and that infection during pregnancy can cause congenital abnormalities (congenital Zika syndrome), preterm births and miscarriage [64–70]. Normocephalic children exposed to ZIKV infection during pregnancy and with no observable Zika-associated birth defects may also present with later neurodevelopmental delay or post-natal microcephaly. The proportion of affected neonates born to mothers infected with ZIKV during pregnancy varies widely between different cohort studies. It varies with trimester of pregnancy at the time of infection and clinical manifestation in the mother [9, 12, 71–76]. Besides intrauterine transmission, intrapartum transmission and transmission through breastfeeding have been suggested. Although infectious ZIKV has been detected in breast milk, there is no irrefutable evidence in the literature for mother-to-infant transmission through breastfeeding [27, 77–79], even though some studies are highly suggestive of the existence of this transmission mode [77, 80–82]. Intrapartum transmission was indicated as a likely transmission mode in the case of French Polynesia [26]. However, in this case, the likelihood of intrapartum transmission versus intrauterine and mosquito-borne transmission has been received with scepticism [81].

Transmission through SoHO. Data on the actual transmission of ZIKV through substances of human origin (SoHO) are limited. Transfusion-transmitted (TT) infection with closely related viruses like DENV and WNV has been described [83, 84]. The risk for TT ZIKV infections will be associated with the percentage of sub-clinical ZIKV infections (estimated to be 50–73% [85]) and donations of patients in the incubation period of infection [86]. ZIKV RNA-positive blood donations have been described during outbreaks with percentages ranging from 0.05% to 0.17% in Campinas, Brazil 2015–2016 [87, 88] via 0.53%–0.9% in 2015–2016 in Puerto Rico [89–91] and 1.8% in Martinique in 2016 [92] to 2.7% in Sao Paolo state, Brazil in 2016 [93] and 2.8% in 2013–2014 in French Polynesia [94]. Reports on ZIKV RNA-positive blood donations in non-endemic regions are rare. Williamson et al. described a prevalence of 0.001% in 2016 in blood donations in US states without autochthonous transmission, and Borena et al. found no molecular evidence for ZIKV in Austrian donors in 2016 [95, 96]. There are no published data on blood donations in the current, post-epidemic era. To date, no cases of clinical ZIKV infection have been attributed to the transfusion of contaminated blood. In scientific literature, three probable cases of platelet transfusion transmitted (TT) ZIKV infection have been reported from Brazil, none of which had any clinical sequelae [97, 98]. All three cases of TT ZIKV were recipients of pre-symptomatic donors. Overall, the available data suggest that the risk of TT (clinical) ZIKV infections is low during outbreaks [99]. The risk of ZIKV transmission through transplantation and in reproductive medicine has been acknowledged [100–103]. Still, cases of ZIKV transmission through other SoHO, like donated tissues, organs, semen and oocytes, have not been reported [104].

16.4 Epidemiology

While the origin of ZIKV has been traced to East Africa, ZIKV is currently widely distributed across Africa, Asia, the Pacific and the Americas (Fig. 16.2) [9, 105]. As of February 2022, 89 countries and territories have had evidence of mosquito-borne ZIKV transmission, while 61 countries and territories have established *Ae. aegypti* populations, but there are no reported cases of ZIKV [9]. The current situation (May 2023) is such that accurate and up-to-date epidemiological data on active ZIKV circulation are limited for many areas in the world, mainly due to the absence or limited availability of routine surveillance, case detection and reporting, and probably worsened in the period 2020–2022 by the SARS-CoV-2 pandemic [9, 12, 106]. In addition, the high percentage of subclinical infections and non-specific, mild

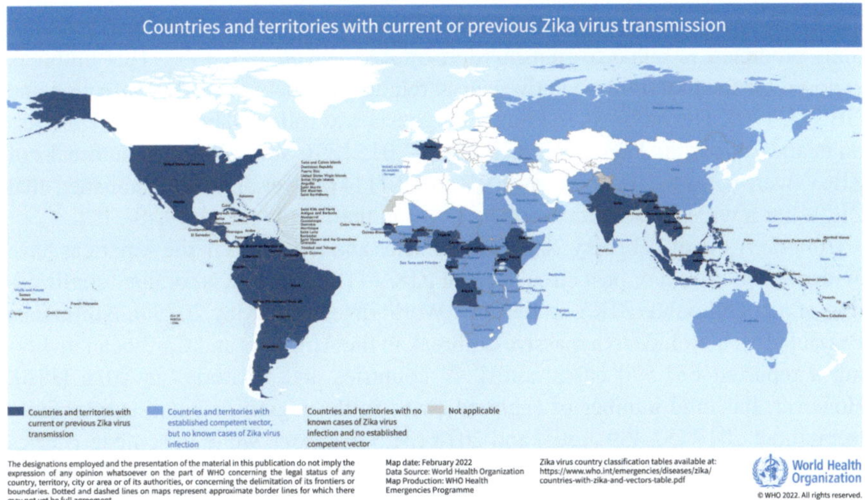

Fig. 16.2 Map of countries and territories with current or previous Zika virus transmission Source WHO: map-of-countries_with_zika_transmission_feb2022.pdf (who.int)

clinical infections will contribute to underreporting of ZIKV circulation. Therefore, data on active ZIKV circulation is often collected outside routine surveillance systems, mostly through traveller cases and research projects.

Continental Europe. Locally acquired ZIKV infections have been reported from Southern France in 2019 [107]. Two mosquito species established in parts of Europe have shown some competence for ZIKV transmission in experimental studies, i.e. *Ae. albopictus* and *Ae. japonicus.* Nevertheless, local or sustained transmission risk is still considered very low as these are less competent vectors [16]. The primary vector, *Ae.aegypti* is present in parts of Georgia, Portugal (Madeira), Spain (Fuerteventura), Russia and Turkey, but none of these European region countries have reported local, mosquito-borne transmission of ZIKV [10, 108]. It is assumed that during late summer and autumn, when temperatures and vector abundances are high, conditions for autochthonous transmission of ZIKV can arise in Southern Europe after the initial introduction of the virus by returning viraemic travellers [12].

South-East Asia and the Pacific region. As of February 2022, 25 countries and territories in South-East Asia and the Pacific region have evidence for past or current circulation of ZIKV [10]. ZIKV, as a cause for human disease outbreaks, became a focus of worldwide attention with the first recognized human outbreak in Yap State, Micronesia [4]. The outbreak was caused by the Asian lineage of ZIKV. The outbreak manifested with mild febrile fever, rash, conjunctivitis and arthralgia. An estimated 73% of the population of 3 years and older in Yap state (total population ~11,500) was estimated to be affected. It lasted a couple of months, and since then, re-occurrence of ZIKV has only been documented once in Micronesia, with a small outbreak of ZIKV in Kosrae state in 2016 [109]. The next documented outbreak of ZIKV started in October 2013 in French Polynesia, affecting in the end an estimated 28,000 cases that sought medical care (~11% of the population) [110–112]. The causing strain was identified as a more recent strain of the Asian lineage with accumulated phenotypically important amino acid substitutions predicted to enhance transmission by *Ae. aegypti* [23, 113]. This outbreak exposed for the first time a putative causal relationship between ZIKV infection and GBS [5, 110]. The outbreak in French Polynesia was followed by smaller outbreaks on Islands across the Pacific region in 2014–2015 [25]. Several limited outbreaks of ZIKV were reported in India in 2017–2018 [114]. Overall, it is established that ZIKV has a widespread circulation in Asia and the Pacific region [9, 10, 12].

Americas. As of February 2022, 49 countries and territories in the Americas have evidence for current or past circulation of ZIKV [10]. The first laboratory confirmation of autochthonous ZIKV in the New World dates from May 2015 in North-East Brazil [115], a prelude to a massive outbreak in the Americas and Caribbean involving a reported 651,590 cases across 49 countries and territories in 2016 [116]. However, the total number of reported cases in the region declined substantially throughout 2017 (57,469 cases) and 2018 (31,576 cases), while in some territories the circulation seems to be interrupted [116]. The clusters of microcephaly cases and other neurological disorders in areas affected by ZIKV resulted in the declaration of a PHEIC by WHO on 1 February 2016. The PHEIC ended on 18 November 2016 [7]. Phylogenetic analysis points to a single introduction event to the region, estimated in May–December 2013 in North-East Brazil, from where ZIKV moved within the Americas while evolving the American sublineage [113]. Recent data have shown that both the Asian and American subgroups of the Asian lineage have outbreak potential, and adverse birth outcomes are not limited to American sublineage-Asian strains [117–119].

Africa. As of February 2022, 14 countries on the African continent have been classified as having current or past ZIKV circulation [10]. Despite the decade-long endemicity in Africa, systematic cohort studies into the teratogenicity of African lineage ZIKV are lacking and much needed. Nevertheless, laboratory evidence is accumulating that African lineage ZIKV might be even more pathogenic in pregnancy than the Asian lineage, causing severe damage resulting in foetal loss rather than birth defects [120–122]. Cases of microcephaly presumptively associated with ZIKV in Guinea-Bissau are assumed to be related to African lineage ZIKV [9] while a case of CZS reported from Angola in 2018 appeared to be caused by an American subgroup-Asian lineage strain that had emerged in Angola [123, 124]. Besides Angola, the American subgroup-Asian lineage ZIKV has emerged in Cabo Verde, causing an outbreak in 2015–2016 with a reported 7580 cases, including 18 microcephaly cases [125]. Overall, data on ZIKV circulation in Africa are very limited [13].

ZIKV and travellers. International travellers are the assumed cause of the rapid geographical expansion of ZIKV [14, 113, 126–131]. Furthermore, travellers can serve as sentinels for active circulation in areas without up-to-date reporting [132, 133]. Retrospective analysis of data in a global travel surveillance system showed that travellers revealed active ZIKV circulation in five Asian countries in the period 2012–2016 before these countries had reported any ZIKV cases [131]. Furthermore, a non-reported outbreak in Cuba in 2017 was uncovered with the same surveillance system [129]. In the case of ZIKV, ZIKV infection of travellers revealed sexual intercourse as a mode of transmission, something that would have remained obscure in countries with mosquito-borne transmission [31, 42, 44–46]. The surveillance atlas of the European Centre for Disease Prevention and Control (ECDC) reported 26 ZIKV cases known to be imported to the EU/EEA for 2015, 1882 for 2016, 249 for 2017, 46 for 2018, 56 for 2019, 21 for 2020 and 7 for 2021 [134]. The US CDC reported 62 ZIKV cases in returning travellers in 2015, 4944 in 2016, 445 in 2017, 74 in 2018, 28 in 2019, 4 in 2020 and 2 in 2021 [135]. A systematic review of PubMed publications indicated 15 cases in returning travellers globally in 2014, 131 cases in 2015 and 799 cases in 2016 [14]. The decline in cases of returning travellers observed in the United States and EU/EEA from 2016 to 2017 directly reflects the waning of the epidemic in the Americas [9, 116].

16.5 Clinical Findings

16.5.1 Adult Infection

Following an average incubation period of 3–14 days, 50–73% of ZIKV infection is asymptomatic [85, 136]. The main clinical symptoms in ZIKV patients are mild fever (65%), maculopapular, often pruritic rash with a centrifugal pattern (90%), myalgia, arthralgia/arthritis (65%), oedema, headache and non-purulent conjunctivitis (55%) [4, 137–139]. Diarrhoea is usually not included in ZIKV case definitions but is nevertheless frequently reported in ZIKV patients [140]. In fact, the clinical picture is similar to that of patients infected with DENV or CHIKV, although it has been suggested that symptoms of a ZIKV infection are milder than other arboviral infections [141, 142]. In contrast to Dengue fever and Chikungunya fever, fever is not always present in ZIKV patients and is generally lower. Furthermore, the febrile period is shorter with around 1–4 days (max. 7 days), and fever is usually monophasic, while it can be biphasic in Dengue fever and persists for a longer period (there up to 1 week to 10 days) [143]. The presence of rash with pruritus is more common in ZIKV infections than in DENV and CHIKV infections and usually present at the onset of symptoms or within the first 2 days of symptoms, in contrast to DENV and CHIKV infections where rash usually appears only during the course of disease around day 4 [140, 142, 144, 145]. The general duration of symptoms in ZIKV infections is around 2–7 days [4]. For an overview of ZIKV infection symptoms compared to DENV and CHIKV infections, see Table 16.1.

Severe or fatal disease following ZIKV infection in adults is rare and is mostly associated with neurological complications, including GBS, myelitis encephalomyelitis, encephalitis, meningoencephalitis, and sensory polyneuropathy [146–148]. For example, the annual incidence rates for GBS ranged from 1/10,000 to 1/17,000 during the ZIKV outbreak [149, 150], while the estimated baseline incidence of GBS worldwide is 0.1/10,000 [151].

Table 16.1 Comparison of selected clinical findings in chikyungunya, dengue and Zika virus infections

Clinical presentation	Zika virus	Dengue virus	Chikungunya virus
Fever	+	+++	+++
Rash	+++	++	++
Myalgia	+	+++	+
Arthralgia	++	+	+++
Oedema	++	–	–
Retro-orbital pain	+	++	+
Conjunctivitis	+++	–	+++
Lymphadenopathy	+	++	++
Hepatomegaly	–	–	+++
Haemorrhage	–	+	–

Table 16.2 Comparison of baseline laboratory findings in chikungunya, dengue and Zika virus infections

Laboratory findings	Zika	Dengue	Chikungunya
Anaemia	−	−	+
Leucopenia	±	+++	++
Neutropenia	−	+++	+
Lymphocytopenia	±	++	+++
Thrombocytopenia	±*	+++	+
Increased CRP	−	+++	++
Increased ALT	−	+++	++

Baseline laboratory findings of ZIKV infections are usually unremarkable compared to DENV and CHIKV infections. If present, leukopenia, lymphopenia and/or mild thrombocytopenia can be seen in a subset of patients. For an overview, see Table 16.2.

16.5.2 Congenital Infection

ZIKV infection during pregnancy can result in pregnancy complications, including foetal loss, stillbirth, and preterm birth [152]. In a recent study in French Guiana, the rate of maternal-foetal transmission is reported to be 26% [74]. Congenital Zika syndrome is a pattern of birth defects associated with ZIKV infection during pregnancy. Congenital ZIKV syndrome has primarily been associated with severe microcephaly, subcortical calcifications, damage to the back of the eye, congenital contractures, such as clubfoot or arthrogryposis and hypertonia restricting body movement soon after birth [153].

Congenital ZIKV syndrome and other birth defects have been reported in 5–15% of babies born from mothers with confirmed ZIKV infection in initial studies [73, 154]. Among foetuses and new-borns infected with ZIKV, 45% did not show any clinical signs, while 20% showed moderate signs, 21% showed severe complications and 14% reported foetal loss [74]. The highest risk of birth defects is from ZIKV infection during the 1st trimester [155, 156].

16.6 Pathogenesis

16.6.1 Virus Life Cycle

Since mosquito-borne transmission is considered the primary transmission mode for ZIKV, following the bite of a female mosquito, cells in the skin are the first to encounter ZIKV [157]. In the skin, a variety of cell types are permissive to ZIKV infection, including dermal fibroblasts, epidermal keratinocytes, and immature dendritic cells [157]. In addition, the saliva of mosquitoes, which is injected along with the virus, is known to modulate the immune response in the skin [158]. The mosquito saliva creates a microenvironment that favours ZIKV replication and recruits immune cells to the bite site, which plays a role in further disseminating the virus. For example, a mosquito saliva protein named neutrophil-stimulating factor 1 (NeSt1) activates neutrophils in the skin to recruit macrophages susceptible to ZIKV infection [159]. Infected dendritic cells and macrophages can subsequently aid the spread of ZIKV to other organs through circulation. In addition, endothelial cells are susceptible to ZIKV infection, which will allow the virus to enter the circulation and cause the observed viremia [160–162].

Following initial replication in the skin and subsequent viremia, ZIKV can infect a variety of organs and tissues. The targeted organs include the joints, eyes, male and female reproductive tract and central nervous system.

16.6.2 Joints

The development of arthralgia is an important clinical symptom reported in several mosquito-borne virus infections, including ZIKV, CHIKV and DENV. Arthralgia has been reported in over 65% of ZIKV cases, including persistent or recurrent arthralgia for more than 30 days has been reported [163, 164]. While several studies have focused on the effect of alphavirus infection (including CHIKV) on bone formation, few studies have focused on orthoflaviviruses. Recently it was shown that ZIKV can infect osteoblasts that are important for bone formation [165, 166]. Upon ZIKV infection, osteoblasts are delayed in their ability to differentiate and mature, and this impaired function can lead to an imbalance in bone homeostasis and induce bone-related disorders such as arthralgia [166].

16.6.3 Eyes

Involvement of the eyes has been reported in both babies and adults and included ocular abnormalities in the retina and choroid [167, 168]. Limited information is available about the pathogenesis of these ocular abnormalities, but in vitro studies have shown that human retinal endothelial, and retinal pigment epithelial cells are highly susceptible to ZIKV infection [169]. ZIKV infection in these cells results in cell death that can lead to the previously reported retinal lesions.

16.6.4 Male Reproductive Tract (MRT)

ZIKV can persist in the male reproductive tract, highlighting the potential for viral transmission over extended periods [170]. The exact cell targets of ZIKV in the male reproductive tract remain unknown, but ZIKV has been shown to infect spermatogonia, primary spermatocytes, Sertoli cells, peritubular myoid cells, Leydig cells, and epithelial cells of the lumen in experimental models [171, 172]. While the effect of ZIKV infection on the male reproductive system seems limited, ZIKV-induced reproductive hormone changes have been reported in men, and findings suggest a possible long-term detrimental effect of ZIKV infection on human male fertility [173]. In experimental animal models, ZIKV can indeed cause progressive testicular atrophy and lead to infertility [174, 175].

16.6.5 Female Reproductive Tract (FRT)

ZIKV infection of the female reproductive tract is considered transient; however, it can play a role in both sexual transmission as well as vertical transmission [176]. Experimental studies have shown that ZIKV can infect through vaginal inoculation [177]. However, little data is available on cell tropism in the FRT. In vitro models show that human endometrial stromal cells can be infected by ZIKV and thereby could play an important role in sexual transmission [178].

16.6.6 Neurotropism

ZIKV is highly neurotropic and has been shown to be harmful to both the adult and developing brain. A broad range of neurological complications have been reported in adults infected with ZIKV, including GBS, acute myelitis encephalomyelitis, encephalitis, meningoencephalitis, and sensory polyneuropathy [149, 179–187]. Little is known about the pathogenesis of ZIKV in the adult brain, but ZIKV seems to primarily infect neurons [188]. Infection of neurons likely leads to inflammation in the brain, resulting in dysfunction of synapses and possible memory impairment [188]. In addition, neural progenitors in stem cell niches in the adult brain of mice are also targeted by ZIKV [189], resulting in a loss of these cell populations. These data suggest that there may be long-term neurological effects of ZIKV infection in adults.

16.6.7 GBS

The main non-congenital neurologic syndrome observed in ZIKV infection is Guillain-Barré
Syndrome (GBS) [183, 190]. GBS is considered a post-infectious autoimmune disease likely resulting from an antigenic stimulus following infection with ZIKV. While the exact mechanism remains unknown, there is evidence that the ZIKV envelope protein shares structural features with a host protein of the classical complement cascade [191]. Antibodies against this complement component C1q are elevated following ZIKV infection in different experimental animal models and have previously been associated with the development of autoimmune diseases [192].

16.6.8　Vertical Transmission

Unlike most orthoflaviviruses, another route of transmission of ZIKV is a human-to-human transmission from mother to foetus [193]. This is of particular concern due to the observed complications during pregnancy. To date, there are at least 2 routes of vertical ZIKV transmission: a placental route observed as early as the first trimester, and a paraplacental route across the chorioamniotic membranes, which is observed from the second trimester [194, 195]. During placental transmission, ZIKV infects invasive cytotrophoblasts of the basal decidua and spreads to the chorionic villi and the foetal circulation. The paraplacental transmission route is characterized by the spread of ZIKV from the maternal blood vessels in the uterus to invasive cytotrophoblasts in the parietal decidua and spreading to the foetal membranes, resulting in the presence of ZIKV in the amniotic fluid and subsequent infection of the foetus. Overall, placentas seem most permissive to ZIKV infection during the first trimester [196]. However, ZIKV-associated congenital abnormalities were reported in cohort studies following infection in all three trimesters [197, 198].

16.6.9　Microcephaly

Microcephaly is a neurodevelopment disorder which is characterized by a reduced head circumference. The reduction of the head circumference can generally result from a reduced brain volume [155]. During neuronal development, neural progenitor cells differentiate into neurons that subsequently migrate basally during the earlier stages of cortical development in a process called 'direct neurogenesis' [199, 200]. During the later stages of cortical development, neural progenitor cells give rise to a second and third pool of neural progenitor cells. These progenitors can produce two identical progenitor cells or two neurons, amplifying the neuronal output from each neural progenitor cell. This process is called 'indirect neurogenesis'. Given these two mechanisms of neurogenesis, the main mechanism of ZIKV-induced microcephaly is believed to be two-fold. First, upon entering the CNS, ZIKV can infect neuronal progenitor cells and block indirect neurogenesis [199]. Second, ZIKV infection also results in neuronal cell death through the induction of apoptosis [199]. These two mechanisms will result in the observed cortical microcephaly.

In addition to a neurodevelopmental disorder, a premature closure of the sutures (craniosynostosis) can also prevent the brain from developing, resulting in microcephaly [201]. This is supported by the observation of very small or apparently closed fontanelles at birth in 25% of neonates born from ZIKV cases [202]. While the mechanism of ZIKV-induced craniosynostosis is unknown, ZIKV has been shown to productively infect cranial neural crest cells, which give rise to cranial bones and influence the developing brain [203, 204]. Experimental data further supports the premature fusion of cranial sutures due to accelerated osteogenesis during ZIKV infection in vitro [205]. However, whether the observed craniosynostosis should be considered a cause or an effect remains unknown.

16.6.10   Antibody-Dependent Enhancement (ADE)

Although ZIKV has been circulating for decades, only recently, major complications have been reported. One hypothesis for this increased pathogenicity is that the circulation of ZIKV in DENV endemic regions will result in antibody-dependent enhancement (ADE) of disease due to the presence of pre-existing antibodies against DENV, which can cross-react with ZIKV [206]. The mechanism behind ADE is that these cross-reactive antibodies can bind ZIKV but do not neutralize the virus. This virus-antibody complex can subsequently bind to the Fc receptor on target cells such as monocytes, macrophages and dendritic cells, thereby increasing the number of virus particles infecting the cell and increasing the number of infected cells. This enhanced infection can result in increased viremia and target cells' altered innate immune response, leading to a cytokine storm and enhanced disease. In addition to enhanced disease, ADE of ZIKV may also result in altered tissue tropism. Specifically, cross-reactive antibodies in the mother could enhance the transmission of ZIKV from mother to child [207]. The complex of cross-reactive antibodies of the mother and ZIKV can cross the placental barrier by binding to the neonatal Fc receptor, which actively transports maternal antibodies to the foetal circulation [208]. This process of maternal antibody transport to the foetus is initiated once the placenta is fully developed, generally occurring by weeks 20–24 of pregnancy. However, while ADE has been extensively studied in experimental models, the evidence of ADE in humans is limited [209]. Katzelnick *et al.* demonstrated that the risk of DENV-2 disease and the DENV-2 and DENV-3 disease severity were enhanced by a prior ZIKV or DENV infection that induced intermediate levels of antibodies. High levels of pre-existing anti-DENV antibodies protected against DENV-1, DENV-3 and ZIKV disease.

16.6.11   Role of Viral Proteins

Several viral proteins are known to play an important role in the pathogenesis of ZIKV infection, including the E protein and the non-structural proteins (NS) 1 and 5.

The ZIKV E protein is important for viral attachment and entry into the host cell, and in vitro studies have identified determinants of ZIKV host tropism. Several amino acid substitutions in E have been identified, which increase the ability of ZIKV to infect primate cells [210]. In addition, in experimental animal models, glycosylation of E was shown to contribute to ZIKV pathogenesis [211].

In addition to its role in ZIKV replication, the NS1 is also secreted from infected cells as a hexamer and is thought to play a role in immune evasion [212, 213]. More recently, studies have shown that NS1 also plays a role in ZIKV pathogenesis by inducing vascular leakage through disruption of the endothelial glycocalyx-like layer [214, 215]. This vascular leakage is tissue-specific and reflects the pathophysiology of ZIKV. For example, ZIKV NS1 increases the permeability of human placentas by reducing the glycosaminoglycans on trophoblasts and chorionic villi, which can lead to placental dysfunction [214].

NS5 plays a role in the evasion of the antiviral immune response by ZIKV. Specifically, ZIKV NS5 blocks the interferon signalling pathway by targeting the IFN-regulated transcriptional activator STAT2 leading to its degradation [216–218]. The ability of ZIKV to evade the interferon response is essential for virulence.

16.7 Laboratory Diagnosis

Although the virus was known for many decades, no commercial diagnostic tests were available at the beginning of the 2015 ZIKV outbreak. In the meantime, several novel assays and methods have been developed that are commercially available, most of them granted emergency use authorization by the FDA or CE-marking [219].

Direct detection methods include virus isolation in cell culture and nucleic acid amplification testing (NAAT) by reverse transcription polymerase chain reaction (rt-PCR) that can be done from all body fluids containing the virus. ZIKV can be detected in various body fluids and tissues such as blood, urine, semen, saliva, breast mild, amniotic fluid, placenta and foetal tissue [92, 220–223]. Serologic methods rely on the detection of IgG, IgM, and recently, IgA antibodies by a variety of methods from serum or plasma [219]. For an overview of the kinetics of viruses and antibodies and diagnostic opportunities in ZIKV infections, see Fig. 16.3.

16.7.1 Virus Culture

ZIKV can be isolated from patient material on mammalian or insect cell lines. They do not play a role in clinical routine diagnostics, but they are the method of choice when the presence of infectious virus particles is of interest. ZIKV is a risk-group-2 pathogen which requires biocontainment precautions at biosafety level 2 (BSL-2) in Europe, the United States and Canada.

16.7.2 Virus Detection by PCR

Most data on ZIKV RNA detection by PCR are obtained in serum or plasma. In general, ZIKV viremia tends to be lower and shorter than in other arboviruses with a similar clinical picture (e.g. dengue, chikungunya). Therefore virus detection by NAAT is more challenging, even with assays that reach high sensitivity. The mean virus titres of ZIKV are 10^4–10^5 copies/ml [224–228], in contrast to DENV with virus titres around 10^5–10^7 and CHIKV with 10^6–10^9. Similar to DENV RNA, ZIKV RNA levels in the blood often reach their maximum before the onset of symptoms. It is usually detectable for around a week and decreases rapidly within a few days in non-pregnant patients. In contrast, in pregnant women, the virus can be detectable for up to 10–12 weeks, extending the diagnostic window for direct virus detection and leading to a different diagnostic algorithm [229]. Testing by NAAT is

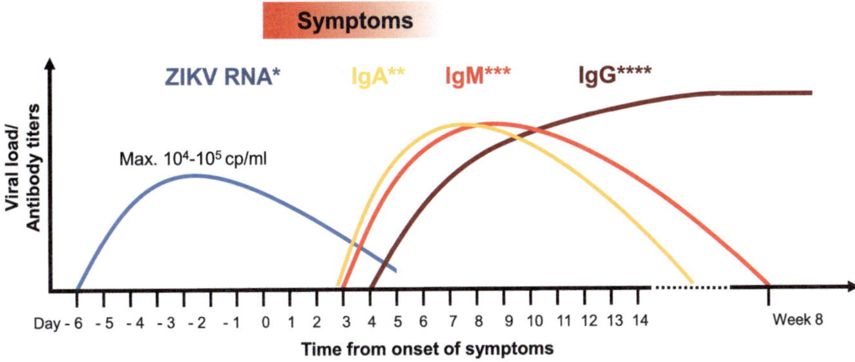

Fig. 16.3 Schematic kinetics of ZIKV RNA and serology for IgA, IgM and IgG in blood in a primary flavivirus infection in symptomatic non-pregnant patients
*Maximum viral copy number of ZIKV in blood as determined in several studies [224–228] Duration of detection is estimated between 7-10 depending on various studies; however, a cut-off of 7 days post-symptom onset for NAAT testing is used in several diagnostic algorithms, for example in the CDC algorithm. Of note, ZIKV load in urine reaches comparable copy numbers but the virus is shed for an extended period
**IgA detection: Detection of IgA is described more or less in parallel with IgM or even earlier. One study found positive IgA in several patients as early as 3 days post-symptom onset. [251]. IgA wanes rapidly and is usually not detectable anymore after day 30 [251] ***IgM detection occurs in the first week of illness, with data from various studies varying from 4-5 after symptom onset and lasting as long as 8 weeks. However, some studies found high rates of positive IgM even beyond 1 year after infection [247]. ****IgG detection: IgG is usually detectable shortly after IgA/IgM detection but can occur at the same time as well. Specific and neutralizing IgGs rise over time and are long-term lasting
Please note that curves are schematic and cover a time range of detection rather than a fixed time point

therefore recommended for both blood and urine for pregnant women within the first 12 weeks post-symptom onset, in parallel to serologic testing.

In whole blood, prolonged detection of ZIKV RNA was observed in comparison to serum and plasma, suggesting whole blood to be the more sensitive sample choice for ZIKV detection, suitable for routine diagnostic detection and expanding the window for direct virus detection for up to 120 days after symptom onset, at least in a small subset of patients [230–233]. Similar findings were obtained for urine, where ZIKV is shed for an extended period of up to 7–20 days, which can improve clinical diagnosis by testing urine as an additional specimen [234]. In semen of men with previous ZIKV infection, ZIKV RNA can be detected by PCR for prolonged periods (see section Transmission). However, routine semen evaluation, neither as a specimen for diagnosing an acute infection nor for assessing a preconception risk, is currently recommended [221, 235, 236]. Diagnosing new-borns and children with suspected congenital ZIKV infection is challenging to date. In cases of congenital ZIKV infection, detection of ZIKV RNA in various fluids or tissues, such as blood, urine or amniotic fluid, was found to be only transient or absent. At the same time, the virus was detected in pregnant women, and amniotic fluid was detected without visible foetal abnormalities [237]. Children with suspected congenital ZIKV infection should be tested by NAAT within the first days of in both blood and urine, and serology, particularly for IgM, should be performed [237].

Of note, antigen detection assays, as they are available for the NS1 protein of DENV, are not an established method for direct detection of ZIKV, which might be not surprising given the low viremia found in patients. Notably, ZIKV non-structural protein 1 (NS1) concentrations were found to be 10-fold lower than that for DENV NS1 in DENV-infected patients [238].

16.7.3 Serology

Serologic tools for detecting ZIKV antibodies are mainly comprised of Enzyme-linked immunosorbent assays (ELISA), immunofluorescence assays (IFA) and plaque-reduction neutralization assays. Similar to other orthoflaviviruses, cross-reactivity and even cross-neutralization of antibodies are observed. This is especially of relevance in patients with previous exposure to other orthoflaviviruses (either residents in areas of endemicity of multiple circulating orthoflaviviruses, e.g. DENV, or after vaccinations against other orthoflaviviruses such as YFV, TBEV, JEV or DENV). Thus, all serological ZIKV tests are prone to false positives and cross-reactivity with other orthoflaviviruses [239].

Serological assays for ZIKV antibody detection are detected against either the envelope (E) protein or the NS1 protein. While it is the E protein against which the main humoral immune response is generated, there is greater specificity among NS-1-based serological assays [219]. Despite a high level of amino acid similarity, the NS1 protein displays a different structure of essential epitope areas in ZIKV compared to DENV [240]. Therefore, the usage of NS1-based assays seems to be especially useful in patients with previous exposure to orthoflavivirus. Furthermore, parallel assessment of both IgM and IgG has shown good sensitivity and specificity in this patient group [241–243].

The gold standard for assessing antibodies against ZIKV and confirming findings obtained from an ELISA is virus neutralization, which will give the highest specificity. However, the need for cell culture and working with live viruses requires a considerable amount of trained personnel and is time-consuming. Since cell-culture-based assays are nowadays abandoned in most diagnostic laboratories, the ability to perform PRNT is mostly with specialized or public health laboratories and is not widely available for routine diagnostics. Nevertheless, some centres such as the American CDC recommend the confirmation of serologic results by PRNT including other orthoflaviviruses of potential exposure.

For diagnostic purposes of acutely diseased patients, detection of ZIKV IgM is of importance, especially in patients that are seen after the detection window for the virus in blood has passed (indicated > 7 days in testing algorithms, such as CDC [239]). IgM antibodies against ZIKV are detectable around 1 week (range 4–12 days) after onset of symptoms and can persist over longer periods of more than 2 months [225, 235, 244, 245]. A negative ZIKV IgM results in blood collected 1–2 weeks after symptom onset argues against a previous ZIKV infection. However, it should be kept in mind that IgM is not always detectable, especially in patients with previous orthoflavivirus exposure (natural or vaccine-based) [237, 245, 246]. On the other hand, the persistence of IgM over an extended period can complicate the diagnosis: a recent study found more than 70% of patients with a previous ZIKV infection still positive for ZIKV IgM after 12–19 months [247]. This can be especially troublesome in pregnant women when IgM of an infection acquired before conception cannot be excluded. One study evaluating the antibody kinetics of pregnant women with ZIKV infection found IgM as early as 2 days post symptom onset, reaching 100% seroprevalence 8–14 days after symptom onset [248]. ZIKV IgG was detectable in this cohort of pregnant women in the 2nd week post-symptom onset and remained positive until delivery in all women [248].

Recently, advances in the detection of ZIKV IgA (directed against NS-1) in blood have been made and additional assessment of IgA can further improve serologic diagnosis of acute ZIKV infection. Although, to date, not many studies have used ZIKV IgA in their diagnostic algorithm, it is suggested that IgA can be assessed at the same time or even before the detection of IgM in the early acute and acute phase of the disease and in contrast to IgM wanes rapidly [249–251]. Furthermore, IgA seems to be of added value in secondary orthoflavivirus infection in the absence of IgM, which is of special importance in endemic areas [249]. Of note, the combined testing of IgA/IgM gives the best results in terms of sensitivity and specificity [249]. No studies on IgA detection specifically in pregnant women or neonates/children exist to date.

16.8 Differential Diagnosis

The differential diagnostics of an acute ZIKV infection are broad and include both infectious and non-infectious causes. In general, the diagnosis of a traveller presenting with fever, rash, myalgia and arthralgia poses a challenge to the clinician due to the unspecific nature of these symptoms. The two main differential diagnoses are DENV and CHIKV infection, which are clinically close to an acute ZIKV infection (see also chapter 'clinical findings' for a more detailed comparison). Other differential diagnoses in the field of infectious diseases include malaria, other arboviruses such as (YFV, WNV, parvovirus B19, measles virus, adenoviruses, enteroviruses, Leptospirosis, Rickettsial infection and others [223, 252]. Non-infectious causes for acute ZIKV infection include, among others, musculoskeletal and autoimmune disorders. Differential diagnoses for congenital ZIKV syndrome include mainly those infections summarized by the acronym TORCH (Toxoplasmosis, other infections, Rubella Cytomegalovirus, Herpesvirus 1 and 2), but also genetic and other non-infectious etiologies [153].

16.9 Management

To date, no antiviral therapy for ZIKV exists; thus treatment is largely supportive and symptomatic [253]. Due to the usually rather mild and self-limiting nature of the disease, in most cases only little treatment, such as analgesics, antipyretics or antihistamines is necessary. The antipyretic drug of choice is acetaminophen, while non-steroidal anti-inflammatory drugs such as Aspirin should be avoided to avoid bleeding complications, especially if the differential diagnosis of a dengue infection cannot be ruled out completely [254]. Since the rash associated with ZIKV usually itches, antihistaminics can provide relief to the patient. Pregnant women with ZIKV infection should be referred to a specialist gynaecological unit for further evaluation and follow-up. Patients developing GBS should be hospitalized and GBS managed according to guidelines [255].

16.10 Prevention and Control

When travelling to areas with active ZIKV circulation, travellers are much more likely to become infected through mosquito-borne transmission than through sexual transmission. Mosquito-borne transmission can be prevented by general measures to avoid mosquito bites. ZIKV is transmitted by active mosquito species during the day, similar to CHIKV, YFV and DENV. Other pathogens like malaria, WNV and JEV are transmitted by active mosquito species from dusk till dawn. As ZIKV circulates in regions where a plethora of mosquito-borne pathogens circulate, the traveller is advised to take precautionary measures to prevent mosquito bites in general (24/7). These include:

- Use of insect repellent, e.g. DEET, icaridin, PMD (availability according to country-specific legislation)
- Cover up, e.g. wear long sleeves, pants, socks
- Block mosquito access, e.g. use of screens for windows/doors, use of mosquito net
- Permethrin treatment of clothing and gear (e.g. mosquito net, tent, socks)

The risk for sexual transmission of ZIKV can be reduced by the consistent and correct use of condoms (male or female during vaginal, anal and oral sex) while the risk can be eliminated by abstinence. The contribution of the prevention of sexual transmission to the overall prevention of infection or travellers will be low. However, in non-endemic ZIKV regions, sexual transmission through infected travellers returning from areas with active virus circulation is the main route of transmission. This is, in particular, important to prevent CZS in case the sexual partner is pregnant or has a pregnancy wish. WHO recommended that returning male travellers should abstain from sex or use condoms for 3 months upon return, while returning female travellers should do so for 2 months. In case the sexual partner of the returning traveller is pregnant, abstinence and condom use are recommended for the whole duration of the pregnancy. As ZIKV infections can be subclinical, these recommendations apply to all returning travellers regardless of the presence of symptoms or not. Pregnant travellers are advised to consider delaying non-essential travel to areas with active ZIKV transmission [9, 12]. As national Public Health authorities may have adapted the WHO recommendations in country-specific guidelines, physicians and travellers are also advised to consult national guidelines on ZIKV prevention.

16.11 Knowledge Gaps That Need to be Addressed

While extensive research has been performed on ZIKV infection, key questions remain unanswered regarding risks and mechanisms of transmission and severe complications. The majority of cohort studies to date use molecular detection of the viral genome to identify ZIKV-infected cases to calculate the risk of maternal-foetal transmission and the development of congenital ZIKV syndrome and other congenital abnormalities. Since the detection window for the ZIKV genome is limited, identification of ZIKV cases by serology should be considered to prevent an underestimation of the number of cases. Unfortunately, to date, confirmation of ZIKV infection by serology has been hampered by the potential cross-reactivity of related orthoflaviviruses such as DENV. The presence of pre-existing immunity to related orthoflaviviruses not only hampers serological diagnostics but also highlights the potential role of pre-existing immunity in the pathogenesis of ZIKV infection. All these key questions require an ability to accurately determine the infection status of individuals, as well as standardized methods to define the clinical outcome of ZIKV infection.

Declaration of Interest We declare no conflict of interest.

References

1. Dick GW, Kitchen SF, Haddow AJ. Zika virus. I. Isolations and serological specificity. Trans R Soc Trop Med Hyg. 1952;46(5):509–20.
2. Schwartz DA. The origins and emergence of Zika virus, the newest TORCH infection: what's old is new again. Arch Pathol Lab Med. 2017;141(1):18–25.
3. Simpson DI. Zika virus infection in man. Trans R Soc Trop Med Hyg. 1964;58:335–8.
4. Duffy MR, Chen TH, Hancock WT, Powers AM, Kool JL, Lanciotti RS, et al. Zika virus outbreak on Yap Island, Federated States of Micronesia. N Engl J Med. 2009;360(24):2536–43.
5. Oehler E, Watrin L, Larre P, Leparc-Goffart I, Lastere S, Valour F, et al. Zika virus infection complicated by Guillain-Barre syndrome—case report, French Polynesia, December 2013. Euro Surveill. 2014;19(9)
6. Cao-Lormeau VM, Blake A, Mons S, Lastere S, Roche C, Vanhomwegen J, et al. Guillain-Barre Syndrome outbreak associated with Zika virus infection in French Polynesia: a case-control study. Lancet. 2016;387(10027):1531–9.
7. WHO. Statement of the Fifth meeting of the Emergency Committee under the International Health Regulations (2005) regarding microcephaly, other neurological disorders and Zika

virus 2016 (Available from: https://www.who.int/news-room/detail/18-11-2016-fifth-meeting-of-the-emergency-committee-under-the-international-health-regulations-(2005)-regarding-microcephaly-other-neurological-disorders-and-zika-virus).

8. Baud D, Gubler DJ, Schaub B, Lanteri MC, Musso D. An update on Zika virus infection. Lancet. 2017;390(10107):2099–109.

9. WHO. Zika epidemiolopgy update: WHO; 2022. (Available from: zika-epidemiology-update_february-2022_clean-version.pdf (who.int)).

10. WHO. Countries and territories with current OR previous Zika virus transmission; data as of February 2022. (Available from: countries-with-zika-and-vectors-table_february-2022.pdf (who.int)).

11. Messina JP, Kraemer MU, Brady OJ, Pigott DM, Shearer FM, Weiss DJ, et al. Mapping global environmental suitability for Zika virus. Elife. 2016;5

12. ECDC. Zika virus transmission world wide: ECDC; 2019. (Available from: https://ecdc.europa.eu/sites/portal/files/documents/zika-risk-assessment-9-april-2019.pdf).

13. Ateutchia Ngouanet S, Wanji S, Yadouleton A, Demanou M, Djouaka R, Nanfack-Minkeu F. Factors enhancing the transmission of mosquito-borne arboviruses in Africa. Virus Dis. 2022;33(4):477–88.

14. Wilder-Smith A, Chang CR, Leong WY. Zika in travellers 1947–2017: a systematic review. J Travel Med. 2018;25(1)

15. ECDC. Surveillance Atlas of infectious diseases—Zika virus infection: ECDC; 2019. (Available from: Surveillance Atlas of Infectious Diseases (europa.eu)).

16. ECDC. Rapid risk assessment: Zika virus disease in Var Department, France. 16 October 2019. Zika virus autochtonous cases, France, 2019 (europa.eu).

17. ICTV. Genus: *Orthoflavivirus*; the Online report of the International Committee on Taxonomy of Viruses 2019 [cited 2023 1805]. Available from: Genus: Orthoflavivirus | ICTV.

18. Musso D, Gubler DJ. Zika virus. Clin Microbiol Rev. 2016;29(3):487–524.

19. Wang A, Thurmond S, Islas L, Hui K, Hai R. Zika virus genome biology and molecular pathogenesis. Emerg Microbes Infect. 2019;6(1):1–6.

20. Kuno G, Chang GJ. Full-length sequencing and genomic characterization of Bagaza, Kedougou, and Zika viruses. Arch Virol. 2007;152(4):687–96.

21. May M, Relich RF. A comprehensive systems biology approach to studying Zika virus. PloS One. 2016;11(9):e0161355.

22. Higuera A, Ramirez JD. Molecular epidemiology of dengue, yellow fever, Zika and Chikungunya arboviruses: an update. Acta Trop. 2019;190:99–111.

23. Pettersson JH, Eldholm V, Seligman SJ, Lundkvist A, Falconar AK, Gaunt MW, et al. How did Zika virus emerge in the Pacific Islands and Latin America? MBio. 2016;7(5)

24. Bernardo-Menezes LC, Agrelli A, Oliveira ASLE, Moura RR, Crovella S, Brandão LAC. An overview of Zika virus genotypes and their infectivity. Rev Soc Bras Med Trop. 2022;55:e02632022.

25. Gubler DJ, Vasilakis N, Musso D. History and emergence of Zika virus. J Infect Dis. 2017;216(Suppl. 10):S860–7.

26. Besnard M, Lastere S, Teissier A, Cao-Lormeau V, Musso D. Evidence of perinatal transmission of Zika virus, French Polynesia, December 2013 and February 2014. Euro Surveill. 2014;19(13)

27. Colt S, Garcia-Casal MN, Pena-Rosas JP, Finkelstein JL, Rayco-Solon P, Weise Prinzo ZC, et al. Transmission of Zika virus through breast milk and other breastfeeding-related bodily-fluids: a systematic review. PLoS Negl Trop Dis. 2017;11(4):e0005528.

28. Leung GH, Baird RW, Druce J, Anstey NM. Zika virus infection in australia following a monkey bite in Indonesia. Southeast Asian J Trop Med Public Health. 2015;46(3):460–4.

29. Runge-Ranzinger S, Morrison AC, Manrique-Saide P, Horstick O. Zika transmission patterns: a meta-review. Trop Med Int Health. 2019;24(5):523–9.

30. Centeno-Tablante E, Medina-Rivera M, Finkelstein JL, Herman HS, Rayco-Solon P, Garcia-Casal MN, Rogers L, Ghezzi-Kopel K, Zambrano Leal MP, Andrade Velasquez JK, Chang

Asinc JG, Peña-Rosas JP, Mehta S. Update on the transmission of Zika virus through breast milk and breastfeeding: a systematic review of the evidence. Viruses. 2021;13(1):123.

31. Gregory CJ, Oduyebo T, Brault AC, Brooks JT, Chung KW, Hills S, et al. Modes of transmission of Zika virus. J Infect Dis. 2017;216(Suppl. 10):S875–83.

32. Boyer S, Calvez E, Chouin-Carneiro T, Diallo D, Failloux AB. An overview of mosquito vectors of Zika virus. Microbes Infect. 2018;20(11-12):646–60.

33. Hunter FF. Linking only aedes aegypti with Zika virus has world-wide public health implications. Front Microbiol. 2017;8:1248.

34. Bueno MG, Martinez N, Abdalla L, Duarte Dos Santos CN, Chame M. Animals in the Zika virus life cycle: what to expect from megadiverse Latin American Countries. PLoS Negl Trop Dis. 2016;10(12):e0005073.

35. Althouse BM, Vasilakis N, Sall AA, Diallo M, Weaver SC, Hanley KA. Potential for Zika virus to establish a sylvatic transmission cycle in the Americas. PLoS Negl Trop Dis. 2016;10(12):e0005055.

36. Gutierrez-Bugallo G, Piedra LA, Rodriguez M, Bisset JA, Lourenco-de-Oliveira R, Weaver SC, et al. Vector-borne transmission and evolution of Zika virus. Nat Ecol Evol. 2019;3(4):561–9.

37. Figueiredo LTM. Human Urban arboviruses can infect wild animals and jump to sylvatic maintenance cycles in South America. Front Cell Infect Microbiol. 2019;9:259.

38. Smartt CT, Stenn TMS, Chen TY, Teixeira MG, Queiroz EP, Souza Dos Santos L, et al. Evidence of Zika virus RNA fragments in aedes albopictus (Diptera: Culicidae) field-collected eggs from Camacari, Bahia, Brazil. J Med Entomol. 2017;54(4):1085–7.

39. Ciota AT, Bialosuknia SM, Ehrbar DJ, Kramer LD. Vertical Transmission of Zika Virus by Aedes aegypti and Ae. albopictus Mosquitoes. Emerg Infect Dis. 2017;23(5):880–2.

40. Izquierdo-Suzan M, Zarate S, Torres-Flores J, Correa-Morales F, Gonzalez-Acosta C, Sevilla-Reyes EE, et al. Natural vertical transmission of Zika virus in larval aedes aegypti populations, Morelos, Mexico. Emerg Infect Dis. 2019;25(8):1477–84.

41. Dahiya N, Yadav M, Yadav A, Sehrawat N. Zika virus vertical transmission in mosquitoes: a less understood mechanism. J Vector Borne Dis. 2022;59(1):37–44.

42. Foy BD, Kobylinski KC, Chilson Foy JL, Blitvich BJ, Travassos da Rosa A, Haddow AD, et al. Probable non-vector-borne transmission of Zika virus, Colorado, USA. Emerg Infect Dis. 2011;17(5):880–2.

43. Cardona MWD, Du Plessis SS, Velilla PA. Semen as virus reservoir? J Assist Reprod Genet. 2016;33(9):1255–6.

44. Davidson A, Slavinski S, Komoto K, Rakeman J, Weiss D. Suspected female-to-male sexual transmission of Zika virus—New York City, 2016. MMWR Morb Mortal Wkly Rep. 2016;65(28):716–7.

45. D'Ortenzio E, Matheron S, Yazdanpanah Y, de Lamballerie X, Hubert B, Piorkowski G, et al. Evidence of sexual transmission of Zika virus. N Engl J Med. 2016;374(22):2195–8.

46. Hastings AK, Fikrig E. Zika virus and sexual transmission: a new route of transmission for mosquito-borne flaviviruses. Yale J Biol Med. 2017;90(2):325–30.

47. Counotte MJ, Kim CR, Wang J, Bernstein K, Deal CD, Broutet NJN, et al. Sexual transmission of Zika virus and other flaviviruses: a living systematic review. PLoS Med. 2018;15(7):e1002611.

48. Brooks RB, Carlos MP, Myers RA, White MG, Bobo-Lenoci T, Aplan D, et al. Likely sexual transmission of Zika virus from a man with no symptoms of infection—Maryland, 2016. MMWR Morb Mortal Wkly Rep. 2016;65(34):915–6.

49. Freour T, Mirallie S, Hubert B, Splingart C, Barriere P, Maquart M, et al. Sexual transmission of Zika virus in an entirely asymptomatic couple returning from a Zika epidemic area, France, April 2016. Euro Surveill. 2016;21(23)

50. Deckard DT, Chung WM, Brooks JT, Smith JC, Woldai S, Hennessey M, et al. Male-to-male sexual transmission of Zika virus—Texas, January 2016. MMWR Morb Mortal Wkly Rep. 2016;65(14):372–4.

51. Moreira J, Peixoto TM, Siqueira AM, Lamas CC. Sexually acquired Zika virus: a systematic review. Clin Microbiol Infect. 2017;23(5):296–305.
52. Turmel JM, Abgueguen P, Hubert B, Vandamme YM, Maquart M, Le Guillou-Guillemette H, et al. Late sexual transmission of Zika virus related to persistence in the semen. Lancet. 2016;387(10037):2501.
53. Arsuaga M, Bujalance SG, Diaz-Menendez M, Vazquez A, Arribas JR. Probable sexual transmission of Zika virus from a vasectomised man. Lancet Infect Dis. 2016;16(10):1107.
54. Mead PS, Duggal NK, Hook SA, Delorey M, Fischer M, Olzenak McGuire D, et al. Zika virus shedding in semen of symptomatic infected men. N Engl J Med. 2018;378(15):1377–85.
55. Paz-Bailey G, Rosenberg ES, Doyle K, Munoz-Jordan J, Santiago GA, Klein L, et al. Persistence of Zika virus in body fluids—final report. N Engl J Med. 2018;379(13):1234–43.
56. Barzon L, Percivalle E, Pacenti M, Rovida F, Zavattoni M, Del Bravo P, et al. Virus and antibody dynamics in travelers with acute Zika Virus Infection. Clin Infect Dis. 2018;66(8):1173–80.
57. da Cruz TE, Souza RP, Pelloso SM, Morelli F, Suehiro TT, Damke E, et al. Case reports: prolonged detection of Zika virus RNA in vaginal and endocervical samples from a Brazilian woman, 2018. Am J Trop Med Hyg. 2019;100(1):183–6.
58. Coelho FC, Durovni B, Saraceni V, Lemos C, Codeco CT, Camargo S, et al. Higher incidence of Zika in adult women than adult men in Rio de Janeiro suggests a significant contribution of sexual transmission from men to women. Int J Infect Dis. 2016;51:128–32.
59. Gao D, Lou Y, He D, Porco TC, Kuang Y, Chowell G, et al. Prevention and control of Zika as a mosquito-borne and sexually transmitted disease: a mathematical modeling analysis. Sci Rep. 2016;6:28070.
60. Allard A, Althouse BM, Hebert-Dufresne L, Scarpino SV. The risk of sustained sexual transmission of Zika is underestimated. PLoS Pathog. 2017;13(9):e1006633.
61. Miller JC. Mathematical models of SIR disease spread with combined non-sexual and sexual transmission routes. Infect Dis Model. 2017;2(1):35–55.
62. Agusto FB, Bewick S, Fagan WF. Mathematical model of Zika virus with vertical transmission. Infect Dis Model. 2017;2(2):244–67.
63. Baca-Carrasco D, Velasco-Hernandez JX. Sex, mosquitoes and epidemics: an evaluation of Zika disease dynamics. Bull Math Biol. 2016;78(11):2228–42.
64. Mlakar J, Korva M, Tul N, Popovic M, Poljsak-Prijatelj M, Mraz J, et al. Zika virus associated with microcephaly. N Engl J Med. 2016;374(10):951–8.
65. Kleber de Oliveira W, Cortez-Escalante J, De Oliveira WT, do Carmo GM, Henriques CM, Coelho GE, et al. Increase in reported prevalence of microcephaly in infants born to women living in areas with confirmed Zika virus transmission during the first trimester of pregnancy—Brazil, 2015. MMWR Morb Mortal Wkly Rep. 2016;65(9):242–7.
66. Driggers RW, Ho CY, Korhonen EM, Kuivanen S, Jaaskelainen AJ, Smura T, et al. Zika virus infection with prolonged maternal viremia and fetal brain abnormalities. N Engl J Med. 2016;374(22):2142–51.
67. van der Eijk AA, van Genderen PJ, Verdijk RM, Reusken CB, Mogling R, van Kampen JJ, et al. Miscarriage associated with Zika virus infection. N Engl J Med. 2016;375(10):1002–4.
68. Rasmussen SA, Jamieson DJ, Honein MA, Petersen LR. Zika virus and birth defects—reviewing the evidence for causality. N Engl J Med. 2016;374(20):1981–7.
69. Brasil P, Nielsen-Saines K. More pieces to the microcephaly–Zika virus puzzle in Brazil. Lancet Infect Dis. 2016;16(12):1307–9.
70. França GVA, Schuler-Faccini L, Oliveira WK, Henriques CMP, Carmo EH, Pedi VD, et al. Congenital Zika virus syndrome in Brazil: a case series of the first 1501 livebirths with complete investigation. Lancet. 2016;388(10047):891–7.
71. Johansson MA, Mier-y-Teran-Romero L, Reefhuis J, Gilboa SM, Hills SL. Zika and the risk of microcephaly. N Engl J Med. 2016;375(1):1–4.
72. Rice ME, Galang RR, Roth NM, Ellington SR, Moore CA, Valencia-Prado M, et al. Vital signs: Zika-associated birth defects and neurodevelopmental abnormalities possibly associated with congenital Zika Virus infection—U.S. Territories and Freely Associated States, 2018. MMWR Morb Mortal Wkly Rep. 2018;67(31):858–67.

73. Shapiro-Mendoza CK, Rice ME, Galang RR, Fulton AC, VanMaldeghem K, Prado MV, et al. Pregnancy outcomes after maternal Zika virus infection during pregnancy - U.S. Territories, January 1, 2016-April 25, 2017. MMWR Morb Mortal Wkly Rep. 2017;66(23):615–21.

74. Pomar L, Vouga M, Lambert V, Pomar C, Hcini N, Jolivet A, et al. Maternal-fetal transmission and adverse perinatal outcomes in pregnant women infected with Zika virus: prospective cohort study in French Guiana. BMJ. 2018;363:k4431.

75. Lessler J, Ott CT, Carcelen AC, Konikoff JM, Williamson J, Bi Q, et al. Times to key events in Zika virus infection and implications for blood donation: a systematic review. Bull World Health Organ. 2016;94(11):841–9.

76. Marbán-Castro E, Goncé A, Fumadó V, Romero-Acevedo L, Bardají A. Zika virus infection in pregnant women and their children: a review. Eur J Obstet Gynecol Reprod Biol. 2021;265:162–8.

77. Giovanetti M, Goes de Jesus J, Lima de Maia M, Junior JX, Castro Amarante MF, Viana P, et al. Genetic evidence of Zika virus in mother's breast milk and body fluids of a newborn with severe congenital defects. Clin Microbiol Infect. 2018;24(10):1111–2.

78. Mann TZ, Haddad LB, Williams TR, Hills SL, Read JS, Dee DL, et al. Breast milk transmission of flaviviruses in the context of Zika virus: a systematic review. Paediatr Perinat Epidemiol. 2018;32(4):358–68.

79. Sampieri CL, Montero H. Breastfeeding in the time of Zika: a systematic literature review. PeerJ. 2019;7

80. Blohm GM, Lednicky JA, Márquez M, White SK, Loeb JC, Pacheco CA, et al. Evidence for mother-to-child transmission of Zika virus through breast milk. Clin Infect Dis. 2018;66(7):1120–1.

81. Siqueira Mello A, Pascalicchio Bertozzi APA, Rodrigues MMD, Gazeta RE, Moron AF, Soriano-Arandes A, et al. Development of secondary microcephaly after delivery: possible consequence of mother-baby transmission of Zika virus in breast milk. Am J Case Rep. 2019;20:723–5.

82. Desgraupes S, Hubert M, Gessain A, Ceccaldi PE, Vidy A. Mother-to-child transmission of arboviruses during breastfeeding: from epidemiology to cellular mechanisms. Viruses. 2021;13(7):1312.

83. Pealer LN, Marfin AA, Petersen LR, Lanciotti RS, Page PL, Stramer SL, et al. Transmission of West Nile virus through blood transfusion in the United States in 2002. N Engl J Med. 2003;349(13):1236–45.

84. Sabino EC, Loureiro P, Lopes ME, Capuani L, McClure C, Chowdhury D, et al. Transfusion-transmitted dengue and associated clinical symptoms during the 2012 epidemic in Brazil. J Infect Dis. 2016;213(5):694–702.

85. Mitchell PK, Mier-y-Teran-Romero L, Biggerstaff BJ, Delorey MJ, Aubry M, Cao-Lormeau V-M, et al. Reassessing serosurvey-based estimates of the symptomatic proportion of Zika virus infections. Am J Epidemiol. 2019;188(1):206–13.

86. Lanteri MC, Kleinman SH, Glynn SA, Musso D, Keith Hoots W, Custer BS, et al. Zika virus: a new threat to the safety of the blood supply with worldwide impact and implications. Transfusion. 2016;56(7):1907–14.

87. Benites BD, Rocha D, Andrade E, Godoy DT, Alvarez P, Addas-Carvalho M. Zika virus and the safety of blood supply in Brazil: a retrospective epidemiological evaluation. Am J Trop Med Hyg. 2019;100(1):174–7.

88. Magnus MM, Espósito DLA, Costa VAD, Melo PSD, Costa-Lima C, Fonseca BALD, et al. Risk of Zika virus transmission by blood donations in Brazil. Hematol Transfus Cell Ther. 2018;40(3):250–4.

89. Kuehnert MJ, Basavaraju SV, Moseley RR, Pate LL, Galel SA, Williamson PC, et al. Screening of blood donations for Zika virus infection—Puerto Rico, April 3–June 11, 2016. MMWR Morb Mortal Wkly Rep. 2016;65(24):627–8.

90. Adams L, Bello-Pagan M, Lozier M, Ryff KR, Espinet C, Torres J, et al. Update: ongoing Zika virus transmission—Puerto Rico, November 1, 2015–July 7, 2016. MMWR Morb Mortal Wkly Rep. 2016;65(30):774–9.

91. Chevalier MS, Biggerstaff BJ, Basavaraju SV, Ocfemia MCB, Alsina JO, Climent-Peris C, et al. Use of blood donor screening data to estimate Zika virus incidence, Puerto Rico, April–August 2016. Emerg Infect Dis. 2017;23(5):790–5.
92. Gallian P, Cabie A, Richard P, Paturel L, Charrel RN, Pastorino B, et al. Zika virus in asymptomatic blood donors in Martinique. Blood. 2017;129(2):263–6.
93. Slavov SN, Hespanhol MR, Rodrigues ES, Levi JE, Ubiali EMA, Covas DT, et al. Zika virus RNA detection in asymptomatic blood donors during an outbreak in the northeast region of Sao Paulo State, Brazil, 2016. Transfusion. 2017;57(12):2897–901.
94. Musso D, Nhan T, Robin E, Roche C, Bierlaire D, Zisou K, et al. Potential for Zika virus transmission through blood transfusion demonstrated during an outbreak in French Polynesia, November 2013 to February 2014. Euro Surveill. 2014;19(14)
95. Williamson PC, Linnen JM, Kessler DA, Shaz BH, Kamel H, Vassallo RR, et al. First cases of Zika virus-infected US blood donors outside states with areas of active transmission. Transfusion. 2017;57(3pt2):770–8.
96. Borena W, Hofer T, Stiasny K, Aberle SW, Gaber M, von Laer D, et al. No molecular or serological evidence of Zikavirus infection among healthy blood donors living in or travelling to regions where Aedes albopictus circulates. PloS One. 2017;12(5):e0178175.
97. Motta IJ, Spencer BR, Cordeiro da Silva SG, Arruda MB, Dobbin JA, Gonzaga YB, et al. Evidence for transmission of Zika virus by platelet transfusion. N Engl J Med. 2016;375(11):1101–3.
98. Barjas-Castro ML, Angerami RN, Cunha MS, Suzuki A, Nogueira JS, Rocco IM, et al. Probable transfusion-transmitted Zika virus in Brazil. Transfusion. 2016;56(7):1684–8.
99. Giménez-Richarte Á, Ortiz de Salazar MI, Giménez-Richarte MP, Collado M, Fernández PL, Clavijo C, Navarro L, Arbona C, Marco P, Ramos-Rincon JM. Transfusion-transmitted arboviruses: update and systematic review. PLoS Negl Trop Dis. 2022;16(10):e0010843.
100. Nogueira ML, Estofolete CF, Terzian AC, Mascarin do Vale EP, da Silva RC, da Silva RF, et al. Zika virus infection and solid organ transplantation: a new challenge. Am J Transplant. 2017;17(3):791–5.
101. Silveira FP, Campos SV. The Zika epidemics and transplantation. J Heart Lung Transplant. 2016;35(5):560–3.
102. FDA. Donor screening recommendations to reduce the risk of transmission of Zika virus by human cells, tissues, and cellular and tissue-based products; 2018 (Available from: https://www.fda.gov/media/96528/download).
103. Heck E, Cavanagh HD, Robertson DM. Zika virus RNA in an asymptomatic donor's vitreous: risk of transmission? Am J Transplant. 2017;17(8):2227–8.
104. Freeman MC, Coyne CB, Green M, Williams JV, Silva LA. Emerging arboviruses and implications for pediatric transplantation: a review. Pediatr Transplant. 2019;23(1):e13303.
105. Gatherer D, Kohl A. Zika virus: a previously slow pandemic spreads rapidly through the Americas. J Gen Virol. 2016;97(2):269–73.
106. Pergolizzi J Jr, LeQuang JA, Umeda-Raffa S, Fleischer C, Pergolizzi J 3rd, Pergolizzi C, Raffa RB. The Zika virus: lurking behind the COVID-19 pandemic? J Clin Pharm Ther. 2021;46(2):267–76.
107. Giron S, Franke F, Decoppet A, Cadiou B, Travaglini T, Thirion L, Durand G, Jeannin C, L'Ambert G, Grard G, Noël H, Fournet N, Auzet-Caillaud M, Zandotti C, Aboukaïs S, Chaud P, Guedj S, Hamouda L, Naudot X, Ovize A, Lazarus C, de Valk H, Paty MC, Leparc-Goffart I. Vector-borne transmission of Zika virus in Europe, southern France, August 2019. Euro Surveill. 2019;24(45):1900655.
108. ECDC. Aedes aegypti-current known distribution: July 2019 (Available from: https://ecdc.europa.eu/en/publications-data/aedes-aegypti-current-known-distribution-july-2019).
109. Taulung LA, Masao C. Situation report #17: Zika virus & dengue fever, Kosrae State, Federated States of Micronesia 2016 (Available from: https://reliefweb.int/report/micronesia-federated-states/situation-report-17-zika-virus-dengue-fever-kosrae-state).
110. Cao-Lormeau V-M, Roche C, Teissier A, Robin E, Berry A-L, Mallet H-P, et al. Zika virus, French Polynesia, South Pacific, 2013. Emerg Infect Dis. 2014;20(6):1084–6.

111. Musso D, Nilles EJ, Cao-Lormeau VM. Rapid spread of emerging Zika virus in the Pacific area. Clin Microbiol Infect. 2014;20(10):O595–6.
112. Musso D, Bossin H, Mallet HP, Besnard M, Broult J, Baudouin L, et al. Zika virus in French Polynesia 2013-14: anatomy of a completed outbreak. Lancet Infect Dis. 2018;18(5):e172–e82.
113. Faria NR, Azevedo R, Kraemer MUG, Souza R, Cunha MS, Hill SC, et al. Zika virus in the Americas: early epidemiological and genetic findings. Science. 2016;352(6283):345–9.
114. Government I. Zika Virus strain that causes microcephaly not found in Rajasthan New Delhi: Press Information Bureau, Government of India, Ministry of Health and Family Welfare; 2018 (Available from: https://pib.gov.in/newsite/PrintRelease.aspx?relid=184586).
115. Zanluca C, Melo VC, Mosimann AL, Santos GI, Santos CN, Luz K. First report of autochthonous transmission of Zika virus in Brazil. Mem Inst Oswaldo Cruz. 2015;110(4):569–72.
116. PAHO. Cases of Zika virus disease by country or Territory 2019 (Available from: http://www.paho.org/data/index.php/en/mnu-topics/zika/524-zika-weekly-en.html).
117. Wongsurawat T, Athipanyasilp N, Jenjaroenpun P, Jun SR, Kaewnapan B, Wassenaar TM, et al. Case of microcephaly after congenital infection with Asian Lineage Zika virus, Thailand. Emerg Infect Dis. 2018;24:9.
118. Lan PT, Quang LC, Huong VTQ, Thuong NV, Hung PC, Huong T, et al. Fetal Zika virus Infection in Vietnam. PLoS Curr. 2017;9
119. Moi ML, Nguyen TTT, Nguyen CT, Vu TBH, Tun MMN, Pham TD, et al. Zika virus infection and microcephaly in Vietnam. Lancet Infect Dis. 2017;17(8):805–6.
120. Duggal NK, Ritter JM, McDonald EM, Romo H, Guirakhoo F, Davis BS, et al. Differential neurovirulence of African and Asian genotype Zika virus isolates in outbred immunocompetent mice. Am J Trop Med Hyg. 2017;97(5):1410–7.
121. Sheridan MA, Balaraman V, Schust DJ, Ezashi T, Roberts RM, Franz AWE. African and Asian strains of Zika virus differ in their ability to infect and lyse primitive human placental trophoblast. PloS One. 2018;13(7):e0200086.
122. Simonin Y, van Riel D, Van de Perre P, Rockx B, Salinas S. Differential virulence between Asian and African lineages of Zika virus. PLoS Negl Trop Dis. 2017;11(9):e0005821.
123. Sassetti M, Ze-Ze L, Franco J, Cunha JD, Gomes A, Tome A, et al. First case of confirmed congenital Zika syndrome in continental Africa. Trans R Soc Trop Med Hyg. 2018;112(10):458–62.
124. Hill SC, Vasconcelos J, Neto Z, Jandondo D, Zé-Zé L, Santana Aguiar R, et al. Emergence of the Zika virus Asian lineage in Angola. Lancet Infect Dis. 2019;19(10):1138–47. bioRxiv
125. Lourenço J, Monteiro M, Tomás T, Monteiro Rodrigues J, Pybus O, Rodrigues Faria N. Epidemiology of the Zika virus outbreak in the Cabo Verde Islands, West Africa. PLoS Curr. 2018. doi: https://doi.org/10.1371/currents.outbreaks.19433b1e4d007451c69 1f138e1e67e8c
126. Faria NR, Quick J, Claro IM, Thézé J, de Jesus JG, Giovanetti M, et al. Establishment and cryptic transmission of Zika virus in Brazil and the Americas. Nature. 2017;546(7658):406–10.
127. Metsky HC, Matranga CB, Wohl S, Schaffner SF, Freije CA, Winnicki SM, et al. Zika virus evolution and spread in the Americas. Nature. 2017;546(7658):411–5.
128. Grubaugh ND, Ladner JT, Kraemer MUG, Dudas G, Tan AL, Gangavarapu K, et al. Genomic epidemiology reveals multiple introductions of Zika virus into the United States. Nature. 2017;546(7658):401–5.
129. Grubaugh ND, Saraf S, Gangavarapu K, Watts A, Tan AL, Oidtman RJ, et al. Travel surveillance and genomics uncover a hidden Zika Outbreak during the waning epidemic. Cell. 2019;178(5):1057–71. e11
130. Grubaugh ND, Faria NR, Andersen KG, Pybus OG. Genomic insights into Zika virus emergence and spread. Cell. 2018;172(6):1160–2.
131. Leder K, Grobusch MP, Gautret P, Chen LH, Kuhn S, Lim PL, et al. Zika beyond the Americas: travelers as sentinels of Zika virus transmission. A GeoSentinel analysis, 2012–2016. PloS One. 2017;12(10):e0185689.

132. Cleton N, Reusken C, Murk JL, de Jong M, Reimerink J, van der Eijk A, et al. Using routine diagnostic data as a method of surveillance of arboviral infection in travellers: a comparative analysis with a focus on dengue. Travel Med Infect Dis. 2014;12(2):159–66.
133. Wilson ME. The traveller and emerging infections: sentinel, courier, transmitter. J Appl Microbiol. 2003;94(Suppl. 1):1S–11S.
134. ECDC. Surveillance atlas of infectious diseases; Zika virus infection: ECDC; access 2023 2405 (Available from: Surveillance Atlas of Infectious Diseases (europa.eu)).
135. CDC. Zika virus; Yearly counts for US states and territories; Access 2023 2405 (Available from: Statistics and Maps I Zika virus I CDC).
136. Krow-Lucal ER, Biggerstaff BJ, Staples JE. Estimated incubation period for Zika virus disease. Emerg Infect Dis. 2017;23(5):841–5.
137. Smithburn KC. Neutralizing antibodies against arthropod-borne viruses in the sera of long-time residents of Malaya and Borneo. Am J Hyg. 1954;59(2):157–63.
138. Grossi-Soyster EN, LaBeaud AD. Clinical aspects of Zika virus. Curr Opin Pediatr. 2017;29(1):102–6.
139. Daudens-Vaysse E, Ledrans M, Gay N, Ardillon V, Cassadou S, Najioullah F, et al. Zika emergence in the French Territories of America and description of first confirmed cases of Zika virus infection on Martinique, November 2015 to February 2016. Euro Surveill. 2016;21(28)
140. Guanche Garcell H, Gutierrez Garcia F, Ramirez Nodal M, Ruiz Lozano A, Perez Diaz CR, Gonzalez Valdes A, et al. Clinical relevance of Zika symptoms in the context of a Zika Dengue epidemic. J Infect Public Health. 2020;13(2):173–6.
141. Stamm LV. Zika virus in the Americas: an obscure arbovirus comes calling. JAMA Dermatol. 2016;152(6):621–2.
142. Pinto Junior VL, Luz K, Parreira R, Ferrinho P. Zika virus: a review to clinicians. Acta Med Port. 2015;28(6):760–5.
143. Waddell LA, Greig JD. Scoping review of the Zika virus literature. PloS One. 2016;11(5):e0156376.
144. Paniz-Mondolfi AE, Blohm GM, Hernandez-Perez M, Larrazabal A, Moya D, Marquez M, et al. Cutaneous features of Zika virus infection: a clinicopathological overview. Clin Exp Dermatol. 2019;44(1):13–9.
145. Garcia E, Yactayo S, Nishino K, Millot V, Perea W, Brianda S. Zika virus infection: global update on epidemiology and potentially associated clinical manifestations. Weekly Epidemiol Record. 2016;91(7):73–88.
146. Soares CN, Brasil P, Carrera RM, Sequeira P, de Filippis AB, Borges VA, et al. Fatal encephalitis associated with Zika virus infection in an adult. J Clin Virol. 2016;83:63–5.
147. Swaminathan S, Schlaberg R, Lewis J, Hanson KE, Couturier MR. Fatal Zika virus infection with secondary nonsexual transmission. N Engl J Med. 2016;375(19):1907–9.
148. Zonneveld R, Roosblad J, Staveren JW, Wilschut JC, Vreden SG, Codrington J. Three atypical lethal cases associated with acute Zika virus infection in Suriname. IDCases. 2016;5:49–53.
149. Styczynski AR, Malta J, Krow-Lucal ER, Percio J, Nobrega ME, Vargas A, et al. Increased rates of Guillain-Barre syndrome associated with Zika virus outbreak in the Salvador metropolitan area, Brazil. PLoS Negl Trop Dis. 2017;11(8):e0005869.
150. Capasso A, Ompad DC, Vieira DL, Wilder-Smith A, Tozan Y. Incidence of Guillain-Barre Syndrome (GBS) in Latin America and the Caribbean before and during the 2015-2016 Zika virus epidemic: a systematic review and meta-analysis. PLoS Negl Trop Dis. 2019;13(8):e0007622.
151. Sejvar JJ, Baughman AL, Wise M, Morgan OW. Population incidence of Guillain-Barre syndrome: a systematic review and meta-analysis. Neuroepidemiology. 2011;36(2):123–33.
152. Chibueze EC, Tirado V, Lopes KD, Balogun OO, Takemoto Y, Swa T, et al. Zika virus infection in pregnancy: a systematic review of disease course and complications. Reprod Health. 2017;14(1):28.
153. Moore CA, Staples JE, Dobyns WB, Pessoa A, Ventura CV, Fonseca EB, et al. Characterizing the pattern of anomalies in congenital Zika syndrome for pediatric clinicians. JAMA Pediatr. 2017;171(3):288–95.

154. Hoen B, Schaub B, Funk AL, Ardillon V, Boullard M, Cabie A, et al. Pregnancy outcomes after ZIKV infection in French territories in the Americas. N Engl J Med. 2018;378(11):985–94.
155. Cauchemez S, Besnard M, Bompard P, Dub T, Guillemette-Artur P, Eyrolle-Guignot D, et al. Association between Zika virus and microcephaly in French Polynesia, 2013–15: a retrospective study. Lancet. 2016;387(10033):2125–32.
156. Reynolds MR, Jones AM, Petersen EE, Lee EH, Rice ME, Bingham A, et al. Vital signs: update on Zika virus-associated birth defects and evaluation of all U.S. infants with congenital Zika virus exposure—U.S. Zika Pregnancy Registry, 2016. MMWR Morb Mortal Wkly Rep. 2017;66(13):366–73.
157. Hamel R, Dejarnac O, Wichit S, Ekchariyawat P, Neyret A, Luplertlop N, et al. Biology of Zika virus infection in human skin cells. J Virol. 2015;89(17):8880–96.
158. Pingen M, Schmid MA, Harris E, McKimmie CS. Mosquito biting modulates skin response to virus infection. Trends Parasitol. 2017;33(8):645–57.
159. Hastings AK, Uraki R, Gaitsch H, Dhaliwal K, Stanley S, Sproch H, et al. Aedes aegypti NeSt1 protein enhances Zika virus pathogenesis by activating neutrophils. J Virol. 2019;93(13)
160. Liu S, DeLalio LJ, Isakson BE, Wang TT. AXL-mediated productive infection of human endothelial cells by Zika virus. Circ Res. 2016;119(11):1183–9.
161. Peng H, Liu B, Yves TD, He Y, Wang S, Tang H, et al. Zika virus induces autophagy in human umbilical vein endothelial cells. Viruses. 2018;10(5)
162. Anfasa F, Goeijenbier M, Widagdo W, Siegers JY, Mumtaz N, Okba N, et al. Zika virus infection induces elevation of tissue factor production and apoptosis on human umbilical vein endothelial cells. Front Microbiol. 2019;10:817.
163. Colombo TE, Estofolete CF, Reis AFN, da Silva NS, Aguiar ML, Cabrera EMS, et al. Clinical, laboratory and virological data from suspected ZIKV patients in an endemic arbovirus area. J Clin Virol. 2017;96:20–5.
164. Chan JF, Choi GK, Yip CC, Cheng VC, Yuen KY. Zika fever and congenital Zika syndrome: an unexpected emerging arboviral disease. J Infect. 2016;72(5):507–24.
165. Colavita F, Musumeci G, Caglioti C. Human osteoblast-like cells are permissive for Zika virus replication. J Rheumatol. 2018;45(3):443.
166. Mumtaz N, Koedam M, van den Doel PB, van Leeuwen J, Koopmans MPG, van der Eerden BCJ, et al. Zika virus infection perturbs osteoblast function. Sci Rep. 2018;8(1):16975.
167. Capiz D, Grossniklaus HE, Yeh S. Pathogenesis of ocular findings in congenital Zika syndrome. JAMA Ophthalmol. 2017;135(10):1077.
168. Manangeeswaran M, Kielczewski JL, Sen HN, Xu BC, Ireland DDC, McWilliams IL, et al. ZIKA virus infection causes persistent chorioretinal lesions. Emerg Microbes Infect. 2018;7(1):96.
169. Singh PK, Guest JM, Kanwar M, Boss J, Gao N, Juzych MS, et al. Zika virus infects cells lining the blood-retinal barrier and causes chorioretinal atrophy in mouse eyes. JCI Insight. 2017;2(4):e92340.
170. Oliveira DBL, Durigon GS, Mendes EA, Ladner JT, Andreata-Santos R, Araujo DB, et al. Persistence and intra-host genetic evolution of Zika virus infection in symptomatic adults: a special view in the male reproductive system. Viruses. 2018;10(11)
171. Siemann DN, Strange DP, Maharaj PN, Shi PY, Verma S. Zika virus infects human sertoli cells and modulates the integrity of the in vitro blood-testis barrier model. J Virol. 2017;91(22)
172. Matusali G, Houzet L, Satie AP, Mahe D, Aubry F, Couderc T, et al. Zika virus infects human testicular tissue and germ cells. J Clin Invest. 2018;128(10):4697–710.
173. Avelino-Silva VI, Alvarenga C, Abreu C, Tozetto-Mendoza TR, Canto C, Manuli ER, et al. Potential effect of Zika virus infection on human male fertility? Rev Inst Med Trop Sao Paulo. 2018;60:e64.
174. Govero J, Esakky P, Scheaffer SM, Fernandez E, Drury A, Platt DJ, et al. Zika virus infection damages the testes in mice. Nature. 2016;540(7633):438–42.
175. Ma W, Li S, Ma S, Jia L, Zhang F, Zhang Y, et al. Zika virus causes testis damage and leads to male infertility in mice. Cell. 2016;167(6):1511–24. e10

176. Visseaux B, Mortier E, Houhou-Fidouh N, Brichler S, Collin G, Larrouy L, et al. Zika virus in the female genital tract. Lancet Infect Dis. 2016;16(11):1220.
177. Carroll T, Lo M, Lanteri M, Dutra J, Zarbock K, Silveira P, et al. Zika virus preferentially replicates in the female reproductive tract after vaginal inoculation of rhesus macaques. PLoS Pathog. 2017;13(7):e1006537.
178. Pagani I, Ghezzi S, Ulisse A, Rubio A, Turrini F, Garavaglia E, et al. Human endometrial stromal cells are highly permissive to productive infection by Zika virus. Sci Rep. 2017;7:44286.
179. Roze B, Najioullah F, Ferge JL, Dorleans F, Apetse K, Barnay JL, et al. Guillain-Barre syndrome associated with Zika virus infection in Martinique in 2016: a prospective study. Clin Infect Dis. 2017;65(9):1462–8.
180. Salinas JL, Walteros DM, Styczynski A, Garzon F, Quijada H, Bravo E, et al. Zika virus disease-associated Guillain-Barre syndrome-Barranquilla, Colombia 2015–2016. J Neurol Sci. 2017;381:272–7.
181. Galliez RM, Spitz M, Rafful PP, Cagy M, Escosteguy C, Germano CS, et al. Zika virus causing encephalomyelitis associated with immunoactivation. Open Forum Infect Dis. 2016;3(4):ofw203.
182. Mecharles S, Herrmann C, Poullain P, Tran TH, Deschamps N, Mathon G, et al. Acute myelitis due to Zika virus infection. Lancet. 2016;387(10026):1481.
183. Munoz LS, Barreras P, Pardo CA. Zika virus-associated neurological disease in the adult: Guillain-Barre syndrome, Encephalitis, and Myelitis. Semin Reprod Med. 2016;34(5):273–9.
184. Brito Ferreira ML, Antunes de Brito CA, Moreira AJP, de Morais Machado MI, Henriques-Souza A, Cordeiro MT, et al. Guillain-Barre syndrome, acute disseminated encephalomyelitis and encephalitis associated with Zika virus infection in Brazil: detection of viral RNA and isolation of virus during late infection. Am J Trop Med Hyg. 2017;97(5):1405–9.
185. Niemeyer B, Niemeyer R, Borges R, Marchiori E. Acute disseminated encephalomyelitis following Zika virus infection. Eur Neurol. 2017;77(1–2):45–6.
186. Pradhan F, Burns JD, Agameya A, Patel A, Alfaqih M, Small JE, et al. Case report: Zika virus meningoencephalitis and myelitis and associated magnetic resonance imaging findings. Am J Trop Med Hyg. 2017;97(2):340–3.
187. Carod-Artal FJ. Neurological complications of Zika virus infection. Expert Rev Anti Infect Ther. 2018;16(5):399–410.
188. Figueiredo CP, Barros-Aragao FGQ, Neris RLS, Frost PS, Soares C, Souza INO, et al. Zika virus replicates in adult human brain tissue and impairs synapses and memory in mice. Nat Commun. 2019;10(1):3890.
189. Li H, Saucedo-Cuevas L, Regla-Nava JA, Chai G, Sheets N, Tang W, Terskikh AV, Shresta S, Gleeson JG. Zika virus infects neural progenitors in the adult mouse brain and alters proliferation. Cell Stem Cell. 2016;19(5):593–8.
190. Dos Santos T, Rodriguez A, Almiron M, Sanhueza A, Ramon P, de Oliveira WK, et al. Zika virus and the Guillain-Barre syndrome—case series from seven countries. N Engl J Med. 2016;375(16):1598–601.
191. Koma T, Veljkovic V, Anderson DE, Wang LF, Rossi SL, Shan C, et al. Zika virus infection elicits auto-antibodies to C1q. Sci Rep. 2018;8(1):1882.
192. Kallenberg CG. Anti-C1q autoantibodies. Autoimmun Rev. 2008;7(8):612–5.
193. Abbasi AU. Zika virus infection; vertical transmission and foetal congenital anomalies. J Ayub Med Coll Abbottabad. 2016;28(1):1–2.
194. Tabata T, Petitt M, Puerta-Guardo H, Michlmayr D, Wang C, Fang-Hoover J, et al. Zika virus targets different primary human placental cells, suggesting two routes for vertical transmission. Cell Host Microbe. 2016;20(2):155–66.
195. Aagaard KM, Lahon A, Suter MA, Arya RP, Seferovic MD, Vogt MB, et al. Primary human placental trophoblasts are permissive for Zika virus (ZIKV) replication. Sci Rep. 2017;7:41389.
196. Tabata T, Petitt M, Puerta-Guardo H, Michlmayr D, Harris E, Pereira L. Zika virus replicates in proliferating cells in explants from first-trimester human Placentas, potential sites for dissemination of infection. J Infect Dis. 2018;217(8):1202–13.

197. Ho CY, Castillo N, Encinales L, Porras A, Mendoza AR, Lynch R, et al. Second-trimester ultrasound and neuropathologic findings in congenital Zika virus infection. Pediatr Infect Dis J. 2018;37(12):1290–3.
198. Werner H, Sodre D, Hygino C, Guedes B, Fazecas T, Nogueira R, et al. First-trimester intra-uterine Zika virus infection and brain pathology: prenatal and postnatal neuroimaging findings. Prenat Diagn. 2016;36(8):785–9.
199. Gladwyn-Ng I, Cordon-Barris L, Alfano C, Creppe C, Couderc T, Morelli G, et al. Stress-induced unfolded protein response contributes to Zika virus-associated microcephaly. Nat Neurosci. 2018;21(1):63–71.
200. Alfano C, Gladwyn-Ng I, Couderc T, Lecuit M, Nguyen L. The unfolded protein response: a key player in Zika virus-associated congenital microcephaly. Front Cell Neurosci. 2019;13:94.
201. Undabeitia J, Pendleton C, Jallo GI, Quinones-Hinojosa A. Operative treatment for micro-cephaly secondary to craniosynostosis at the turn of the twentieth century. Childs Nerv Syst. 2011;27(11):1995–8.
202. Del Campo M, Feitosa IM, Ribeiro EM, Horovitz DD, Pessoa AL, Franca GV, et al. The phenotypic spectrum of congenital Zika syndrome. Am J Med Genet A. 2017;173(4):841–57.
203. Bayless NL, Greenberg RS, Swigut T, Wysocka J, Blish CA. Zika virus infection induces cranial neural crest cells to produce cytokines at levels detrimental for neurogenesis. Cell Host Microbe. 2016;20(4):423–8.
204. Yan Y, Zhang XT, Wang G, Cheng X, Yan Y, Fu YJ, et al. Zika virus induces abnormal cranial osteogenesis by negatively affecting cranial neural crest development. Infect Genet Evol. 2019;69:176–89.
205. Mumtaz N, Dudakovic A, Nair A, Koedam M, van Leeuwen JPTM, Koopmans MPG, Rockx B, van Wijnen AJ, van der Eerden BCJ. Zika virus alters osteogenic lineage progression of human mesenchymal stromal cells. J Cell Physiol. 2023;238(2):379–92.
206. Dejnirattisai W, Supasa P, Wongwiwat W, Rouvinski A, Barba-Spaeth G, Duangchinda T, et al. Dengue virus sero-cross-reactivity drives antibody-dependent enhancement of infection with zika virus. Nat Immunol. 2016;17(9):1102–8.
207. Rathore APS, Saron WAA, Lim T, Jahan N, St John AL. Maternal immunity and antibodies to dengue virus promote infection and Zika virus-induced microcephaly in fetuses. Sci Adv. 2019;5(2):eaav3208.
208. Zimmerman MG, Quicke KM, O'Neal JT, Arora N, Machiah D, Priyamvada L, et al. Cross-reactive dengue virus antibodies augment Zika virus infection of human placental macro-phages. Cell Host Microbe. 2018;24(5):731–42. e6
209. Katzelnick LC, Narvaez C, Arguello S, Lopez Mercado B, Collado D, Ampie O, Elizondo D, Miranda T, Bustos Carillo F, Mercado JC, Latta K, Schiller A, Segovia-Chumbez B, Ojeda S, Sanchez N, Plazaola M, Coloma J, Halloran ME, Premkumar L, Gordon A, Narvaez F, de Silva AM, Kuan G, Balmaseda A, Harris E. Zika virus infection enhances future risk of severe dengue disease. Science. 2020;369(6507):1123–8.
210. Setoh YX, Amarilla AA, Peng NYG, Griffiths RE, Carrera J, Freney ME, et al. Determinants of Zika virus host tropism uncovered by deep mutational scanning. Nat Microbiol. 2019;4(5):876–87.
211. Carbaugh DL, Baric RS, Lazear HM. Envelope protein glycosylation mediates Zika virus pathogenesis. J Virol. 2019;93(12)
212. Asif A, Manzoor S, Tuz-Zahra F, Saalim M, Ashraf M, Ishtiyaq J, et al. Zika virus: immune evasion mechanisms, currently available therapeutic regimens, and vaccines. Viral Immunol. 2017;30(10):682–90.
213. Xia H, Luo H, Shan C, Muruato AE, Nunes BTD, Medeiros DBA, et al. An evolutionary NS1 mutation enhances Zika virus evasion of host interferon induction. Nat Commun. 2018;9(1):414.
214. Puerta-Guardo H, Tabata T, Petitt M, Dimitrova M, Glasner DR, Pereira L, et al. Zika virus non-structural protein 1 disrupts glycosaminoglycans and causes permeability in developing human placentas. J Infect Dis. 2020;221(2):313–24.

215. Puerta-Guardo H, Glasner DR, Espinosa DA, Biering SB, Patana M, Ratnasiri K, et al. Flavivirus NS1 triggers tissue-specific vascular endothelial dysfunction reflecting disease tropism. Cell Rep. 2019;26(6):1598–613. e8
216. Bowen JR, Quicke KM, Maddur MS, O'Neal JT, McDonald CE, Fedorova NB, et al. Zika virus antagonizes Type I interferon responses during infection of human dendritic cells. PLoS Pathog. 2017;13(2):e1006164.
217. Grant A, Ponia SS, Tripathi S, Balasubramaniam V, Miorin L, Sourisseau M, et al. Zika virus targets human STAT2 to inhibit Type I interferon signaling. Cell Host Microbe. 2016;19(6):882–90.
218. Kumar A, Hou S, Airo AM, Limonta D, Mancinelli V, Branton W, et al. Zika virus inhibits type-I interferon production and downstream signaling. EMBO Rep. 2016;17(12):1766–75.
219. Theel ES, Hata DJ. Diagnostic testing for Zika virus: a postoutbreak update. J Clin Microbiol. 2018;56(4)
220. Gourinat AC, O'Connor O, Calvez E, Goarant C, Dupont-Rouzeyrol M. Detection of Zika virus in urine. Emerg Infect Dis. 2015;21(1):84–6.
221. Atkinson B, Hearn P, Afrough B, Lumley S, Carter D, Aarons EJ, et al. Detection of Zika virus in semen. Emerg Infect Dis. 2016;22(5):940.
222. Musso D, Roche C, Nhan TX, Robin E, Teissier A, Cao-Lormeau VM. Detection of Zika virus in saliva. J Clin Virol. 2015;68:53–5.
223. Calvet G, Aguiar RS, Melo ASO, Sampaio SA, de Filippis I, Fabri A, et al. Detection and sequencing of Zika virus from amniotic fluid of fetuses with microcephaly in Brazil: a case study. Lancet Infect Dis. 2016;16(6):653–60.
224. Musso D, Rouault E, Teissier A, Lanteri MC, Zisou K, Broult J, et al. Molecular detection of Zika virus in blood and RNA load determination during the French Polynesian outbreak. J Med Virol. 2017;89(9):1505–10.
225. Lanciotti RS, Kosoy OL, Laven JJ, Velez JO, Lambert AJ, Johnson AJ, et al. Genetic and serologic properties of Zika virus associated with an epidemic, Yap State, Micronesia, 2007. Emerg Infect Dis. 2008;14(8):1232–9.
226. Waggoner JJ, Gresh L, Vargas MJ, Ballesteros G, Tellez Y, Soda KJ, et al. Viremia and clinical presentation in Nicaraguan patients infected with Zika virus, Chikungunya virus, and dengue virus. Clin Infect Dis. 2016;63(12):1584–90.
227. Corman VM, Rasche A, Baronti C, Aldabbagh S, Cadar D, Reusken CB, et al. Assay optimization for molecular detection of Zika virus. Bull World Health Organ. 2016;94(12):880–92.
228. Bozza FA, Moreira-Soto A, Rockstroh A, Fischer C, Nascimento AD, Calheiros AS, et al. Differential shedding and antibody kinetics of Zika and Chikungunya viruses, Brazil. Emerg Infect Dis. 2019;25(2):311–5.
229. Meaney-Delman D, Oduyebo T, Polen KN, White JL, Bingham AM, Slavinski SA, et al. Prolonged detection of Zika virus RNA in pregnant women. Obstet Gynecol. 2016;128(4):724–30.
230. Rossini G, Gaibani P, Vocale C, Cagarelli R, Landini MP. Comparison of Zika virus (ZIKV) RNA detection in plasma, whole blood and urine—case series of travel-associated ZIKV infection imported to Italy, 2016. J Infect. 2017;75(3):242–5.
231. Joguet G, Mansuy JM, Matusali G, Hamdi S, Walschaerts M, Pavili L, et al. Effect of acute Zika virus infection on sperm and virus clearance in body fluids: a prospective observational study. Lancet Infect Dis. 2017;17(11):1200–8.
232. Mansuy JM, Mengelle C, Pasquier C, Chapuy-Regaud S, Delobel P, Martin-Blondel G, et al. Zika virus infection and prolonged viremia in whole-blood specimens. Emerg Infect Dis. 2017;23(5):863–5.
233. Voermans JJC, Pas SD, van der Linden A, GeurtsvanKessel C, Koopmans M, van der Eijk A, et al. Whole-blood testing for diagnosis of acute Zika virus infections in routine diagnostic setting. Emerg Infect Dis. 2019;25(7):1394–6.
234. Bingham AM, Cone M, Mock V, Heberlein-Larson L, Stanek D, Blackmore C, et al. Comparison of test results for Zika virus RNA in urine, serum, and saliva specimens from persons with travel-associated Zika virus disease—Florida, 2016. MMWR Morb Mortal Wkly Rep. 2016;65(18):475–8.

235. Paz-Bailey G, Rosenberg ES, Sharp TM. Persistence of Zika virus in body fluids—final report. N Engl J Med. 2019;380(2):198–9.
236. Pyke AT, Daly MT, Cameron JN, Moore PR, Taylor CT, Hewitson GR, et al. Imported zika virus infection from the cook islands into Australia, 2014. PLoS Curr. 2014;6
237. Schaub B, Vouga M, Najioullah F, Gueneret M, Monthieux A, Harte C, et al. Analysis of blood from Zika virus-infected fetuses: a prospective case series. Lancet Infect Dis. 2017;17(5):520–7.
238. Bosch I, de Puig H, Hiley M, Carre-Camps M, Perdomo-Celis F, Narvaez CF, et al. Rapid antigen tests for dengue virus serotypes and Zika virus in patient serum. Sci Transl Med. 2017;9(409)
239. Prevention CfDCa. (Available from: https://www.cdc.gov/pregnancy/zika/testing-follow-up/testing-and-diagnosis.html).
240. Song H, Qi J, Haywood J, Shi Y, Gao GF. Zika virus NS1 structure reveals diversity of electrostatic surfaces among flaviviruses. Nat Struct Mol Biol. 2016;23(5):456–8.
241. Kadkhoda K, Gretchen A, Racano A. Evaluation of a commercially available Zika virus IgM ELISA: specificity in focus. Diagn Microbiol Infect Dis. 2017;88(3):233–5.
242. Sloan A, Safronetz D, Makowski K, Barairo N, Ranadheera C, Dimitrova K, et al. Evaluation of the Diasorin Liaison(R) XL Zika Capture IgM CMIA for Zika virus serological testing. Diagn Microbiol Infect Dis. 2018;90(4):264–6.
243. Huzly D, Hanselmann I, Schmidt-Chanasit J, Panning M. High specificity of a novel Zika virus ELISA in European patients after exposure to different flaviviruses. Euro Surveill. 2016;21(16)
244. Organization WH. WHO Statement on the First Meeting of the International Health Regulations (2005) (IHR 2005) Emergency Committee on Zika virus and observed increase in neurological disorders and neonatal malformations; 2016.
245. Rabe IB, Staples JE, Villanueva J, Hummel KB, Johnson JA, Rose L, et al. Interim guidance for interpretation of Zika virus antibody test results. MMWR Morb Mortal Wkly Rep. 2016;65(21):543–6.
246. Landry ML, St George K. Laboratory diagnosis of Zika virus infection. Arch Pathol Lab Med. 2017;141(1):60–7.
247. Griffin I, Martin SW, Fischer M, Chambers TV, Kosoy O, Falise A, et al. Zika virus IgM detection and neutralizing antibody profiles 12–19 months after illness. Onset Emerg Infect Dis. 2019;25(2):299–303.
248. Hoen B, Carpentier M, Gaete S, Tressieres B, Herrmann-Storck C, Vingadassalom I, et al. Kinetics of anti-Zika virus antibodies after acute infection in pregnant women. J Clin Microbiol. 2019;57(11):e01151-19.
249. Warnecke JM, Lattwein E, Saschenbrecker S, Stocker W, Schlumberger W, Steinhagen K. Added value of IgA antibodies against Zika virus non-structural protein 1 in the diagnosis of acute Zika virus infections. J Virol Methods. 2019;267:8–15.
250. Zhao LZ, Hong WX, Wang J, Yu L, Hu FY, Qiu S, et al. Kinetics of antigen-specific IgM/IgG/IgA antibody responses during Zika virus natural infection in two patients. J Med Virol. 2019;91(5):872–6.
251. Amaro F, Sanchez-Seco MP, Vazquez A, Alves MJ, Ze-Ze L, Luz MT, et al. The application and interpretation of IgG avidity and IgA ELISA tests to characterize Zika virus infections. Viruses. 2019;11(2)
252. Eckerle I, Briciu VT, Ergonul O, Lupse M, Papa A, Radulescu A, et al. Emerging souvenirs-clinical presentation of the returning traveller with imported arbovirus infections in Europe. Clin Microbiol Infect. 2018;24(3):240–5.
253. CDC. Recognizing, managing, and reporting Zika virus infections in travelers returning from Central America, South America, the Caribbean, and Mexico. CDC; 2016. (Available from: https://www.emergency.cdc.gov/han/han00385.asp)
254. Sampathkumar P, Sanchez JL. Zika virus in the Americas: a review for clinicians. Mayo Clin Proc. 2016;91(4):514–21.
255. Hasan S, Saeed S, Panigrahi R, Choudhary P. Zika virus: a global public health menace: a comprehensive update. J Int Soc Prev Community Dent. 2019;9(4):316–27.

West Nile Virus Infection in Travellers

17

Francesco Castelli, Corneliu Petru Popescu, and Lina Rachele Tomasoni

Abstract

West Nile virus is a widespread arboviral flavivirus infection occurring nearly everywhere around the globe. It is transmitted by the bite of several mosquitoes, the most epidemiologically relevant of whom belong to the Genus *Culex*. The natural reservoirs of the infection are several sylvatic birds, where the infection may be mild or life-threatening. Mammals, including humans and equids, are accidentally infected and are considered dead-end hosts, as viraemia does not reach high enough levels to infect biting mosquitoes. In humans, the infection may be asymptomatic (75–80%), mild (essentially febrile syndrome with myalgia, 20–25%) or severe with neurological involvement (1%), with lethal cases especially occurring in immunocompromised and older hosts. Individuals may be infected during travel and the travel medicine doctors must suspect diagnosis promptly among the many viral and bacterial causes of encephalitis and meningitis. Confirmation of West Nile virus (WNV) infection may benefit from molecular tools in the early phase of

F. Castelli (✉)
Department of Infectious and Tropical Diseases, University of Brescia and ASST Spedali Civili of Brescia, Brescia, Italy

ESCMID Study Group for Infections in Travelers and Migrants, Basel, Switzerland

UNESCO Chair Training and empowering human resources of health development in resource-limited countries, UNESCO, Brescia, Italy
e-mail: francesco.castelli@unibs.it

C. P. Popescu
ESCMID Study Group for Infections in Travelers and Migrants, Basel, Switzerland

Carol Davila University of Medicine and Pharmacy, Bucharest, Romania

Dr Victor Babes Clinical Hospital of Infectious and Tropical Diseases, Bucharest, Romania

L. R. Tomasoni
Unit for Tropical Diseases, ASST Spedali Civili of Brescia, Brescia, Italy

© The Author(s), under exclusive license to Springer Nature Switzerland AG 2024
H. Leblebicioglu et al. (eds.), *Emerging and Re-emerging Infections in Travellers*, https://doi.org/10.1007/978-3-031-49475-8_17

the infection. Serology is also a useful tool, although cross-reactions may occur. No vaccine nor specific treatment exists so far and prevention of mosquito bites (covering clothes, repellents, mosquito nets) still represents the best preventive measure for the traveller, especially if at risk of severe infection.

17.1 Background

West Nile virus (WNV) is a neurotropic virus that belongs to the Family *Flaviviridae*, Genus *Flavivirus*. It has first been isolated in 1937 in a feverish patient in the West Nile District of Uganda [1]. WNV has subsequently moved to southern and Mediterranean Europe in the last half of the twentieth century, reaching the United States of America in 1999. The cycle of the infection involves both mosquito vectors (mainly *Culex* spp.) and wild bird (active reservoir of the virus), while mammals (in particular, but not limited to, equids and humans) may be clinically affected but do not act as reservoir of the infection as they do not develop significant viraemia. They are therefore defined as dead-end hosts. Asymptomatic (75–80%) or pauci-symptomatic febrile (20–25%) infections greatly exceed clinically significant neurological symptoms that occur in nearly 1% of cases when the virus invades the central nervous system (neuroinvasive diseases leading to meningitis, encephalitis of acute flaccid paralysis), mainly in immunosuppressed or elderly patients and patients with renal diseases. The epidemiological burden of the infection in humans is increasingly relevant. During the 2018 transmission season in Europe (June–October), as many as 2083 human cases were reported in Europe [2], a very significant increase in comparison to previous years. In the USA, the 2018 count of WNV symptomatic cases was 2647, representing 94% of domestic arboviral diseases [3].

The continuous spreading of the disease, also interesting Asia [4], the climate changes influence on the vector geographical distribution [5] and competence in addition to its public health impact on the blood transfusion supplies and on travellers make West Nile virus infection an emerging threat requiring careful surveillance activity and diagnostic skills [6].

17.2 Aetiology and Transmission

West Nile virus is a single-stranded positive-sense enveloped RNA arthropod-borne virus (arbovirus) belonging to the Family *Flaviviridae*, Genus *Flavivirus*. Its genome codes for 3 structural and 7 non-structural (NS) proteins. Two major WNV lineages are presently known, with lineage 1 virus (WNVL-1) (mainly present in Africa, Europe, North America and Australia) and lineage 2 virus (WNVL-2) causing outbreaks especially in southern Africa [7] and, quite recently, in central Europe. WNVL-1 has long been considered more pathogenic for animals and humans than WNVL-2, but last decade European neuroinvasive cluster by WNL-2 disproved this theory [8]. Changing in WNVL-2 virulence has been linked to six amino acid substitutions at the level of the E (V159I), NS1 (L338T), NS2A (A126S), NS3 (N421S),

NS4B (L20P) and NS5 (Y254F) proteins [9]. The two lineages can co-circulate, as it has been demonstrated during the current, early and intense transmission season in northern Italy, after the appearance of a new L1 strain in 2021 [10]. Other 7 lineages exist [11, 12], but their epidemiological impact is limited so far. Given the common transmission pattern and reservoir, West Nile virus and Usutu virus are sometimes identified in the same vector and in the same area, especially in Europe [13].

Ornithophilic *Culex* mosquito vectors biting wild birds, both resident and migratory, that act as amplifying hosts, mainly sustain the enzootic cycle in nature. Identified receptive birds vary with geographical area and include crows, sparrows, finches, robins and grackles. Clinical presentation in wild birds varies with species from asymptomatic infection to mild neurological manifestations to fatal cases, especially among *Corvidae* (crows) that are often regarded as the sentinel species. The virus has been isolated in many *Culex* spp., *Culex pipiens* (eastern USA, southern Europe), *Culex tarsalis* (western USA) and *Culex quinquefasciatus* and *Culex tarsalis* (southern USA) [14], as well as *Culex univittatus* and *Culex tritaeniorhynchus* in Africa [15] being the major WNV vectors. Although free from autochthonous WNV, England hosts *Culex modestus*, a competent bridge vector between wild birds and humans. Competent *Culex pipiens* mosquitoes are also present in northern Europe and may become an important WNV bridge vector should temperature raise in this area [16].*Aedes albopictus* is also a potential competent vector for West Nile virus [17], but its epidemiological relevance is yet to be defined. In contrast, *Aedes koreicus* seems susceptible but not competent for it [18].

Mammals, including humans and equids, are incidentally infected but viraemia is short, transient and usually non-significant enough to allow mosquito infection. Their role in maintaining the cycle in nature is therefore negligible and they are referred to as "dead-end hosts". Equally, the role of ticks in the enzootic cycle of West Nile virus is yet to be defined [19].

Environmental factors (climate, humidity) have been demonstrated to have a significant effect on the intensity of WNV transmission in a given area [20]. Warmer temperature can increase the vectors' feeding frequency and shorten the development time of the virus [21]. Higher humidity favours the larval habitat leading to a larger population of vectors. Infection persistence in overwintering mosquitoes [22, 23] and vertical transmission from female mosquitoes to progeny (eggs-larvae) [24, 25] can explain the maintenance of endemicity in a given area. However a non-vector bird-to-bird direct transmission way is suggested, to justify bird infections and deaths happening in midwinter [26, 27]. Enteral transmission has been demonstrated experimentally [28].

Apart from vector transmission, other transmission routes may also play a role even for humans, including blood transfusion [29] and organ transplantation [30]. In exceptional circumstances, in utero and breastfeeding transmission have also been demonstrated [31, 32]. Given the frequently asymptomatic clinical picture of the infection, blood and organ transmission represents an issue of the upmost public health importance and requires appropriate epidemiological and serological screening procedures [33, 34].

17.3   Epidemiology

Since it was first recognized in 1937 in Uganda, West Nile virus has spread to most regions of the world. The migratory pattern of wild birds from affected areas is regarded as one of the main mechanism WNV infection is spreading in the western hemisphere [35], even if molecular and serological surveys on migratory birds led to not univocal results. [36, 37]

17.3.1 Africa

Phylogenetic analysis suggests WNV evolution from an ancestor virus (tMRCA) between the sixteenth and the seventeenth century in Africa [38]. The presence of WNV has been documented throughout Africa, from South Africa to northern and western Africa, and about 30 species of birds have been reported to be involved, often without clinical symptoms thus assuring an excellent reservoir. WNV-L1, only clade A, has been reported in Algeria, Central African Republic, Egypt, Côte d'Ivoire, Kenya, Morocco, Tunisia, Senegal, and South Africa; WNV-L2, all clades, has been reported in Botswana, Central African Republic, Congo, Djibouti, Madagascar, Mozambique, Namibia, Senegal, South Africa, Tanzania, and Uganda [12]. Lineage 2 is usually responsible for sporadic human and zoonotic cases, although South Africa experienced human outbreaks since 1974 [39].

17.3.2 Europe and the Mediterranean Region

The first neurological case in Israel dates back to 1957 [40]. The first outbreak in humans in European countries was registered in 1962–1963 in the Camargue area, France [41]. Mediterranean and Eastern Europe, including former Soviet Union States, witnessed zoonotic and human outbreaks in the 1990s. Romania was severely affected in 1996 with 352 neuroinvasive cases and 17 deaths [42]. Russia experienced an outbreak in 1999 [43]. In both cases lineage 1 virus was involved, with high degree of similarity between the two episodes. Lineage 1 was also implicated in most sporadic cases reported in Europe until 2004 when, in Hungary, WNV lineage 2 firstly appeared outside Africa [44]. This so called central-southern European clade of WNV-L2 then caused outbreaks in humans in Austria, Greece, Serbia, and Italy in 2013 [45]. Meanwhile a different WNV-L2, named Russian/Romanian clade, circulated in eastern Europe, in Russia (2004–2007) and in Romania (2010). Here, data from a large single-centre retrospective survey [46] suggests an increased morbidity and fatality rate of this clade. European areas with human autochthonous infection cases in the last decade are shown in Fig. 17.1, as reported at the European Surveillance System (TESSy) managed by ECDC.

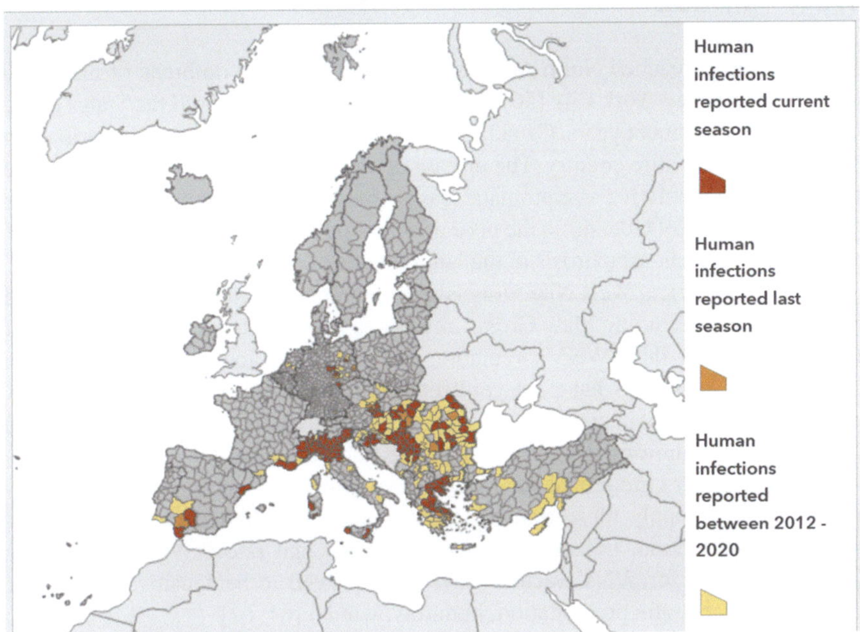

Fig. 17.1 European areas with human infections reported between 2012 and 2020
Source: ECDC. https://gis.ecdc.europa.eu/portal/apps/opsdashboard/index.html#/305f1b279cb04
dddac3d4833b770a620

In 2018, European WNV transmission season started earlier than in previous years, with first reported disease onset on 31 May in Greece [47], and cases reached the number of 2083, 7.2-fold increase mainly in Bulgaria (15-fold), France (13.5-fold) and Italy (10.9-fold) [48]. Eight years after the last outbreak of WNV-1 in Italy, in 2021 a newly introduced WNV-1a strain was demonstrated [49]. Compared to the co-circulating WN-L2, it was predominant in symptomatic cases. [50] In 2022, more than half of the 965 WNV European cases occurred in Italy (n. 586) with 73 deaths [51].

17.3.3 Asia

The presence of West Nile virus in the animal reservoir and in humans has been documented in many places of interest to travellers in Asia, such as Sri Lanka [52], India [53], China [54] and Turkey [55], alone or in association with other flaviviruses. Data on the epidemiology of WNV in Central Asia are limited, but reports of febrile WNV from south-western Russia, Tajikistan, Kazakhstan, Turkmenistan and the Caucasus exist [4].

17.3.4 Americas

West Nile virus reached North America in 1999, causing an outbreak of meningo-encephalitis in New York City [56] and rapidly spreading across all the States of the USA in the subsequent years. Canada reported its first cases in 2001 in Ontario, then spreading to the entire country. The disease is now endemic in the USA, with more than 52,000 cumulative symptomatic cases, half of them neuroinvasive disease cases, and about 2500 deaths in the period 1999–2020 [57], a figure that ranks WNV as the most relevant arbovirosis in the United States [3].

In South America, West Nile virus is now endemic in equids and birds in some States of Brazil including Mato Grosso and Parà and other States of touristic interest [58]. Serosurveys show WNV circulation among humans too [59]; however, large human WNV outbreaks have not yet been reported in South American countries. Among various explanations, other highly circulating flaviviruses may provide cross-protection limiting the number of deaths and outbreaks due to WNV [60].

Climate changes are one of the factors driving the epidemiology of some infectious diseases, mainly those transmitted by vectors [5], by expanding their geographical distribution, transmission activity period and rate of virus replication. This is true also for WNV vectors, have been proved to be sensitive to weather changes (temperature, precipitation, humidity, winds) [61, 62].

Climate changes have been reported to have increased the suitability of WNV ecology in many regions of the world, including Southern Europe, Eastern Mediterranean, Western Asia and Northern America (USA and Canada) [63]. The possible impact of future climate and environmental changes on the vectorial capacity of competent WNV invasive mosquitoes present in Europe is cause of concern [64, 65]. Besides climate changes, the immune status of the receptive avian population, serving as reservoir population, is an important driver of transmission and risk for humans in a given area [66].

17.4 Pathogenesis

Once inoculated into the skin of the human host, WNV infects the keratinocytes and Langheran's dendritic cells and it is transported to local draining lymph nodes; what follows is a viraemia at first and an invasion of liver, spleen, kidney and, possibly brain. Central nervous system infection has been demonstrated shortly after viraemia, especially in immunodepressed animal models, and persists after viral clearance from blood and many peripheral tissues [67]. Multiple mechanisms of WNV neuroinvasion have been hypothesized: as free virions or inside CNS infiltrating immune cells; with and without disruption of blood-brain barrier; by haematogenous or by trans-neural way; by infection of olfactory neurons and rostral spread and by direct axonal retrograde transport [68, 69]. Most affected CNS regions are the brainstem (medulla and pons), deep grey matter nuclei (*substantia nigra* of the basal ganglia and thalamus), and cerebellum grey matter as revealed by autoptic studies and by neuroimaging. In the spinal cord, the anterior horns (ventral horns) and anterior spinal nerve roots may be involved too [70, 71].

Brain and spinal cord histopathology shows perivascular inflammation, microglial nodules, neuronophagia, and necrosis and neuronal loss, but also demyelination, gliosis, and perivascular infiltrates [72]. Damage has been explained by viral direct effect but also by activation of innate immune response [73]. Even if cell disruption due to plasma membrane damage by intracellular viral progeny stack has been described [74], neuronal apoptosis seems to play a major role [75–77].

A recent study [78] has shown higher levels of inflammatory cytokines, in particular IL1β, IL1α, IL4, IL8, IL10, IL13, IL17, and CCL2, IFNα and IFNγ, not only in cerebrospinal-fluid (CSF) but also in serum of patients affected by WNV neurological diseases. However, although cytokines and chemokines act in preventing viral growth and clearing the infection in the CNS, they contribute to multiple pathogenic condition too. Models using minocyclin [79] or rosiglitazone [80], both inhibitors of microglia activation, to study the role of neuroinflammation response in viral clearance and, on the other hand, in tissue damage led to contradictory results. Further studies are required to clarify if increased and/or persistent, both innate and induced, adaptive immunity is indicator of uncontrolled viral replication or the cause of disease itself [81].

17.5 Clinical Findings

Most infections with West Nile virus are asymptomatic and only around 20–25% of the cases are clinically expressed. After an incubation period of 2–14 days or even longer in immunosuppressed patients, the onset is abrupt with the most frequent clinical manifestation—fever accompanied by chills, myalgia, arthralgia, generalized weakness, malaise, headache, nausea, vomiting, diarrhoea, cough or sore throat and sometimes by a transient diffuse maculopapular rash. The rash seems to be present more frequently in young persons and in mild cases than in older persons and severe cases [82]. Myocardial, pancreatic, hepatic, renal or ocular disorders have been described in West Nile virus infections, especially in severe cases. This clinical syndrome without neurological manifestations has been called "West Nile fever" (WNF), affects all ages and usually is mild, leading to severe clinical course with poor outcome and death only in few cases.

Less than 1% of infected persons experience neurological manifestations. Neurological impairment can take different forms, such as encephalitis, meningitis, meningoencephalitis and acute flaccid paralysis (AFP) or less common forms such as ataxia, extrapyramidal signs, polyradiculitis, seizures, and eye neuritis.

West Nile virus meningitis has an abrupt onset with fever, headache, nausea, vomiting, photophobia and positive neck stiffness, Kernig and Brudzinski signs. Evolution is generally self-limited with good outcome and a case fatality rate around 1–2% [83]. Encephalitis and meningoencephalitis cases are more severe with a case fatality rate from 4% to 40% [46]. Some population groups are exposed to a greater risk to have severe neurological disease in West Nile virus infection with evolution to coma and death—elderly, immunocompromised persons, male with cardiovascular diseases, neoplasms, renal failure or diabetes mellitus [45]. Recipients of solid organ transplantations due to immunosuppressed status have an increased risk for WNV neuroinvasive disease, up to 40-fold increase in some studies, often with severe forms and poor outcome [84, 85]. Several studies showed that some clinical signs could be associated with a severe evolution of the disease: sleepiness, confusion, obtundation, depressed deep tendon reflexes and coma [46, 82]. WNV encephalitis due to brainstem and basal ganglia damage may present with extrapyramidal disorders, especially in the upper extremities, such as tremor (up to 90% of patients), rigidity, spasm, bradykinesia or myoclonus [86]. These extrapyramidal manifestations are suggestive for WNV infection in patients from endemic WNV areas. Muscle weakness are more frequent in WNV encephalitis in contrast with other encephalitis [85]. Seizures may appear in 3–30% of cases [46, 56]. Cranial neuropathies are related in almost 20% of WNV encephalitis especially with unilateral or bilateral peripheral facial palsy [85].

Acute flaccid paralysis can present with isolated anterior horn cells involvement or associated with encephalitis and mortality rate can reach 50% when respiratory failure due to neuromuscular paralysis occurs. Survivors' recovery is usually with sequelae [87]. In some studies, the incidence of paralysis was comparable to that seen during epidemics of poliovirus infection [88]. The AFP onset is characterized by fasciculations of muscles with evolution from monoplegia to quadriplegia and brainstem involvement and respiratory failure that requires mechanical ventilation [89]. Sometimes, bowel and bladder function can be also affected [90]. Early dysarthria and dysphagia may be predictors of subsequent respiratory failure and poor outcome [88]. WNV infection in children is mostly asymptomatic, but severe cases of encephalitis, AFP and hepatitis have been described [91]. Usually WNV neuroinvasive disease in children consist in self-limited meningitis.

Neurologic sequelae are common in case of neuroinvasive WNV disease and the survivors may have cognitive impairment including difficulties with attention and concentration, movement disorders, parkinsonism, weakness, persistent headaches, paralysis [82, 92]. Neuropsychiatric symptoms, as depression and severe anxiety, have been reported even months and years after WNV encephalitis [82, 93]. Some studies revealed that patients with "milder" illness including those with only WNV fever demonstrated equivalent rates of depression, abnormalities in executive functions and memory input on 1 year follow-up comparative with neuroinvasive WNV patients [94].

17.6 Laboratory Diagnosis

The laboratory methods commonly used for the diagnosis of WNV infection are serology and viral detection [95]. In current practice, serology (immunofluorescence assay—IF and enzyme-linked immunosorbent assays—ELISA) is the primary method of diagnosing WNV infection due to its rapidity, reproducibility and lower cost in comparison with viral detection methods. The detection of a specific IgM immune response in the cerebrospinal fluid (CSF) is confirmatory for the diagnosis. Unfortunately, the use of serology is hindered by cross-reactivity with other flavivirus infections or vaccinations, especially viruses from the same serocomplex [96, 97]. The plaque reduction neutralization technique may discriminate between real WNV infection or cross-reaction, but it requires viable virus isolates and must be performed under BSL3 safety conditions [95]. Several different tools are presently available to detect the virus, including viral isolation and molecular methods. Viral isolation is used mostly in research because of technical difficulties and safety that requires BSL3 laboratory. Molecular methods differ in the clinical diagnostic setting (infected patients usually have high of viral RNA loads in blood, CSF or urine) or in the screening setting for blood and organ from asymptomatic infected donors, where low viral loads are expected. In the latter case, high sensitivity tests detecting as low as less than 100 genome copies/mL must be used [97–99]. RNA viral detection in blood or CSF is usually positive early after the onset of the disease, confirming the infection but in many cases, mostly in travellers who may come to hospital after the viraemia has cleared, WNV diagnosis is based on serological methods with detection of IgM antibodies from serum or CSF. Sometimes the serological diagnosis can be delayed because of inability to produce antibodies in immunosuppressed patients even if they have immunosuppressed diseases or immunosuppressive treatments. Cases of patients with rheumatoid arthritis treated with rituximab have been described and in these cases the diagnosis requires the detection of viral nucleic acid [100, 101]. Search for IgG and IgM antibodies in a second serum sample drawn 10 days after onset could be useful for diagnosis. Viruria of WNV can be detected even years after infection [102].

The European Commission [103] has set the criteria for the laboratory diagnosis of a confirmed case of WNV infection when one of the following criteria is met:

- isolation of WNV from blood or CSF;
- detection of WNV nucleic acid in blood or CSF;
- WNV-specific antibody response (IgM) in CSF;
- WNV IgM high titre AND detection of WNV IgG AND confirmation by neutralization.

CSF analysis shows elevated proteins, normal glucose and moderate pleocytosis (<500 cells/µL) with a possible early neutrophilic predominance followed by lymphocytosis [87].

17.7 Differential Diagnosis

Clinicians should be aware of the risk of WNV infection in travellers returning from WNV endemic countries during the whole transmission season, especially during late summer and early autumn [46]. The differential diagnosis of WNV infection may be approached by separating patients in two groups with or without neurological manifestations.

Due to non-specific clinical picture of West Nile virus fever (fever, myalgia, arthralgia, cough, rash, nausea, vomiting) in patients without neurological manifestations differential diagnosis includes other arboviruses (Dengue, Chikungunya, Zika), rickettsial diseases, leptospirosis, enteroviral or respiratory virus infections.

Patients with neurological manifestation could also be split into subgroups: those with or without acute flaccid paralysis [104]. It is important to discriminate between WNV and herpes virus (HSV) encephalitis, for which an effective good aetiological treatment with acyclovir is available. The sensitive molecular diagnosis by HSV-DNA from CSF and specific lesions on cerebral MRI in temporal lobes may help in the diagnosis of HSV encephalitis. Other encephalitis aetiology, viral, bacterial or fungal must be verified and the area where the patient has travelled should be considered. Considering that most cases of encephalitis are in the elderly and in patients with underlying diseases, in addition to HSV, clinicians must consider testing patients for *Listeria monocytogenes*.

Neuroinvasive viral infections with limited geographical distribution should be considered according to which the destination of the trip was. In the Mediterranean area, fleboviruses such as Toscana virus should be considered. In Central Europe, tick-borne encephalitis virus and the less common Usutu virus could be implicated in the aetiology of encephalitis in travellers. Japanese encephalitis virus, Enterovirus 71 and Nipah virus are present in South-Eastern and Murray Valley encephalitis is present in Australia. For the Americas, St. Louis encephalitis virus, encephalitis from the California group, Equine encephalitis group or new emerging Powassan virus must be considered. Rabies remains an important differential diagnosis for travellers with encephalitis. In case of acute flaccid paralysis differential diagnosis is usually with poliomyelitis or polio-like enteroviruses and Guillain-Barré syndrome [104].

In case of extrapyramidal manifestations, even in the absence of changes in mental status, the suspicion of neurological infection with WNV must be raised. Brain imaging may help clinicians to suspect diagnosis of encephalitis, even if sometimes MRI can be normal even in severe cases. Pathological cerebral MRI results have been reported from 20% to 70% cases with changes in the basal ganglia, thalami, brainstem, and cerebellum and higher sensitivity in T2 and FLAIR sequences [46, 105, 106]. These changes are described for other flavivirus infections too. Cerebral CT scan has a much lower sensitivity but in absence of MRI, in severe cases, can be used to exclude contraindications to lumbar puncture.

17.8 Management

There is no specific treatment for WNV infections. Most patients with WNF do not require hospitalization and receive symptomatic treatment for fever control or rehydration in case of vomiting. However, elderly patients, immunosuppressants or those with underlying diseases require careful monitoring because of the possibility of severe disease progression.

There are only few antiviral treatments in viral encephalitis. The administration of acyclovir in all cases of encephalitis should not be forgotten until confirmation of its aetiology or exclusion of herpes simplex or varicella-zoster virus infections. In most countries, diagnosis of WNV infection is made in reference laboratories and may be delayed so that acyclovir treatment should be continued while waiting for the results.

In the absence of antiviral treatment, management of WNV infection remains supportive and in severe cases admission into intensive care unit is required. Hydro-electrolytic and acid-basic equilibrium correction with infusion solutions may also be needed. Acute neuromuscular respiratory failures need a rapidly and prolonged ventilatory support.

Anecdotal cases treated with several antiviral agents, nucleic acid analogues, missense sequences, immunomodulating agents and angiotensin-receptor blockers have also been reported. However, no randomized clinical trial is available so that they are not included in the treatment guidelines of the WNV infection [82]. In patients infected with WNV or St. Louis encephalitis virus, interferon alpha treatment cases has also been suggested to provide a potential benefit [107], but there are no controlled clinical trials to support these observations. Other attempts to use interferon alpha in the treatment of WNV encephalitis have failed [108]. Chimeric peptide molecules with antiviral properties against flaviviruses are patented but future clinical trials are needed [109].

Encephalopathy and cerebral oedema are frequently associated with increased intracranial pressure clinically manifested through loss of consciousness, respiratory or cardiovascular disorders, or seizures. In such situations, decreased cerebral oedema is an emergency and the use of corticosteroids could be considered to lower cerebral oedema [110], even if no consensus exists. In some reported cases using of high doses of corticosteroids showed rapid improvement of clinical conditions and may suggest a pro-inflammatory state rather than neuronal loss [111, 112]. The control of seizures is also of the upmost importance. Recovery after WNV encephalitis or AFP may require time and a multidisciplinary approach (neurology, psychiatry, nursing), as well as social support, is needed.

17.9 Public Health Responses around Management of an Individual Case

As humans (and mammals in general) do not develop a sufficient viraemia to permit the maintenance of the transmission chain (dead-end host), isolation is not required for patients affected by West Nile virus infection. The caring health staff require standards protection measures, as WNV is not usually present in biological fluids even in clinical cases. However, a careful epidemiological and screening investigation is required for patient's contacts potentially exposed in the two previous weeks in sporadic cases. Given the rarity of milk transmission, breastfeeding is not discouraged in lactating mothers in endemic areas [113]. Screening of blood products and organ donors by nucleic acid amplification tests is recommended in endemic settings during transmission season. As viral circulation starts earlier in mosquitoes and birds than in humans [114], integrated entomological, ornithological, equine surveillance programme, as the one adopted in some Italian regions, allows to postpone the beginning of blood sample tests until the first positive specimen. This approach avoids significant costs without losing in safety [115].

17.10 Prevention and Advice for Travellers

Given the prevalence of WNV in highly attractive touristic and commercial destinations in North America, Europe and Asia, it is no surprise that West Nile virus infection has been the subject of surveillance in the travelling population returning from these areas. The large GeoSentinel database, populated by over 70 Infectious Diseases clinics around the world reports only two cases of symptomatic WNV infection in 1222 travellers to the USA in 1997–2016 [116]. However, the GeoSentinel network only reports ill travellers reporting to the network Clinics, likely under appreciating the large proportion of asymptomatic or poorly symptomatic WNV infected travellers. A similar retrospective study from Belgium identified 5 cases of WNV infection (4 confirmed, 1 probable; 3 neuroinvasive diseases) in a cohort of 899 ill travellers who reported back to an outpatient clinic for travellers after return. The presumed place of infection in the 4 confirmed cases were Senegal, Democratic Republic of the Congo, South Sudan and Greece [117]. WNV infected travellers from Israel to the Netherlands have been suspected on the basis of the ongoing outbreak in 2010 [118]. Ill returning travellers from South Africa to the UK were recently reported with WNV infection [119]. A literature review identified 39 cases of documented travel-related WNV disease. [120] Intra-European imported cases have been described: from Hungary to Belgium [121]; from Austria to Germany [122].

Serological surveys in travellers are lacking. A recent paper from southern Italy showed the presence of IgG or IgM antibodies in 9/156 returning travellers who agreed to be tested. However, no information about the yellow-fever vaccination status is provided and all the 9 positive patients also showed the presence of Dengue virus antibodies, suggesting possible cross-reactivity. Neutralization test was not performed [123]. Epidemiological worldwide surveillance of arboviruses may help prompt diagnosis and treatment of WNV infected returning travellers. On the other side, given the large distribution of competent vectors in many travellers sending countries, concern about the possible role of travellers to disseminate the infection has been raised.

In the absence of an effective human vaccine against WNV and most other vector-borne diseases, prevention in travellers essentially consists in adequate counselling of personal preventive measures to prevent mosquito bites in the endemic destination areas, even in the western world [124]. Travellers at risk of the most severe forms of the disease, including immunosuppressed individuals, older patients and patients with chronic renal diseases, need to be addressed by specific and intensive counselling. Interestingly, however, when risk studies have been carried out in the US, the perception of West Nile infective risk when travelling abroad was significantly lower than Dengue, Zika virus and Chikungunya, correlating to a lower attitude to use personal preventive behaviours (covering clothes, repellents and mosquito coils/lights) [125].

Apart from environmental interventions to reduce the intensity of vector replication, prevention of mosquito bites relies on personal preventive measures, such as wearing long-sleeve shirts and pants, light and pyrethroid spray cloths, use of insecticide repellents using nets and eliminating all possible breeding sites in the surroundings (especially important for *Aedes* spp.). Culex mosquitoes' biting habits are usually from dusk to dawn, requiring strict adherence to protection especially during evening and night time. The review by Nguyen and co-workers (2018) reaffirms the excellent activity of *N,N*-diethyl-3-methylbenzamide (DEET) to prevent *Culex* spp. bites, with broad spectrum and long protection time at the usual concentration of 10–35% [126]. DEET skin repellents are considered safe in the second and third trimester of pregnancy and in children over 2 years, provided that the manufacturers' instructions are strictly adhered to [126]. Other active insect repellents are Picaridin (KBR 3023 or icaridin), IR3535, Oil of lemon eucalyptus (OLE), Para-menthane-diol (PMD), and 2-undecanone (CDC, 2019). Permethrin-impregnated clothes may also be considered to avoid mosquito bites but permethrin should not be applied directly on the skin [127].

Other mosquito control measures include the use of window screens, of air conditioners and of mosquito nets. Cleaning of environment suitable breeding sites for mosquito eggs and larval reproduction (such as tyres, flowerpots, and trash containers) may help reducing the potential vector population around the houses.

17.11 Gaps in Knowledge that Need to be Addressed

Data about spread and introduction of WNV in Europe or USA are limited and many questions remain without answer. The neurotropism of WNV and poor prognosis especially for elderly are partially explained, but many other questions about pathogenesis of WNV strains with different phenotypic mutations remain unexplained. These mutations can modulate WNV pathogenicity in humans with increase virulence or adaptation to host, especially birds, and may explain the different epidemiological patterns from Europe and USA.

On the other hand, co-circulation of several arboviruses in the same geographic region raises questions about viruses' interactions and immune response of the hosts. In Europe, co-circulation of Usutu virus and West Nile virus may change the immune response and patients with atypical immune response to WNV have been reported [85]. Moreover, apart from other flaviviruses, the simultaneous circulation of different WNV viral strains (from lineage 1 and 2) may lead to more virulent and neuroinvasive strains with increasing mortality and severity of the disease.

In the context of increasing life expectancy and ageing population, more cases of severe West Nile virus neuroinvasive infections are to be expected and the lack of specific treatment and of human vaccines constitutes an important gap in the mitigation of WNND [128]. Cross-reactivity in serological diagnostic tests with other flaviviruses remains an important problem for diagnosis of WNV since detection of IgM and IgG antibodies is the main diagnostic test for WNV. The development and production of multiplex nucleic acid tests for simultaneous detection of flaviviruses is under research and would bring major benefits in diagnosis.

In this period with climate changes a "one health" approach in WNV epidemiology and infection is necessary to understand relations between vectors, hosts, virus strains, and humans.

Disclosure The Author is responsible for the views contained in this article and for opinion expressed therein, which are not necessarily those of UNESCO and do not commit the Organization.

References

1. Smithburn KC, Hughes TP, Burka AW, Paul JH. A neurotropic virus isolated from the blood of a native from Uganda. Am J Trop Med. 1940;20:471–92.
2. ECDC. Communicable diseases threats report, 4–10 August 2019, week 32. Available at https://ecdc.europa.eu/en/publications-data/communicable-disease-threats-report-4-10-august-2019-week-32 (accessed August 9, 2019).
3. McDonald E, Martin SW, Landry K, Gould CV, Lehman J, Fischer M, Lindsey NP. West Nile virus and other domestic nationally notifiable arboviral diseases—United States, 2018. Morb Mortal Wkly Rep. 2019;68(31):673–8.
4. Atkinson B, Hewson R. Emerging arboviruses of clinical importance in Central Asia. J Gen Virol. 2018;99:1172–84.
5. Semenza JC, Suk JE. Vector-borne diseases and climate changes: a European perspective. FEMS Microbiol Lett. 2018;365:fnx244.
6. Johnson N, de Marco MF, Giovannini A, Ippoliti C, Danzetta ML, Svartz G, et al. Emerging mosquito-borne threats and the response from European and eastern Mediterranean countries. Int J Environ Res Public Health. 2018;15:2775. https://doi.org/10.3390/ijerph15122775.
7. Sejvar JJ. West Nile virus infection. Microbiol Spectrum. 2016;4:3. https://doi.org/10.1128/microbiolspec.EI10-0021-2016.
8. Napp S, Petrić D, Busquets N. West Nile virus and other mosquito-borne viruses present in Eastern Europe. Pathog Glob Health. 2018;112(5):233–48. https://doi.org/10.1080/20477724.2018.1483567.
9. McMullen AR, Albayrak H, May FJ, Davis CT, Beasley DWC, Barrett ADT. Molecular evolution of lineage 2 West Nile virus. J Gen Virol. 2013;94(Pt 2):318–25. https://doi.org/10.1099/vir.0.046888-0.
10. Barzon L, Montarsi F, Quaranta E, Monne I, Pacenti M, Michelutti A, Toniolo F, Danesi P, Marchetti G, Gobbo F, Sinigaglia A, Riccetti S, Dal ME, Favero L, Russo F, Capelli G. Early start of seasonal transmission and co-circulation of West Nile virus lineage 2 and a newly introduced lineage 1 strain, northern Italy, June 2022. Euro Surveill. 2022;27(29) pii=2200548 https://doi.org/10.2807/1560-7917.ES.2022.27.29.2200548.
11. Fall G, Di Paola N, Faye M, Dia M, Freire CCM, Loucoubar C, Zanotto PMA, Faye O, Sall AA. Biological and phylogenetic characteristics of west African lineages of West Nile virus. PLoS Negl Trop Dis. 2017;11(11):e0006078. https://doi.org/10.1371/journal.pntd.0006078.

12. Mencattelli G, Ndione MHD, Rosà R, Marini G, Diagne CT, Diagne MM, Fall G, Faye O, Diallo M, Faye O, Savini G, Rizzoli A. Epidemiology of West Nile virus in Africa: an underestimated threat. PLoS Negl Trop Dis. 2022;16(1):e0010075. https://doi.org/10.1371/journal.pntd.0010075.

13. Vilibic-Cavlek T, Savic V, Petrovic T, Toplak I, Barbic L, Petric D, Tabain I, Hrnjakovic-Cvjetkovic I, Bogdanic M, Klobucar A, Mrzljak A, Stevanovic V, Dinjar-Kujundzic P, Radmanic L, Monaco F, Listes E, Savini G. Emerging trends in the epidemiology of West Nile and Usutu virus infections in southern Europe. Front Vet Sci. 2019;6:437. https://doi.org/10.3389/fvets.2019.00437.

14. Saxena V, Bolling BG, Wang T. West Nile virus. Clin Lab Med. 2017;37:243–52.

15. Sule WF, Oluwayelu DO, Hernández-Triana LM, Fooks AR, Venter M, Johnson N. Epidemiology and ecology of West Nile virus in sub-Saharan Africa. Parasit Vectors. 2018;11:414. https://doi.org/10.1186/s13071-018-2998-y.

16. Fros JJ, Geertsema C, Vogels CB, et al. West Nile virus: high transmission rate in northwestern European mosquitoes indicates its epidemic potential and warrants increased surveillance. PLoS Negl Trop Dis. 2015;9:e0003956.

17. Zhang YM, Guo XX, Jiang SF, Li CX, Xing D, Zhang HD, Dong YD, Zhao TY. The potential vector competence and overwintering of West Nile virus in vector Aedes Albopictus in China. Front Microbiol. 2022;13:888751. https://doi.org/10.3389/fmicb.2022.888751.

18. Jansen S, Cadar D, Lühken R, Pfitzner WP, Jöst H, Oerther S, Helms M, Zibrat B, Kliemke K, Becker N, Vapalahti O, Rossini G, Heitmann A. Vector competence of the invasive mosquito species Aedes koreicus for arboviruses and interference with a novel insect specific virus. Viruses. 2021;13(12):2507. https://doi.org/10.3390/v13122507.

19. Flores FS, Zanluca C, Guglielmone AA, Duarte Dos Santos CN, Labruna MB, Diaz A. Vector competence for West Nile virus and St. Louis encephalitis virus (Flavivirus) of three tick species of the genus Amblyomma (Acari: Ixodidae). Am J Trop Med Hyg. 2019;100(5):1230–5. https://doi.org/10.4269/ajtmh.18-0134.

20. Lorenz C, de Azevedo TS, Chiaravalloti-Neto F. Impact of climate change on West Nile virus distribution in South America. Trans R Soc Trop Med Hyg. 2022;116:trac044. https://doi.org/10.1093/trstmh/trac044.

21. Reisen WK. Landscape epidemiology of vector-borne diseases. Annu Rev Entomol. 2010;55:461–83.

22. Rudolf I, Betášová L, Blažejová H, Venclíková K, Straková P, Šebesta O, Mendel J, Bakonyi T, Schaffner F, Nowotny N, Hubálek Z. West Nile virus in overwintering mosquitoes, Central Europe. Parasit Vectors. 2017;10(1):452. https://doi.org/10.1186/s13071-017-2399-7.

23. Kampen H, Tews BA, Werner D. First evidence of West Nile virus overwintering in mosquitoes in Germany. Viruses. 2021;13(12):2463. https://doi.org/10.3390/v13122463.

24. Nelms BM, Fechter-Leggett E, Carroll BD, Macedo P, Kluh S, Reisen WK. Experimental and natural vertical transmission of West Nile virus by California Culex (Diptera: Culicidae) mosquitoes. J Med Entomol. 2013;50(2):371–8. https://doi.org/10.1603/me12264.

25. Anderson JF, Main AJ, Ferrandino FJ. Horizontal and vertical transmission of West Nile virus by Aedes vexans (Diptera: Culicidae). J Med Entomol. 2020;57(5):1614–8. https://doi.org/10.1093/jme/tjaa049.

26. Mencattelli G, Iapaolo F, Polci A, Marcacci M, Di Gennaro A, Teodori L, Curini V, Di Lollo V, Secondini B, Scialabba S, Gobbi M, Manuali E, Cammà C, Rosà R, Rizzoli A, Monaco F, Savini G. West Nile virus lineage 2 overwintering in Italy. Trop Med Infect Dis. 2022;7(8):160. https://doi.org/10.3390/tropicalmed7080160.

27. Hinton MG, Reisen WK, Wheeler SS, Townsend AK. West Nile virus activity in a winter roost of American crows (Corvus brachyrhynchos): is bird-to-bird transmission important in persistence and amplification? J Med Entomol. 2015;52(4):683–92. https://doi.org/10.1093/jme/tjv040.

28. Banet-Noach C, Simanov L, Malkinson M. Direct (non-vector) transmission of West Nile virus in geese. Avian Pathol. 2003;32:489–94.

29. Pisani G, Cristiano K, Pupella S, Liumbruno GM. West Nile virus in Europe and safety of blood transfusion. Transfus Med Hemother. 2016;43:158–67.
30. Iwamoto M, Jernigan DB, Guasch A, Trepka MJ, Blackmore CG, Hellinger WC, et al. Transmission of West Nile virus from an organ donor to four transplant recipients. N Engl J Med. 2003;348:2196–203.
31. Centers for Disease Control and Prevention (CDC). Intrauterine West Nile virus infection: New York, 2002. MMWR Morb Mortal Wkly Rep. 2002;51:1135–6.
32. Centers for Disease Control and Prevention (CDC). Possible West Nile virus transmission to an infant through breast-feeding: Michigan, 2002b. MMWR Morb Mortal Wkly Rep. 2002;51:877–8.
33. Garzon Jimenez RC, Lieshout-Krikke RW, Janssen MP. West Nile virus and blood transfusion safety: a European perspective. Vox Sang. 2021;116(10):1094–101. https://doi.org/10.1111/vox.13112.
34. Russell WA, Custer B, Brandeau ML. Optimal portfolios of blood safety interventions: test, defer or modify? Health Care Manag Sci. 2021;24(3):551–68. https://doi.org/10.1007/s10729-021-09557-1.
35. Rappole JH, Derrickson SR, Hubálek Z. Migratory birds and spread of West Nile virus in the western hemisphere. Emerg Infect Dis. 2000;6:319–28.
36. Mancuso E, Cecere JG, Iapaolo F, Di Gennaro A, Sacchi M, Savini G, Spina F, Monaco F. West Nile and Usutu virus introduction via migratory birds: a retrospective analysis in Italy. Viruses. 2022;14:416. https://doi.org/10.3390/v14020416.
37. Grisenti M, Arnoldi D, Rizzolli F, Giacobini M, Bertolotti L, Rizzoli A. Lack of identification of flaviviruses in oral and cloacal swabs from long- and short distance migratory birds in Trentino-Alto Adige (North-Eastern Italy). Virology J. 2013;10:306.
38. McIntosh BM, Jupp PG, dos Santos I, Meenehan GM. Epidemics of West Nile and Sindbis viruses in South Africa with Culex (Culex) univittatus Theobald as vector. S Afr J Sci. 1976;72:295–300.
39. Zaayman D, Venter M. West Nile virus neurologic disease in humans, South Africa, September 2008–May 2009. Emerg Infect Dis. 2012;18(12):2051–4. https://doi.org/10.3201/eid1812.111208.
40. Spigland I, Jasinska-Klingberg W, Hofshi E, Goldblum N. Clinical and laboratory observations in an outbreak of West Nile fever in Israel in 1957. Harefuah. 1958;54:275–80. (in French)
41. Joubert L, Oudar J, Hannoun C, Beytout D, Corniou B, Guillon JC, et al. Epidemiology of the West Nile virus: study of a focus in Camargue. IV. Meningo-encephalomyelitis of the horse. Ann Inst Pasteur (Paris). 1970;118(2):239–47.
42. Tsai TF, Popovici F, Cernescu C, Campbell GL, Nedelcu NI. West Nile encephalitis epidemic in southeastern Romania. Lancet. 1998;352:767–71.
43. Platonov AE. West Nile encephalitis in Russia 1999–2001: were we ready? Are we ready? Ann N Y Acad Sci. 2001;951:102–16.
44. Bakonyi T, Ivanics E, Erdélyi K, Ursu K, Ferenczi E, Weissenböck H, et al. Lineage 1 and 2 strains of encephalitic West Nile virus, Central Europe. Emerg Infect Dis. 2006;12:618–23. https://doi.org/10.3201/eid1204.051379.
45. Barzon L, Pacenti M, Franchin E, Lavezzo E, Masi G, Squarzon L, Pagni S, Toppo S, Russo F, Cattai M, et al. Whole genome sequencing and phylogenetic analysis of West Nile virus lineage 1 and lineage 2 from human cases of infection, Italy, August 2013. Eur Secur. 2013;18:20591.
46. Popescu CP, Florescu SA, Cotar AI, Badescu D, Ceianu CS, Zaharia M, et al. Re-emergence of severe West Nile virus neuroinvasive disease in humans in Romania, 2012 to 2017—implications for travel medicine. Trav Med Infect Dis. 2018;22:30–5.
47. Haussig JM, Young JJ, Gossner CM, Mezei E, Bella A, Sirbu A, Pervanidou D, Drakulovic MB, Sudre B. Early start of the West Nile fever transmission season 2018 in Europe. Euro Surveill. 2018;23(32):1800428. https://doi.org/10.2807/1560-7917.ES.2018.23.32.1800428.

48. ECDC. Epidemiological update: West Nile virus transmission season in Europe, 2018. https://www.ecdc.europa.eu/en/news-events/epidemiological-update-west-nile-virus-transmission-season-europe-2018

49. Barzon L, Montarsi F, Quaranta E, Monne I, Pacenti M, Michelutti A, Toniolo F, Danesi P, Marchetti G, Gobbo F, Sinigaglia A, Riccetti S, Dal Molin E, Favero L, Russo F, Capelli G. Early start of seasonal transmission and co-circulation of West Nile virus lineage 2 and a newly introduced lineage 1 strain, northern Italy, June 2022. Euro Surveill. 2022;27(29):2200548. https://doi.org/10.2807/1560-7917.ES.2022.27.29.2200548.

50. Barzon L, Pacenti M, Montarsi F, Fornasiero D, Gobbo F, Quaranta E, Monne I, Fusaro A, Volpe A, Sinigaglia A, Riccetti S, Molin ED, Satto S, Lisi V, Gobbi F, Galante S, Feltrin G, Valeriano V, Favero L, Russo F, Mazzucato M, Bortolami A, Mulatti P, Terregino C, Capelli G. Rapid spread of a new West Nile virus lineage 1 associated with increased risk of neuro-invasive disease during a large outbreak in northern Italy, 2022: one health analysis. J Travel Med. 2022:taac125. https://doi.org/10.1093/jtm/taac125. Epub ahead of print

51. ECDC. Weekly updates: 2022 West Nile virus transmission season https://www.ecdc.europa.eu/en/west-nile-fever/surveillance-and-disease-data/disease-data-ecdc

52. Lohitharajah J, Malavige N, Arambepola C, Wanigasinghe J, Gamage R, Gunaratne P, et al. Viral aetiologies of acute encephalitis in a hospital-based south Asian population. BMC Infect Dis. 2017;17(1):303. https://doi.org/10.1186/s12879-017-2403-z.

53. Balakrishnan A, Thekkekare RJ, Sapkal G, Tandale BV. Seroprevalence of Japanese encephalitis virus & West Nile virus in Alappuzha district, Kerala. Indian J Med Res. 2017;146(Suppl. 1):S70–5. https://doi.org/10.4103/ijmr.IJMR_1638_15.

54. Cao L, Fu S, Lu Z, Tang C, Gao X, Li X, et al. Detection of West Nile virus infection in viral encephalitis cases, China. Vector Borne Zoonotic Dis. 2019;19(1):45–50. https://doi.org/10.1089/vbz.2018.2275.

55. Ergünay K, Litzba N, Brinkmann A, Günay F, Sarıkaya Y, Kar S, et al. Co-circulation of West Nile virus and distinct insect-specific flaviviruses in Turkey. Parasit Vectors. 2017;10(1):149. https://doi.org/10.1186/s13071-017-2087-7.

56. Nash D, Mostashari F, Fine A, Miller J, O'Leary D, Murray K, et al. The outbreak of West Nile virus infection in the New York City area in 1999. New Engl J Med. 2001;344(24):1807–14.

57. ArboNET, Arboviral Diseases Branch, Centers for Disease Control and Prevention. West Nile virus final cumulative maps & data for 1999–2020. https://www.cdc.gov/westnile/statsmaps/cumMapsData.html#one

58. Fujita DM, Salvador FS, Nali LHDS. The silent spread of West Nile virus in Brazil: non-human positive case in a beach tourist destination-Espirito Santo. J Travel Med. 2018;25(1) https://doi.org/10.1093/jtm/tay052.

59. Salgado BB, de Jesus Maués FC, Pereira RL, Chiang JO, de Oliveira Freitas MN, Ferreira MS, Martins LC, da Costa Vasconcelos PF, Ganoza C, Lalwani P. Prevalence of arbovirus antibodies in young healthy adult population in Brazil. Parasit Vectors. 2021;14(1):403. https://doi.org/10.1186/s13071-021-04901-4.

60. Lorenz C and Chiaravalloti-Neto F. Why are there no human West Nile virus outbreaks in South America? The lancet regional health—Americas 2022;12: 100276.

61. Morin CW, Comrie AC. Regional and seasonal response of a West Nile virus vector to climate change. Proc Natl Acad Sci U S A. 2013;110(39):15620–5.

62. Wimberly MC, Davis JK, Hildreth MB, Clayton JL. Integrated forecasts based on public health surveillance and meteorological data predict West Nile Virus in a high-risk Region of North America. Environ Health Perspect. 2022;130(8):87006. https://doi.org/10.1289/EHP10287.

63. Paz S. Climate changes impact on West Nile virus transmission in a global context. Phil Trans R Soc B. 370:20130561. https://doi.org/10.1098/rstb.2013.0561.

64. Baylis M. Potential impact of climate change on emerging vector-borne and other infections in the UK. Environ Health. 2017;16(Suppl. 1):112. https://doi.org/10.1186/s12940-017-0326-1.

65. Watts MJ, i Monteys VS, Mortyn PG, Kotsila P. The rise of West Nile virus in southern and southeastern Europe: a spatial-temporal analysis investigating the combined effects of climate, land use and economic changes. One Health. 2021;13:100315. https://doi.org/10.1016/j.onehlt.2021.100315.

66. Montgomery RR, Murray KO. Risk factors for West Nile virus infection and disease in populations and individuals. Expert Rev Anti-Infect Ther. 2015;3:317–25. https://doi.org/10.1586/14787210.2015.1007043.

67. Diamond MS, Shrestha B, Marri A, Mahan D, Engle M. B cells and antibody play critical roles in the immediate defense of disseminated infection by West Nile encephalitis virus. J Virol. 2003;77(4):2578–86. https://doi.org/10.1128/jvi.77.4.2578-2586.2003.

68. Cain MD, Salimi H, Diamond MS, Klein RS. Mechanisms of pathogen invasion into the central nervous system. Neuron. 2019;103(5):771–83. https://doi.org/10.1016/j.neuron.2019.07.015.

69. Mustafá YM, Meuren LM, Coelho SVA, de Arruda LB. Pathways exploited by Flaviviruses to counteract the blood-brain barrier and invade the central nervous system. Front Microbiol. 2019;10:525. https://doi.org/10.3389/fmicb.2019.00525.

70. Byas AD, Ebel GD. Comparative pathology of West Nile virus in humans and non-human animals. Pathogens. 2020;9(1):48. https://doi.org/10.3390/pathogens9010048.

71. Ali M, Safriel Y, Sohi J, Llave A, Weathers S. West Nile virus infection: MR imaging findings in the nervous system. AJNR Am J Neuroradiol. 2005;26(2):289–97.

72. Hayes EB, Sejvar JJ, Zaki SR, et al. Virology, pathology, and clinical manifestations of West Nile virus disease. Emerg Infect Dis. 2005;11(8):1174–9. https://doi.org/10.3201/eid1108.050289b.

73. Cho H, Diamond MS. Immune responses to West Nile virus infection in the central nervous system. Viruses. 2012;4(12):3812–30. https://doi.org/10.3390/v4123812.

74. Chu JJH, Ng ML. The mechanism of cell death during West Nile virus infection is dependent on initial infectious dose. J Gen Virol. 2003;84(Pt 12):3305–14. https://doi.org/10.1099/vir.0.19447-0.

75. Ramanathan MP, Chambers JA, Pankhong P, Chattergoon M, Attatippaholkun W, Dang K, Shah N, Weiner DB. Host cell killing by the West Nile virus NS2B–NS3 proteolytic complex: NS3 alone is sufficient to recruit caspase-8-based apoptotic pathway. Virology. 2006;345:56–72.

76. del Carmen Parquet M, Kumatori A, Hasebe F, Morita K, Igarashi A. West Nile virus-induced bax-dependent apoptosis. FEBS Lett. 2001;500:17–24.

77. Peng BH, Wang T. West Nile virus induced cell death in the central nervous system. Pathogens. 2019;8(4):215. https://doi.org/10.3390/pathogens8040215.

78. Constant O, Barthelemy J, Nagy A, Salinas S, Simonin Y. West Nile virus Neuroinfection in humans: peripheral biomarkers of Neuroinflammation and neuronal damage. Viruses. 2022;14:756. https://doi.org/10.3390/v14040756.

79. Kapadia R, Yi JH, Vemuganti R. Mechanisms of anti-inflammatory and neuroprotective actions of PPAR-gamma agonists. Front Biosci. 2008;13:1813–26. https://doi.org/10.2741/2802.

80. Clarke P, Leser JS, Tyler KL. Intrinsic innate immune responses control viral growth and protect against neuronal death in an ex vivo model of West Nile virus-induced central nervous system disease. J Virol. 2021;95(18):e0083521. https://doi.org/10.1128/JVI.00835-21.

81. Graham JB, Swarts JL, Thomas S, Voss KM, Sekine A, Green R, Ireton RC, Gale M, Lund JM. Immune correlates of protection from West Nile virus Neuroinvasion and disease. J Infect Dis. 2019;219(7):1162–71. https://doi.org/10.1093/infdis/jiy623.

82. Sejvar JJ. Clinical manifestations and outcomes of West Nile virus infection. Viruses. 2014;6:606–23.

83. Ceausu E, Erscoiu S, Calistru P, Ispas D, Dorobat O, Homos M, et al. Clinical manifestations in the West Nile virus outbreak. Rom J Virol. 1997;48:3–11.

84. Zannoli S, Sambri V. West Nile virus and Usutu virus co-circulation in Europe: epidemiology and implications. Microorganisms. 2019;7(7):184. https://doi.org/10.3390/microorganisms7070184.

85. Kleinschmidt-DeMasters BK, Marder BA, Levi ME, Laird SP, McNutt JT, Escott EJ, et al. Naturally-acquired West Nile virus encephalomyelitis in transplant recipients: clinical, laboratory, diagnostic and neuropathological features. Arch Neurol. 2004;61:1210–20.

86. Debiasi RL, Tyler KL. West Nile virus meningoencephalitis. Nat Clin Pract Neurol. 2006;2(5):264–75. https://doi.org/10.1038/ncpneuro0176.

87. Bradshaw MJ, Venkatesan A. Emergency evaluation and management of encephalitis and myelitis in adults. Semin Neurol. 2019;39:82–101.

88. Hart J Jr, Tillman G, Kraut MA, Chiang HS, Strain JF, Li Y, Agrawal AG, et al. West Nile virus neuroinvasive disease: neurological manifestations and prospective longitudinal outcomes. BMC Infect Dis. 2014;14:248.

89. Sejvar JJ, Bode AV, Marfin AA, Campbell GL, Ewing D, Mazowiecki M, et al. West Nile virus-associated flaccid paralysis. Emerg Infect Dis. 2005;11(7):1021–7. https://doi.org/10.3201/eid1107.040991.

90. Maramattom BV, Philips G, Sudheesh N, Arunkumar G. Acute flaccid paralysis due to West Nile virus infection in adults: a paradigm shift entity. Ann Indian Acad Neurol. 2014;17(1):85–8. https://doi.org/10.4103/0972-2327.128561.

91. Leis AA, Stokic DS. Neuromuscular manifestations of West Nile virus infection. Front Neurol. 2012;3:37.

92. Hawkes MA, Carabenciov ID, Wijdicks EFM, Rabinstein AA. Outcomes in patients with severe West Nile neuroinvasive disease. Crit Care Med. 2018;46(09):e955–8.

93. Murray KO, Resnick M, Miller V. Depression after infection with West Nile virus. Emerg InfectDis. 2007;13:479–81. https://doi.org/10.3201/eid1303.060602.

94. Carson PJ, Konewko P, Wold KS, Mariani P, Goli S, Bergloff P, et al. Long-term clinical and neuropsychological outcomes of West Nile virus infection. Clin Infect Dis. 2006;43(6):723–30. https://doi.org/10.1086/506939.

95. Sambri V, Capobianchi M, Charrel R, Fyodorova M, Gaibani P, Gould E, et al. West Nile virus in Europe: emergence, epidemiology, diagnosis, treatment, and prevention. Clin Microbiol Infect. 2013;19(8):699–704.

96. Dauphin G, Zientara S. West Nile virus: recent trends in diagnosis and vaccine development. Vaccine. 2007;25:5563–76.

97. Sambri V, Capobianchi MR, Cavrini F, Charrel R, Donoso-Mantke O, Escadafal C, et al. Diagnosis of West Nile virus human infections: overview and proposal of diagnostic protocols considering the results of external quality assessment studies. Viruses. 2013;5:2329–48. https://doi.org/10.3390/v5102329.

98. Grazzini G, Liumbruno GM, Pupella S, Silvestri AR, Randi V, Pascarelli N, et al. West Nile virus in Italy: a further threat to blood safety, a further challenge to the blood system. Blood Transfus. 2008;6:235–7.

99. Lim SM, Koraka P, Osterhaus AD, Martina BE. West Nile virus: immunity and pathogenesis. Viruses. 2011;3:811–28.

100. Goates C, Tsuha S, Working S, Carey J, Spivak ES. Seronegative West Nile virus infection in a patient treated with rituximab for rheumatoid arthritis. Am J Med. 2017;130(6):e257–8. https://doi.org/10.1016/j.amjmed.2017.01.014.

101. Abdalla AA, Fanciullo J, Ateeli H. Delayed diagnosis of West Nile meningoencephalitis in a patient receiving rituximab for rheumatoid arthritis. Cureus. 2022;14(10):e30221. https://doi.org/10.7759/cureus.30221.

102. Murray K, Walker C, Herrington E, Lewis JA, McCormick J, Beasley DW, et al. Persistent infection with West Nile virus years after initial infection. J Infect Dis. 2010;201:2–4.

103. European Commission. Commission Decision of 28 April 2008 amending Decision 2002/253/EC laying down case definitions for reporting communicable diseases to the Community network under Decision No 2119/98/EC of the European Parliament and of

the Council. 18.06.2008:L 159. Available from: http://ec.europa.eu/health/ph_threats/com/docs/1589_2008_en.pdf.

104. Cunha BA. Differential diagnosis of West Nile encephalitis. Curr Opin Infect Dis. 2004;17:413–20.

105. Chowers MY, Lang R, Nassar F, Ben-David D, Giladi M, Rubinshtein E, et al. Clinical characteristics of the West Nile fever outbreak, Israel, 2000. Emerg Infect Dis. 2001;7(4):675–8. https://doi.org/10.3201/eid0704.010414.

106. Davis LE, Beckham JD, Tyler KL. North American encephalitic arboviruses. Neurol Clin. 2008;26:727–57. https://doi.org/10.1016/j.ncl.2008.03.012.

107. Kalil AC, Devetten MP, Singh S, Lesiak B, Poage DP, Bargenquast K, et al. Use of interferon-alpha in patients with West Nile encephalitis: report of 2 cases. Clin Infect Dis. 2005;40:764–6.

108. Chan-Tack KM, Forrest G. Failure of interferon alpha-2b in a patient with West Nile virus meningoencephalitis and acute flaccid paralysis. Scand J Infect Dis. 2005;37:944–6.

109. Mousavi Maleki MS, Sardari S, Ghandehari Alavijeh A, Madanchi H. Recent patents and FDA-approved drugs based on antiviral peptides and other peptide-related antivirals. Int J Pept Res Ther. 2023;29(1):5. https://doi.org/10.1007/s10989-022-10477-z. Epub 2022 Nov 25

110. Solomon T, Michael BD, Smith PE, Sanderson F, Davies NW, Hart IJ, et al. Management of suspected viral encephalitis in adults—association of British Neurologists and British Infection Association national guidelines. J Infect. 2012;64:347–73.

111. Leis AA, Sinclair DJ. Lazarus effect of high dose corticosteroids in a patient with West Nile virus encephalitis: a coincidence or a clue? Front Med (Lausanne). 2019;6:81. https://doi.org/10.3389/fmed.2019.00081.

112. Kal S, Beland A, Hasan M. West Nile Neuroinvasive disease treated with high-dose corticosteroids. Cureus. 2022;14(11):e31971. https://doi.org/10.7759/cureus.31971.

113. Staples E, Fisher M. West Nile virus disease. In: Heyman D, editor. Control of communicable diseases manual. 20th ed. American Public Health Association (APHA) Press; 2015. p. 675–9.

114. Report West Nile Disease (WND) Year 2015. DG Welfare-Lombardy Region, IZLER and Regional Blood Center. Lombardy Region. 2016. Available online: https://www.regione.lombardia.it/wps/wcm/connect/32f70896-0d84-4b85-88b2-ed726cc5fa84/report_ WND_2015.pdf?MOD=AJPERES&CACHEID=ROOTWORKSPACE-32f70896-0d84-4b85-88b2-ed726cc5fa84-lGjaM5.

115. Defilippo F, Dottori M, Lelli D, Chiari M, Cereda D, Farioli M, Chianese R, Cerioli MP, Faccin F, Canziani S, Trogu T, Sozzi E, Moreno A, Lavazza A, Restelli U. Assessment of the costs related to West Nile virus monitoring in Lombardy region (Italy) between 2014 and 2018. Int J Environ Res Public Health. 2022;19(9):5541. https://doi.org/10.3390/ijerph19095541.

116. Stoney RJ, Esposito DH, Kozarsky P, Hamer DH, Grobusch MP, Gkrania-Klotsas E, et al. Infectious diseases acquired by international travelers visiting the United States. J Travel Med. 2018;25(1) https://doi.org/10.1093/jtm/tay053.

117. Van den Bossche D, Cnops I, Meersman K, Domingo C, Van Gompel A, Van Esbroeck M. Chikungunya virus and West Nile virus infections imported into Belgium, 2007–2012. Epidemiol Infect. 2015;143:2227–36. https://doi.org/10.1017/s0950268814000685.

118. Aboutaleb N, Beersma MF, Wunderink HF, Vossen AC, Visser LG. Case report: West-Nile virus infection in two Dutch travellers returning from Israel. Euro Surveill. 2010;15(34):19649. Available online: http://www.eurosurveillance.org/ViewArticle.aspx?ArticleId=19649

119. Parkash V, Woods K, Kafetzopoulou L, Osborne J, Aarons E, Cartwright K. West Nile virus infection in travelers returning to United Kingdom from South Africa. Emerg Infect Dis. 2019;25(2):367–9.

120. Jani C, Kakoullis L, Abdallah N, Mouchati C, Page S, Colgrove R, Chen LH. West Nile virus: another emerging arboviral risk for travelers? Curr Infect Dis Rep. 2022;24(10):117–28. https://doi.org/10.1007/s11908-022-00783-4.

121. Wollants E, Smolders D, Naesens R, Bruynseels P, Lagrou K, Matthijnssens J, Van Ranst M. Use of next-generation sequencing for diagnosis of West Nile virus infection in patient returning to Belgium from Hungary. Emerg Infect Dis. 2018;24(12):2380–2. https://doi.org/10.3201/eid2412.180494.
122. Pietsch C, Trawinski H, Lübbert C, Liebert UG. Short communication: West Nile fever imported from Austria to Germany. Transbound Emerg Dis. 2019;66(2):1033–6. https://doi.org/10.1111/tbed.13079.
123. Loconsole D, Metallo A, De Robertis AL, Morea A, Quarto M, Chironna M. Seroprevalence of dengue virus, West Nile virus, chikungunya virus, and Zika virus in international travelers attending a travel and migration center in 2015–2017, southern Italy. Vector-Borne Zoonotic Dis. 2018;18(6):331. https://doi.org/10.1089/vbz.2017.2260.
124. Hayes EB. Looking the other way: preventing vector-borne disease among travelers to the United States. Trav Med Infect Dis. 2010;8:277e284.
125. Omodior O, Luetkeb MC, Nelson EJ. Mosquito-borne infectious disease, risk-perceptions, and personal protective behavior among U.S. international travellers. Prev Med Rep. 2018;12:336–42.
126. Nguyen Q-BD, Vu M-AN, Hebert AA. Insect repellents: an updated review for the clinician. J Am Acad Dermatol. 2018;88:123. https://doi.org/10.1016/j.jaad.2018.10.053.
127. Centers for Disease Control and Prevention (CDC). West Nile prevention. https://www.cdc.gov/westnile/prevention/index.html (accessed 12 August 2019) (CDC 2019).
128. Rizzoli A, Jiménez-Clavero MA, Barzon L, Cordioli P, Figuerola J, Koraka P, Martina B, Moreno A, Nowotny N, Pardigon N, Sanders N, Ulbert S, Tenorio A. The challenge of West Nile virus in Europe: knowledge gaps and research priorities. Eurosurveillance. 2015;20(20) pii=21135 https://doi.org/10.2807/1560-7917.ES2015.20.20.21135.

Meningococcal Diseases in Travellers

18

Hasip Kahraman, Hüseyin Aytaç Erdem,
and Oğuz Reşat Sipahi

Abstract

Today, the importance of easily transmissible and serious diseases has increased due to the widespread human movements such as travel and migration. Invasive meningococcal diseases remain a considerable public health problem, causing small clusters in industrialized countries and large outbreaks in developing countries. Since meningococcal diseases are endemic in many countries, international travelers may transport the bacterial agent during their journeys and spread it across the countries. Herein, we aimed to summarize meningococcal diseases and travel-associated infections.

18.1 Background

Gaspard Vieusseux reported the first meningococcal meningitis epidemic with a series comprising 33 fatal cases and made a comprehensive clinical description in 1805 in Geneva, Switzerland [1]. In 1887, Anton Weichselbaum isolated the micro-organism from the cerebrospinal fluid and named it *Diplococcus intracellularis* meningitis. In 1913, Simon Flexner introduced a treatment option for meningococcal diseases by treating 1300 meningitis patients during an epidemic with

H. Kahraman
Department of Infectious Diseases and Clinical Microbiology, Osmangazi University Faculty of Medicine, Eskişehir, Turkey
e-mail: hasip.kahraman@ogu.edu.tr

H. A. Erdem (✉) · O. R. Sipahi
Department of Infectious Diseases and Clinical Microbiology, Ege University Faculty of Medicine, Bornova, Izmir, Turkey
e-mail: huseyin.aytac.erdem@ege.edu.tr; Oguz.resat.sipahi@ege.edu.tr

281

H. Leblebicioglu et al. (eds.), *Emerging and Re-emerging Infections in Travellers*, https://doi.org/10.1007/978-3-031-49475-8_18

intrathecal equine meningococcal antiserum, reducing mortality to 31%. Later, antimicrobial therapy was first reported with the use of sulfonamides in 1937 by Francois Schwentker [2]. Meningococcal meningitis had a mortality rate of 80% before the antibiotic era, which decreased to 3–10% with appropriate treatment regimens [3, 4].

Neisseria meningitidis may lead to fatal clinical conditions such as central nervous system involvement, bacteremia, and septicemia [5]. Invasive meningococcal diseases (IMD) remain an important public health problem, still causing small clusters in industrialized countries and large outbreaks in developing countries [6, 7].

Today, the importance of easily transmitted and serious diseases has increased due to the widespread human movements such as travel and migration. Since meningococcal diseases are endemic in many countries, international travelers may transport the bacterial agent during their journeys and spread it across the countries [8]. Herein, we aimed to summarize meningococcal diseases and travel-associated infections.

18.2 Aetiology

N. meningitidis is an aerobic, Gram-negative diplococcus. Almost all the strains causing invasive diseases have a polysaccharide capsule, one of the major virulence factors [9]. Meningococci are fastidious bacteria and cannot survive on inanimate surfaces. A temperature of 35 °C–37 °C and CO_2 concentration of 5–10% are required for optimal growth. Blood agar, trypticase soy agar, supplemented chocolate agar, and Mueller–Hinton agar may be used for bacteriological culture [10].

Meningococci can be classified in terms of serotype, serosubtype, and immunotypes according to outer membrane protein (OMP) antigens and lipooligosaccharide (LOS) structures. Serogroups constitute the basis for the determination of meningococcal epidemiology and control of the disease. As a result, currently, *N. meningitidis* is classified into 13 serogroups according to the immunogenetic and capsule structure, as A, B, C, D, X, Y, Z, 29 E, W-135, H, I, K, and L [10, 11]. However, only six of these serogroups (A, B, C, W-135, X, and Y) cause life-threatening diseases [10].

18.3 Transmission

The only reservoir of *N. meningitidis* is humans. It cannot survive in nature [12, 13]. Meningococci may be found asymptomatically in the upper respiratory tract mucosa of approximately 10–35% of healthy young adults [14]. These asymptomatic carriers have a major role in spreading the bacteria, which may be transmitted by droplets among people living close to each other for the long term or by direct contact through kissing or sexual intercourse [13]. Therefore, people who live in crowded places such as schools, dormitories, or barracks or share the same dwelling with asymptomatic carriers have a greater risk of transmission [15]. Theoretically and practically, big and crowded international travel vehicles such as airplanes or cruise ships may also disseminate meningococci. Stefanelli et al. described four cases of IMDs that occurred on a cruise ship sailing along the Italian coast in October 2012. All four cases were hospitalized with severe illness, and one of them died [16]. Likewise, O'Connor et al. identified two cases of meningococcal disease in passengers who travelled on the same international flight. Both cases were serogroup B positive with the same allelic profile [17]. Moreover, another case of air-travel-associated meningococcal disease was reported in 2001 as a patient who met the case definition of meningococcal disease, i.e. occurrence within 14 days of travel on a flight of at least 8 h duration [18].

18.4 Epidemiology

Approximately 500,000–1,200,000 IMD cases are seen annually, resulting in 50,000–135,000 deaths worldwide [19]. The number of cases differs between countries and regions. While the incidence of annual IMD is <1/100,000 in developed countries, sub-Saharan Africa, named the meningitis belt, has an incidence of 10–1000/100,000 [6, 7].

Over time, there have been significant differences in the dominant serogroup distribution or epidemiology of meningococcal infections among different regions of the world. Serogroup A was the most commonly isolated serotype from the pre-World War I period to the 1970s. Then serogroup B emerged as the most common serotype in Europe after 1970 and in South America during the post-1980s. Later, due to the outbreaks in the twenty-first century, serogroup W-135 and Y became the dominant serogroups, especially in South Africa and Europe and among the pilgrims returning from the Hajj in Saudi Arabia [20–23].

Today, in most parts of Europe and North America, the dominant serogroups are B, C, and Y. Furthermore, in Africa, there is no significant difference in the distribution of serogroups, and serogroup A remains to be the causative agent in most infections. Although cases of serogroup C, W, and X are still reported in this region, a ten-fold reduction in the frequency of meningococcal epidemics has been achieved since 2010 via the introduction of serogroup A vaccine in sub-Saharan Africa [24–26]. Although large epidemics of serogroup A were previously observed in Asia, serogroup B and C are still the causes of most cases. Furthermore, since the 1990s, serogroup W has been reported to be the most common causative agent of IMDs in pilgrims and persons in close contact [10]. Although recent outbreaks of serogroup W have been reported in some South American countries, serogroup B and C are the dominant serogroups in this region [27]. However, interestingly, the distribution of these serogroups is also affected by age. While there is a decrease in the frequency of serogroup C infections in the adolescent age group, serogroup Y is increasing in elderly patients [24].

IMD is more common in children aged <1 year due to decreasing level of maternal antibodies. It is also common in adolescents and young adults (15–25 years) due to relatively high nasopharyngeal carriage rates [19, 28]. Apart from these, those living in crowded accommodation facilities such as schools, dormitories, immigrant camps, and military facilities, where close contact is intense, are at risk for epidemics. Additionally, complement system defects and asplenia are other important risk factors for IMDs [7].

The above-mentioned epidemiology of meningococci naturally poses a danger for travellers. Rapp et al. evaluated travel-related cerebro-meningeal infections during 8 years in a French infectious diseases unit. Fortunately, only one of the 56 cases was attributable to *N. meningitidis*. The reported outbreaks and case reports published in PubMed-indexed journals between 2009 and November 2022 (search strategy [(travel) AND (meningococci or "*Neisseria meningitidis*")]) have been summarized in Table 18.1. The table shows that meningococci affect not only developing countries but also developed countries such as England, Ghana, France, India, Japan, South Africa, and Italy.

Since accommodation in crowded settings is important in epidemiology, migrants resting in large immigrant centres are also at risk. Tafuri et al. evaluated the prevalence of *N. meningitidis* carriers in 253 African refugee residents in the Asylum Seeker Centre of Bari, Italy, and 13 subjects (5.1%) were identified as carriers of meningococci [39]. Furthermore, Stefanelli et al. reported three meningococci meningitis cases in two migrants and a worker in the immigrant centre, necessitating the need for vaccinating refugees and workers in the immigrant centres [40].

Table 18.1 The reported outbreaks and case reports published in PubMed-indexed journals between 2009 and November 2022

Origin country	Year	Number of cases	Dominant/case serotype	Reference
Japan	2022	1 case from Argentina	B&W/W135	[29]
Malaysia	2020	1 case related to the recent Kingdom of Saudi Arabia travel	W/?	[30]
England	2019	3 cases related to recent Kingdom of Saudi Arabia travel	W/non-groupable strain	[31]
Jirapa-Ghana	2016	233 meningitis cases	A/W135	[32]
United States	2016	1 case report related to travel to Romania	?/B	[33]
Japan	2015	4 cases from Scotland, 2 cases from Sweden	B&C(Scotland)-Y(Sweden)/W	[34]
France	2012	16 cases, 8 related to African travel	A/W135	[35]
France	2012	6 cases, all related to recent African travel	A/W135	[36]
International	2012	4 cases related to cruise ship travel	–/C	[16]
Japan	2011	1 case report related to a prior France visit	B/B	[37]
Italy	2009	1 case report related to travel to India	A/A	[38]

Finally, to make a short addition in terms of COVID-19, Brueggemann et al. found a significant and sustained reduction in invasive meningococcal diseases in early 2020 (Jan 1 to May 31, 2020), coinciding with the introduction of COVID-19 containment measures [41].

18.5 Pathogenesis

There are many structural and biological factors affecting the virulence of *N. meningitidis,* such as the capsular polysaccharide structure, surface adhesion proteins (the OMPs including pili, porins Por A and B, and adhesion molecules Opa and Opc), LOS, iron sequestration mechanisms, endotoxins, and the genotype of bacteria. The capsule and LOS structure provide resistance to complement-related lysis and phagocytosis. The pili and other OMPs facilitate the adherence of bacteria to the endothelial surfaces [42].

Meningococcal infection begins with the colonization of the bacteria in the upper respiratory tract [13]. The symptoms start after an incubation period of 1–14 days [43]. The first stage of meningococcal colonization is the adhesion of the bacterium to membrane cofactor protein (CD46) in the nasopharyngeal epithelium by type 4 pili [44]. The adhesion process is completed via opacity proteins such as Opa and Opc [45]. Polysaccharide capsules and IgA protease are the most important virulence factors of bacteria. Moreover, factors that inhibit ciliary activity help to preclude phagocytosis and the host immune system [7, 46]. Meningococci must reach the submucosal layer to develop invasive infection after colonization, but this process is not fully understood [13, 46]. After this stage, bacteria reach the bloodstream, causing meningococcemia. It may occur because of the systemic inflammatory response stimulated by rapid bacterial proliferation, and later, may cause invasive disease by reaching the pericardium, joints, and especially the central nervous system causing meningitis [13].

Specific antibodies against the bacteria are most crucial for the prevention of IMDs. Although specific antibodies have a priority role in prevention, there is evidence for the protective effects of natural immunity, especially in the window period between colonization and the start of meningococci-specific antibody synthesis. Classical antibody-mediated, properdin, and lectin complement pathways are protective against meningococcal diseases. Evidently, recurrent infections are more common in patients with complement system disorders such as properdin deficiency [46].

Many bacteria-related factors activate the host immune system [46]. LOS dissemination from the proliferation or disintegration of meningococci stimulates the immune system potently and has a significant role in the development of inflammatory processes in meningococcal meningitis and meningococcemia [43]. In addition, meningococcal LOS levels in the bloodstream are associated with the severity of meningococcal sepsis [42]. LOS molecules are transported to receptor complexes in macrophages, monocytes, and neutrophils by lipopolysaccharide-binding protein [43]. The endothelial surface is damaged due to the inflammatory proteins, proteases, and other enzymes that are induced by the stimulation of immune system cells. As a result, increased vascular permeability, pathological vasodilatation, development of vasoconstriction, excessive stimulation of the coagulation system, and intravascular coagulation may develop, causing septic shock and multiorgan failure [46].

18.6 Clinical Findings

Meningococci may cause various clinical manifestations, such as meningitis with or without septicemia, mild bacteremia, fulminant meningococcemia, meningoencephalitis, pneumonia, and septic arthritis [9]. Moreover, fulminant disease, multiorgan insufficiency or death may be seen during clinical follow-up, even in the patients initially presenting mild symptoms [47]. Meningitis and sepsis are the most common manifestations of meningococcal infections, and both may be exhibited in some cases [6]. Clinical symptoms differ by age and diagnosis may be missed, especially in young children who do not manifest classical symptoms.

Initially, IMDs may manifest as upper respiratory tract infections, colds such as pharyngitis, fever, loss of appetite, nausea, vomiting, and headache. However, in children aged <5 years, lethargy or irritability may be predominant and miscible with non-specific viral infections [6, 47, 48]. Meningitis or sepsis-specific findings may be absent at onset, and clinical manifestations may become evident with disease progression [47].

The presence of multiple purpuric lesions, extreme ages, primary meningococcal pneumonia, shock, hypotension, tachycardia, coma, convulsion, disturbances in consciousness, absence of nuchal rigidity, and hyperventilation are reported to be associated with poor prognosis in meningococcal infections. Furthermore, laboratory and microbiological variables such as leukopenia, thrombocytopenia, serogroup C or W infection, presence of isolated bacteremia, elevated and continuous endotoxinemia, metabolic acidosis, lactate levels above 4 mmol/L, and neutrophil count below $100/\text{mm}^3$ in the CSF may worsen the prognosis [13].

18.6.1 Meningitis

IMDs manifest most commonly as meningitis due to the characteristic tropism of meningococci, and approximately 30–60% of all IMD cases are meningitis [42]. Moreover, meningococci may be accountable for up to approximately 50% of the meningitis cases in the paediatric age group and 27% in the adult age group [49]. Meningococcal meningitis has similar clinical findings to community-acquired meningitis caused by other etiological agents [7]. However, clinical findings may vary in different age groups. While infants present with high fever, hypothermia, malnutrition, vomiting, persistent crying, increased size of fontanel, irritability, lethargy, and coma, older children manifest with fever, vomiting, photophobia, headache, signs of meningeal irritation, and neck stiffness. Moreover, adults often present with signs of classical meningeal irritation, with only a few presenting the classical meningitis triad of fever, mental status change, and neck stiffness. Furthermore, in elderly patients, although disturbances in consciousness and focal neurological deficits are more common than in young adults, nuchal stiffness and headache are rarely reported [13, 50]. Focal neurological deficits are present in app. 20% of the cases. Atypical rashes, distinctive from the septicemia lesions, can be seen in 26% of the cases [13, 47]. Increased cerebral inflammation and edema may result in increased intracranial pressure, causing cerebral herniation and death [51]. Meningococcal meningitis has lower mortality (5–18%) and morbidity rates than meningococcemia. Sensorineural hearing loss, spasticity, seizures, attention disorders, and intellectual disability are the most common sequelae of meningococcal meningitis [7].

18.6.2 Septicemia

Septicemia is another serious clinical condition, frequent in IMD patients, and may be seen in 20–30% of the cases [47]. Sudden onset of fever, petechial, purpuric or maculopapular rash, hypotension, disseminated intravascular coagulation (DIC), osteonecrosis, septic shock, and multiple organ dysfunction syndrome may develop in meningococcemia [52]. The early indicators of sepsis in children and adolescents are cold distal extremities as well as painful and pale skin [48]. The classical hemorrhagic rash associated with meningococcemia occurs in 42–70% of the cases and usually develops after non-specific symptoms [7, 48]. Although rashes are usually severe on the extremities, they may involve the whole body, including the sclera and mucous membranes [43]. Waterhouse–Friderichsen syndrome is a form of meningococcemia with skin rashes and adrenal haemorrhage. It is an indicator of fulminant meningococcemia and may cause thrombotic lesions on the skin, kidneys, choroid plexus, lungs, and extremities [52].

Meningococcemia is characterized by severe and persistent septic shock, resulting in the collapse of the circulatory system and serious coagulopathy. Different clinical trials have indicated the mortality rate of meningococcemia between 20–80%. Moreover, approximately 10% of the survivors may require limb or finger amputation due to ischemia, skin necrosis, or infarction [53].

18.6.3 Meningitis and Septicemia

The concurrent occurrence of meningitis and septicemia has been reported in 12% of IMD cases [48]. The mortality rate in such cases is lower than that in the patients with only meningococcemia (26.3% vs. 6.7%,) [54].

18.6.4 Other Clinical Forms of Meningococcal Diseases

Primary pneumonia develops in 5–10% of the cases and more frequently in adult cases. Approximately 45% of the pneumonia cases are related to serogroup Y. The prognosis of primary pneumonia related to meningococci is relatively poor, and elderly patients demonstrate a mortality rate of 16% [9, 13].

The prognosis of meningococcal arthritis, a complication in app. 7.5% of the IMD cases, is good. Primary meningococcal arthritis is rare and accounts for about 2% of all meningococcal infection cases [55].

Chronic meningococcemia, an unusual clinical presentation of meningococcal diseases, is characterized by fever, maculopapular exanthema, arthralgia, or arthritis and may persist for weeks or months. Meningitis may develop and cause mortality in these cases [13].

Primary pericarditis, associated with serogroup C and W, occurs in adolescents and adult patients. Cardiac tamponade may develop in some cases due to high pericardial effusion [13]. Other rare clinical presentations of meningococcal infections are conjunctivitis, peritonitis, panophthalmitis, epiglottitis, sinusitis, otitis, orbital cellulitis, osteomyelitis, endocarditis, salpingitis, urethritis, and proctitis [13].

18.7 Laboratory Diagnosis

Due to the high mortality rates laboratory tests should not be awaited to start an antimicrobial therapy in suspected IMD cases [56]. Diagnostic tests may be initiated with a complete blood count, coagulation tests, and two sets of blood cultures. Additionally, CSF sampling should be performed in suspected cases of meningitis [57]. The increasing leukocyte and C-reactive protein levels, usually observed in bacterial infections, may be normal in the first 12–24 h, especially in severe and rapid-onset IMD cases [56].

Bacterial culture is the gold standard for microbiological diagnosis [58]. Etiologic agents can be isolated from cultures of blood, CSF, skin lesions, and throat secretions [56]. The sensitivity of blood culture in cases that did not receive antibiotic therapy ranges between 25–50% [59]. Moreover, latex agglutination tests are other diagnostic tools, which can detect bacterial agents rapidly [49]. Blood, CSF, and urine samples can be used for this diagnostic method. However, the sensitivity in meningococci infections varies between 22–93% [50, 56]. Lastly, meningococcal DNA can be detected in the blood or CSF samples with high sensitivity and specificity by polymerase chain reaction (PCR) method [56].

Diagnosis of meningococcal meningitis is usually based on clinical findings and CSF examination. If clinical signs and symptoms suggest meningitis and there is no contraindication, lumbar puncture should be performed immediately. CSF opening pressure is usually around 180 mm-H_2O in acute bacterial meningitis (ABM), while it may range between 200–500 mm-H_2O. CSF has a leukocyte count of 0–10 cells/mm^3 and a clear appearance in healthy individuals. However, in ABM, it exhibits a blurred colour. The leukocyte count ranges between 1000–5000 cells/mm^3, and most cells are polymorphonuclear leukocytes [60]. On biochemical examination, the CSF glucose/serum glucose <40% and CSF protein value >50 mg/dl are diagnostic for ABM [57].

Gram stain is also a fast, effective, and inexpensive method for diagnosing ABM, with a sensitivity of about 75% in untreated meningococcal meningitis cases [60, 61]. CSF cultures are positive in about 82% of meningococcal meningitis cases; however, this is reduced significantly after antibiotic use [49]. The positive culture of the bacterial agent in blood or CSF allows an etiological diagnosis as well as the application of antimicrobial susceptibility tests [13]. The sensitivity of PCR assays for detecting *N. meningitidis* ranges between 91–100% [62].

These diagnostic tests have various advantages and disadvantages over each other. For example, while the ability to determine antibiotic susceptibility and being inexpensive is aligned with the advantages of the gold-standard bacterial cultures, its lengthy procedure and property to get affected by previous antibiotic treatment (similar to the latex agglutination tests and Gram stain) are considered as the disadvantages. On the other hand, high sensitivity and specificity, no requirement of live bacteria, yield of results within 2 h, and a property to be affected less by previous antibiotic treatment are enumerated as the advantages of PCR. However, its limitations include the inability to allow antibiotic susceptibility tests, the need for an experienced staff and the laboratory equipment, and high cost [49, 50, 59].

Computed tomography scan and magnetic resonance imaging can be used especially in cases with clinical conditions such as meningococcal meningitis with focal neurologic deficit, clinically suspected cranial abscesses, a history of chronic recurrent otitis, coma or epileptic seizure that persists for 72 h during treatment, and those under immunosuppressive therapy or with a history of recurrent meningoencephalitis [13].

Biopsy specimens from cutaneous lesions may be useful in IMD diagnosis, but the sensitivity and specificity are relatively low (34–47%). Culture may be positive until about 13 h after the beginning of antibiotic treatment, which may take up to 45 h for Gram stain of the skin lesions. Yet, negative culture from the skin lesions cannot exclude the disease [13].

18.8 Differential Diagnosis

CSF examination is required to confirm the diagnosis of meningococcal meningitis. Viral meningoencephalitis, intracranial suppurative diseases, and other bacterial agents (*S. pneumoniae, H. influenzae, Listeria monocytogenes,* etc.) that cause meningoencephalitis and cerebrovascular conditions should be included in the differential diagnosis of IMD [13, 49]. Also for the diagnosis of meningococcemia, conditions such as sepsis, diffuse gonococcemia, infective endocarditis, Rocky Mountain spotted fever, typhoid fever, leukocytoclastic vasculitis, hemorrhagic dengue, and other exanthematous viruses (enteroviruses, infectious mononucleosis, rubella, measles), ehrlichiosis, anaplasmosis, borreliosis (Lyme disease), neoplasms, collagen vascular diseases, thrombotic thrombocytopenic purpura, idiopathic thrombocytopenic purpura, and Henoch-Schonlein purpura should be excluded. Some of these diagnoses, such as dengue and borreliosis, are among major travel-associated etiologic agents [13, 63].

18.9 Management

IMD cases may progress rapidly unless they receive appropriate antibiotic treatment in the early period and develop life-threatening complications and mortality. The definition of an effective treatment for IMD includes assessment and management of antibiotic therapy, sepsis, and/or increased intracranial pressure [64].

Early and appropriate intravenous (IV) antibiotic therapy stops bacterial growth, sterilizes the CSF within 3–4 h, reduces endotoxin levels by 50% in 2 h, and helps in reducing plasma cytokine and chemokine levels. Furthermore, antibiotic treatment blocks the release of high levels of meningococcal endotoxin and increase in the inflammatory response (Herxheimer reaction) [43].

18.9.1 Antibiotic Therapy

Third-generation cephalosporins (ceftriaxone or cefotaxime) may be preferred in IMDs until the results of antibiotic susceptibility tests are obtained [60]. Ceftriaxone is, however, not favoured in the neonatal period because of the risk of hyperbilirubinemia and kernicterus [65]. After the susceptibility of the microorganism to penicillins is determined, it is recommended to step down the therapy with penicillin G or ampicillin, which has a lower cost and narrow spectrum [49, 60]. Chloramphenicol is recommended in cases with a history of penicillin allergy. If chloramphenicol is not available, aztreonam, meropenem, and moxifloxacin are other preferable options [13, 66]. The suggested duration of IMD treatment is 5–7 days, but this may be modified according to the patient's clinical response [49, 66]. The antibiotics recommended for treatment are summarized in Table 18.2.

Table 18.2 Antibiotics recommended for the treatment of IMD cases [49, 67]

	Recommended treatment	Alternative treatment
Cases suspicious of IMD	Third-generation cephalosporin Meropenem	Penicillin G, ampicillin, chloramphenicol, fluoroquinolone, aztreonam
Culture-confirmed case of IMD		
– Penicillin minimum inhibitory concentration (MIC) <0.1 µg/ml	Penicillin G or ampicillin	Third-generation cephalosporin, chloramphenicol
– Penicillin MIC = 0.1–1 µg/ml	Third-generation cephalosporin	Chloramphenicol, fluoroquinolone, meropenem

18.9.2 Hypotension and Shock Treatment

All cases with suspected IMDs should be evaluated in terms of shock findings, and cases with no evidence of increased intracranial pressure must be started with IV fluid support. In paediatric patients with shock symptoms, 20 ml/kg of 0.9% sodium chloride should be given as an IV bolus in 5–10 min, and immediately after, the patient should be reevaluated. If signs of shock persist despite the initial treatment, it is advised to give 20 ml/kg of 0.9% sodium chloride or 4.5% human albumin solution in 5–10 min. If the shock does not improve despite the 40 ml/kg IV fluid treatment, it is recommended to re-administer 20 ml/kg of 0.9% sodium chloride IV bolus or 4.5% human albumin solution. However, in adult cases, it is suggested to administer 30 ml/kg crystalloid fluid within the first 3 h. Vasopressor agents should be added to the treatment according to the local, national, or international protocols. Patients should be monitored for fluid overload, hypoglycemia, and electrolyte imbalance [68, 69].

18.9.3 Glucocorticoid Treatment

The usage of steroids in meningococcemia, especially in patients with concomitant purpura fulminans or Waterhouse–Friderichsen syndrome, is controversial [13]. However, IV hydrocortisone may be considered in patients who are unresponsive to IV fluid therapy and vasoactive agents [70].

Steroid therapy has been shown to reduce hearing loss and neurological sequelae in ABM, but there has been no significant improvement in mortality. On the other hand, it has been noted in the subgroup analysis that steroid usage decreased mortality in pneumococcal meningitis but not in meningitis caused by other agents [49]. High-dose dexamethasone should be initiated before the first antibiotic dose or within 12 h, at the latest, in cases with suspected ABM. Dexamethasone is recommended in a dose of 0.15 mg/kg four times daily for 2–4 days. Since high-dose corticosteroids may worsen the prognosis in adult meningococcemia without meningitis, it is considered to be contraindicated [64].

18.9.4 Treatment of Brain Oedema

Osmotic agents such as glycerol, mannitol, and hypertonic saline may be used in various neurological diseases with increased intracranial pressure and central nervous system infections. However, so far, there are no therapeutic agents with proven efficacy [49]. Although the efficacy is controversial in patients with increased intracranial pressure, mannitol may be administered as an initial dose of 0.5–1 g/kg and repeated maintenance doses of 0.25–0.30 g/kg every 4 h. Furthermore, it is recommended to keep the head position above 30° and avoid hyperextension of the head [13].

18.9.5 Additional Treatments

Activated protein C and unfractionated heparin treatments have been tried in IMD cases with DIC and/or purpura fulminans or other severe sepsis cases, but none have exhibited clinical benefit [13]. In a randomized controlled trial, anti-endotoxin antibody (HA-1A) was administered in children with meningococcemia, but there was no significant reduction in mortality [71]. In another study investigating recombinant bactericidal permeability-increasing protein (rBPI21), which has a binding and neutralizing effect on endotoxins, fewer amputation rates, fewer blood product transfusions, and improved functional outcomes were found in the patients, as compared to placebo. However, the study's strength was insufficient to demonstrate a reduction in mortality [72]. Plasmapheresis, blood exchange, and extracorporeal membrane oxygenation have been tried in a small number of patients, and positive results have been observed; however, controlled studies are needed [73].

18.10 Complications and Sequelae

Long-term complications and sequelae occur in approximately 11–19% of surviving IMD cases [66]. Acute respiratory distress syndrome, complicated bleeding, anuria, and skin and extremity necrosis may develop in meningococcemia. Increased intracranial pressure can cause brain edema, blood flow deterioration, and rarely fatal brain herniation in cases with meningococcal meningitis. However, neurological sequelae are less than those in pneumococcal meningitis [53]. The most common sequelae in meningococcal infections are chronic pain, skin scarring, and neurological deficits. Hearing, visual, and behavioural disorders, motor deficits, seizures, septic arthritis, conjunctivitis, and chronic meningococcemia are other reported complications. Hearing loss and amputations are seen in approximately 3% of the IMD cases [66, 74].

18.11 Prevention

Seeking a medical opinion at least 1 month before the planned travel date is a general concept, yet poorly applied by tourists. This one-month period allows time for proper immunoprophylaxis and antimicrobial prophylaxis, if needed. Furthermore, hand hygiene is critical for the prevention of many travel-associated infections.

18.11.1 Antimicrobial Chemoprophylaxis

In terms of Public Health, the priority step in preventing the spread of IMD is to block meningococcal carriage by administering antibacterial drugs to persons in close contact with the index case(s). Thus, dissemination of the disease to the susceptible population is prevented [75]. The ideal chemoprophylaxis application period is within 24 h after detection of the index case, and the contribution of prophylaxis administered after 14 days is limited [66]. Chemoprophylaxis may fail due to late administration, misapplication, or noncompliance of the persons [53]. Moreover, chemoprophylaxis is recommended prior to discharge in IMD cases treated with antibiotics other than ceftriaxone or cefotaxime, to prevent nasopharyngeal carriage [66].

Household members, roommates, being close up to 1 m long (≥ 8 h) to the index case, people sitting next to the index case on long-term journeys, daycare centre contacts, exposure to oral secretions of the patient in the last week (kissing, endotracheal tube management etc.) should be considered to be close contacts [43, 75]. Routine chemoprophylaxis is not recommended for health personnel not meeting these criteria [66]. Due to the lack of 100% vaccine protection, chemoprophylaxis is recommended for close contact with persons who are previously vaccinated against meningococci [75].

Rifampin (600 mg q12 h for 48 h in adults) or ciprofloxacin (500 mg single dose in adults) or ceftriaxone (250 mg single dose in adults) are the medications that may be used for chemoprophylaxis. When considering ciprofloxacin for prophylaxis in travel medicine, it's important to note the reported cases of ciprofloxacin-resistant meningococci in Canada, China, and India [64, 76].

18.11.2 Immunoprophylaxis

Meningococcal vaccines help to protect the population and control outbreaks of various serogroups [75]. It has been shown that serogroup C carriage and meningococcal disease incidence decreased by more than 50% in the non-vaccine population after MenC vaccination. It has been shown that serogroup C carriage and meningococcal disease incidence decreased by more than 50% in the non-vaccine population after MenC vaccination [43].

Many vaccines may be used for the prevention of meningococcal serogroups. There are three different conjugated vaccines against serogroups A, C, W, and Y (MenACWY-DT Menactra, MenACWY-CRM Menveo, MenACWY-TT Nimenrix) and two different vaccines for serogroup B (MenB-FHbp, Trumenba and MenB-4C, Bexsero). Additionally, vaccines are available for protection from serogroup C (Meningitec, Menjugate, and NeisVac C) and serogroup A (MenAfriVac and PsA-TT) [77, 78]. Meningococcal vaccines are recommended in persons with a higher risk of meningococcal infection (Table 18.3). However, vaccination does not form the basis of post-contact protection since adequate antibody levels develop within 10–14 days [75].

Practice and recommendations for meningococcal vaccines differ according to the specific characteristics of the country and region (dominant serogroup, individual policies, outbreak prevalence, economic conditions, etc.) [78]. In the United States, MenACWY vaccine is recommended for all adolescents aged between 11 and 18, in addition to the MenB vaccine in the ≥ 10-year-old population at risk for developing IMD [77]. Recommendations for vaccination and related age groups vary among European countries. While MenC vaccine is recommended in Germany,

Table 18.3 Recommended vaccination for increased risk of meningococcal disease [77, 79]

First-year college students living in a residence hall and are not up to date with this vaccine
Microbiologists routinely exposed to *Neisseria meningitidis* isolates
Military recruits
Anatomic and functional asplenia or complement system defects
Persons who use complement inhibitors
Travelling to areas where *N. meningitidis* is hyperendemic or epidemic (sub-Saharan Africa and Saudi Arabia)
Persons living with HIV infection
People living in areas with meningococcal disease epidemic
Men who have sex with men
Being a part of a community experiencing a serogroup A, C, W or Y meningococcal disease outbreak

Table 18.4 Recommendations for routine meningococcal vaccination [77, 83]

Meningococcal vaccines	Age groups		
	Child	Adolescent	Adult
– MenA conjugate	9 months through 18 months, single dose	Single dose 1–29 years of age	Single dose 1–29 years of age
– MenB-4C		Two doses 1 month apart 10–25 years of age	Two doses 1 month apart 10–25 years of age
– MenB-FHbp		Two doses 1 month apart or 2 doses at 0 and 6 months 10–25 years of age	Two doses 1 month apart or 2 doses at 0 and 6 months 10–25 years of age
– MenC conjugate	2 doses in infancy, booster in the second year of life or 1 dose at ≥12 months	Single dose	Single dose
– MenACWY	9 months through 23 months 2 doses	Single dose	Single dose

MenB-4C Four-component meningococcal group B vaccine, *MenB-FHbp* meningococcal group B factor H binding protein vaccine

France, Hungary, Spain, Portugal, Poland, and Iceland, MenB, MenC, and MenACWY are advised in Austria, Greece, Ireland, Italy, and the United Kingdom [80]. The routine meningococcal vaccination scheme is presented in Table 18.4.

The Advisory Committee on Immunization Practices recommends quadrivalent (serogroup A, C, W, or Y) meningococcal vaccination prior to travel while visiting sub-Saharan Africa during the dry season. However, The Men B vaccine administration is not recommended for people who visit the meningitis belt region due to the low incidence of serogroup B infections. Moreover, it is necessary to document that a quadrivalent (serogroup A, C, W, or Y) meningococcal vaccine has been administered to those visiting the Kingdom of Saudi Arabia or the Hajj or Umrah prior to the trip. Men B vaccine is not recommended routinely for other international passengers if there are no active outbreaks in the visited region [81].

Furthermore, while travelling to Saudi Arabia for Hajj and Umrah, vaccination with quadrivalent (ACYW) conjugate vaccine is recommended by the WHO (according to a publication provided by Saudi Health Authorities) for the domestic pilgrims, residents of the two holy cities (Makkah and Medina), and any person who may get in contact with pilgrims including personnel in healthcare settings and other authorities [82].

Although the protection provided by the meningococcal vaccines is adequate, the success of vaccination lags behind conjugated *S. pneumoniae* and *H. influenzae* type B vaccines. The reason for relatively lower efficacy is reported to be due to the facts that i) tetravalent vaccines do not contain serogroup B, ii) the dominant meningococci serogroups vary between countries/regions, and iii) it is not easy to implement routine childhood vaccination against all serogroups in every country [75].

Finally, the US Centers for Disease Control and Prevention published guidelines in 2001 for managing persons potentially exposed to meningococcus during air travel. These guidelines may be used for the management of mass transport vehicles (airplanes, cruise ships, etc.) associated cases [84].

18.11.3 Other Precautions

Transmission of the IMD continues during the first 24 h after the start of appropriate antibiotic treatment. Therefore, healthcare workers should pay attention to droplet precautions [44]. Patients should be hospitalized and monitored in isolated rooms. If this is not possible, there should be a minimum distance of 1.5 m between the patient beds [11]. Microbiologists working with *N. meningitidis* isolates may rarely develop meningococcal disease, but the probability is several times higher than in the normal population. Meningococcal disease was associated with the manipulation of meningococcal isolates outside the safety cabinet. Therefore, it is recommended to use a laboratory with biosafety level 2 to reduce the risk of contamination [52].

18.11.4 Gaps in Knowledge That Need to be Addressed

IMD is a typical preventable disease. Data are needed (i) to delineate the role and cost-effectiveness of vaccination in decreasing travel-associated IMDs and (ii) to further clarify the role of chemoprophylaxis during travel and/or after exposure in larger cohorts. Furthermore, prevention strategies against possibly drug-resistant meningococci should be developed. Uniting all meningococcal serogroups in one affordable vaccine may be a feasible methodology to decrease the global number of cases. Finally, medical education programs would be more inclusive and elaborative about travel medicine and vaccination strategies against meningococci [85, 86].

Declaration of Interest We declare no conflict of interest.

References

1. M. V. Memoire sur la maladie qui a régné à Genéve au printemps de 1805. J Med Clin Pharm. 1805;11:163–82.
2. Tyler KL. Chapter 28: a history of bacterial meningitis. Handb Clin Neurol. 2010;95:417–33.
3. Swartz MN. Bacterial meningitis—a view of the past 90 years. N Engl J Med. 2004;351(18):1826–8.
4. Thigpen MC, Whitney CG, Messonnier NE, Zell ER, Lynfield R, Hadler JL, et al. Bacterial meningitis in the United States, 1998-2007. N Engl J Med. 2011;364(21):2016–25.
5. Rosenstein NE, Perkins BA, Stephens DS, Popovic T, Hughes JM. Meningococcal disease. N Engl J Med. 2001;344(18):1378–88.
6. Bosis S, Mayer A, Esposito S. Meningococcal disease in childhood: epidemiology, clinical features and prevention. J Prev Med Hyg. 2015;56(3):E121.
7. Dwilow R, Fanella S. Invasive meningococcal disease in the 21st century—an update for the Clinician. Curr Neurol Neurosci Rep. 2015;15(3):2.
8. Memish ZA. Meningococcal disease and travel. Clin Infect Dis. 2002;34(1):84–90.
9. Harrison LH. Prospects for vaccine prevention of meningococcal infection. Clin Microbiol Rev. 2006;19(1):142–64.
10. Rouphael NG, Stephens DS. Neisseria meningitidis: biology, microbiology, and epidemiology. Neisseria meningitidis. Springer; 2012. p. 1–20.
11. Khatami A, Pollard AJ. The epidemiology of meningococcal disease and the impact of vaccines. Expert Rev Vaccines. 2010;9(3):285–98.
12. Yazdankhah SP, Caugant DA. Neisseria meningitidis: an overview of the carriage state. J Med Microbiol. 2004;53(9):821–32.
13. Batista RS, Gomes AP, Gazineo JLD, Miguel PSB, Santana LA, Oliveira L, et al. Meningococcal disease, a clinical and epidemiological review. Asian Pac J Trop Med. 2017;10(11):1019–29.
14. Caugant DA, Tzanakaki G, Kriz P. Lessons from meningococcal carriage studies. FEMS Microbiol Rev. 2007;31(1):52–63.
15. Meyer SA, Kristiansen PA. Household transmission of Neisseria meningitidis in the meningitis belt. Lancet Glob Health. 2016;4(12):e885–e6.
16. Stefanelli P, Fazio C, Neri A, Isola P, Sani S, Marelli P, et al. Cluster of invasive Neisseria meningitidis infections on a cruise ship, Italy, October 2012. Eur Secur. 2012;17(50):20336.
17. Chant K, McAnulty J, O'Connor B, Maidment CA, Binotto E, Maywood P. Meningococcal disease-probable transmission during an international flight. Commun Dis Intell Q Rep. 2005;29(3):312.
18. CfD C, Prevention. Exposure to patients with meningococcal disease on aircrafts--United States, 1999-2001. MMWR Morb Mortal Wkly Rep. 2001;50(23):485.
19. Gabutti G, Stefanati A, Kuhdari P. Epidemiology of Neisseria meningitidis infections: case distribution by age and relevance of carriage. J Prev Med Hyg. 2015;56(3):E116.
20. Broker M, Jacobsson S, Kuusi M, Pace D, Simoes MJ, Skoczynska A, et al. Meningococcal serogroup Y emergence in Europe Update 2011. Hum Vacc Immunother. 2012;8(12):1907–11.
21. Fine A, Layton M, Hakim A, Smith P. Serogroup W-135 meningococcal disease among travelers returning from Saudi Arabia—United States, 2000 (Reprinted from MMWR, vol 49, pg 345-346, 2000). JAMA J Am Med Assoc. 2000;283(20):2647.
22. von Gottberg A, du Plessis M, Cohen C, Prentice E, Schrag S, de Gouveia L, Coulson G, de Jong G, Klugman K. Group for enteric, respiratory and meningeal disease surveillance in South Africa. Clin Infect Dis. 2008;46(3):377.
23. Krone M, Gray S, Abad R, Skoczyńska A, Stefanelli P, van der Ende A, et al. Increase of invasive meningococcal serogroup W disease in Europe, 2013–2017. Euro Surveill. 2019;24(14)
24. Abio A, Neal KR, Beck CR. An epidemiological review of changes in meningococcal biology during the last 100 years. Taylor & Francis; 2013.

25. Borrow R, Caugant DA, Ceyhan M, Christensen H, Dinleyici EC, Findlow J, et al. Meningococcal disease in the Middle East and Africa: Findings and updates from the Global Meningococcal Initiative. J Infect. 2017;75(1):1–11.
26. Greenwood BM, Aseffa A, Caugant DA, Diallo K, Kristiansen PA, Maiden MCJ, et al. Narrative review of methods and findings of recent studies on the carriage of meningococci and other Neisseria species in the African Meningitis Belt. Trop Med Int Health. 2019;24(2):143–54.
27. Sáfadi MAP, O'ryan M, Bravo MTV, Brandileone MCC, Gorla MCO, De Lemos APS, et al. The current situation of meningococcal disease in Latin America and updated Global Meningococcal Initiative (GMI) recommendations. Vaccine. 2015;33(48):6529–36.
28. Yue M, Xu J, Yu J, Shao Z. Carriage prevalence of Neisseria meningitidis in China, 2005-2022: a systematic review and meta-analysis. BMC Infect Dis. 2022;22(1):594.
29. Ito H, Okamoto K, Ariyoshi T, Yamamoto S, Yamashita M, Kanno Y, et al. Neisseria meningitidis serogroup W135 in a traveler visiting Japan from Argentina, 2019. J Infect Chemother. 2022;28(8):1180–1.
30. Meningococcal pneumonia, a case report—ClinicalKey. [cited 2023 Mar 20]. Available from: https://www.clinicalkey.com/#!/content/playContent/1-s2.0-S1201971220311206?returnurl=https:%2F%2Flinkinghub.elsevier.com%2Fretrieve%2Fpii%2FS1201971220311206%3Fshowall%3Dtrue&referrer=https:%2F%2Fwww.ijidonline.com%2F
31. Willerton L, Lucidarme J, Campbell H, Caugant DA, Claus H, Jacobsson S, et al. Geographically widespread invasive meningococcal disease caused by a ciprofloxacin resistant non-groupable strain of the ST-175 clonal complex. J Infect. 2020;81(4):575–84.
32. Domo NR, Nuolabong C, Nyarko KM, Kenu E, Balagumyetime P, Konnyebal G, et al. Uncommon mixed outbreak of pneumococcal and meningococcal meningitis in Jirapa District, Upper West Region, Ghana, 2016. Ghana Med J. 2017;51(4):149–55.
33. Crawford E, Drennon M, Winston T. Notes from the Field: Pediatric Death from Meningococcal Disease in a Family of Romani Travelers - Sarasota, Florida, 2015. MMWR Morb Mortal Wkly Rep. 2016;65(37):1017. https://doi.org/10.15585/mmwr.mm6537a7.
34. Smith-Palmer A, Oates K, Webster D, Taylor S, Scott KJ, Smith G, et al. Outbreak of Neisseria meningitidis capsular group W among scouts returning from the World Scout Jamboree, Japan, 2015. Eur Secur. 2016;21(45)
35. du Chatelet PI, Barboza P, Taha M. W135 invasive meningococcal infections imported from Sub-Saharan Africa to France, January to April 2012. Eurosurveillance. 2012;17(21):100–1.
36. Taha M-K, Kacou-N'Douba A, Hong E, Deghmane AE, Giorgini D, Okpo SL, et al. Travel-related Neisseria meningitidis serogroup W135 infection, France. Emerg Infect Dis. 2013;19(6):1030.
37. Nakayama A, Takahashi H, Ohkusu K, Yamanaka K, Shintani C, Hayakawa S, et al. A Case of Sepsis and Meningitis Caused by Probable Travel-Related Neisseria meningitidis Serogroup B Infection: the First Report of N. meningitidis ST-4893 in Japan. Jpn J Infect Dis. 2011;64(1):61–2.
38. Lapadula G, Vigano F, Fortuna P, Dolara A, Bramati S, Soria A, et al. Imported ciprofloxacin-resistant Neisseria meningitidis. Emerg Infect Dis. 2009;15(11):1852.
39. Tafuri S, Prato R, Martinelli D, Germinario C. Prevalence of carriers of Neisseria meningitidis among migrants: is migration changing the pattern of circulating meningococci? J Travel Med. 2012;19(5):311–3.
40. Stefanelli P, Fazio C, Neri A, Rezza G, Severoni S, Vacca P, et al. Imported and Indigenous cases of Invasive Meningococococcal Disease W:P1.5,2:F1-1: ST-11 in migrants' reception centers. Italy, June-November 2014. Adv Exp Med Biol. 2016;897:81–3.
41. Brueggemann AB, van Rensburg MJJ, Shaw D, McCarthy ND, Jolley KA, Maiden MC, et al. Changes in the incidence of invasive disease due to Streptococcus pneumoniae, Haemophilus influenzae, and Neisseria meningitidis during the COVID-19 pandemic in 26 countries and territories in the Invasive Respiratory Infection Surveillance Initiative: a prospective analysis of surveillance data. Lancet Digital Health. 2021;3(6):e360–e70.

42. Stephens DS. Biology and pathogenesis of the evolutionarily successful, obligate human bacterium Neisseria meningitidis. Vaccine. 2009;27(Suppl. 2):B71–7.
43. Stephens DS, Greenwood B, Brandtzaeg P. Epidemic meningitis, meningococcaemia, and Neisseria meningitidis. Lancet. 2007;369(9580):2196–210.
44. Carbonnelle E, Helaine S, Nassif X, Pelicic V. A systematic genetic analysis in Neisseria meningitidis defines the Pil proteins required for assembly, functionality, stabilization and export of type IV pili. Mol Microbiol. 2006;61(6):1510–22.
45. Pizza M, Rappuoli R. Neisseria meningitidis: pathogenesis and immunity. Curr Opin Microbiol. 2015;23:68–72.
46. Pathan N, Faust SN, Levin M. Pathophysiology of meningococcal meningitis and septicaemia. Arch Dis Child. 2003;88(7):601–7.
47. Pace D, Pollard AJ. Meningococcal disease: clinical presentation and sequelae. Vaccine. 2012;30:B3–9.
48. Thompson MJ, Ninis N, Perera R, Mayon-White R, Phillips C, Bailey L, et al. Clinical recognition of meningococcal disease in children and adolescents. Lancet. 2006;367(9508):397–403.
49. van de Beek D, Cabellos C, Dzupova O, Esposito S, Klein M, Kloek AT, et al. ESCMID guideline: diagnosis and treatment of acute bacterial meningitis. Clin Microbiol Infect. 2016;22(Suppl 3):S37–62.
50. Brouwer MC, Tunkel AR, van de Beek D. Epidemiology, diagnosis, and antimicrobial treatment of acute bacterial meningitis. Clin Microbiol Rev. 2010;23(3):467–92.
51. Neuman HB, Wald ER. Bacterial meningitis in childhood at the Children's Hospital of Pittsburgh: 1988-1998. Clin Pediatr. 2001;40(11):595–600.
52. Takada S, Fujiwara S, Inoue T, Kataoka Y, Hadano Y, Matsumoto K, et al. Meningococcemia in adults: a review of the literature. Intern Med. 2016;55(6):567–72.
53. Van Deuren M, Brandtzaeg P, van der Meer JW. Update on meningococcal disease with emphasis on pathogenesis and clinical management. Clin Microbiol Rev. 2000;13(1):144–66.
54. Horino T, Kato T, Sato F, Sakamoto M, Nakazawa Y, Yoshida M, et al. Meningococcemia without meningitis in Japan. Intern Med. 2008;47(17):1543–7.
55. Ricci S, Montemaggi A, Nieddu F, Serranti D, Indolfi G, Moriondo M, et al. Is primary meningococcal arthritis in children more frequent than we expect? Two pediatric case reports revealed by molecular test. BMC Infect Dis. 2018;18(1):703.
56. Nadel S, Kroll JS. Diagnosis and management of meningococcal disease: the need for centralized care. FEMS Microbiol Rev. 2007;31(1):71–83.
57. Strelow VL, Vidal JE. Invasive meningococcal disease. Arq Neuropsiquiatr. 2013;71(9b):653–8.
58. Moore JE. Meningococcal Disease Section 3: Diagnosis and Management: MeningoNI Forum (see page 87 (2) 83 for full list of authors). Ulster Med J. 2018;87(2):94.
59. Bourke TW, Fairley DJ, Shields MD. Rapid diagnosis of meningococcal disease. Expert Rev Anti-Infect Ther. 2010;8(12):1321–3.
60. Tunkel AR, Hartman BJ, Kaplan SL, Kaufman BA, Roos KL, Scheld WM, et al. Practice guidelines for the management of bacterial meningitis. Clin Infect Dis. 2004;39(9):1267–84.
61. Dunbar SA, Eason RA, Musher DM, Clarridge JE. Microscopic examination and broth culture of cerebrospinal fluid in diagnosis of meningitis. J Clin Microbiol. 1998;36(6):1617–20.
62. Brouwer MC, Thwaites GE, Tunkel AR, van de Beek D. Dilemmas in the diagnosis of acute community-acquired bacterial meningitis. Lancet. 2012;380(9854):1684–92.
63. Siddiqui JA, Ameer MA, Gulick PG. Meningococcemia. 2018.
64. Nadel S. Treatment of meningococcal disease. J Adolesc Health. 2016;59(Suppl. 2):S21–8. https://doi.org/10.1016/j.jadohealth.2016.04.013.
65. Donnelly PC, Sutich RM, Easton R, Adejumo OA, Lee TA, Logan LK. Ceftriaxone-associated biliary and cardiopulmonary adverse events in neonates: a systematic review of the literature. Pediatr Drugs. 2017;19(1):21–34.
66. Khurana KK, Garcia JA, Tendulkar RD, Stephenson AJ. Multidisciplinary management of patients with localized bladder cancer. Surg Oncol Clin N Am. 2013;22(2):357–73.

67. Stephens DS. Neisseria meningitidis. In: Bennett JE, Dolin R, Blaser MJ, editors. Mandell, Douglas, and Bennett's principles and practice of infectious diseases. 9th ed. Philadelphia: WB Saunders; 2020.

68. Evans L, Rhodes A, Alhazzani W, Antonelli M, Coopersmith CM, French C, et al. Executive summary: surviving sepsis campaign: international guidelines for the management of sepsis and septic shock 2021. Crit Care Med. 2021;49(11):1974–82.

69. Excellence NIfC. Meningitis (bacterial) and meningococcal septicaemia in under 16s: recognition, diagnosis and management CG102; 2015.

70. Rhodes A, Evans LE, Alhazzani W, Levy MM, Antonelli M, Ferrer R, et al. Surviving sepsis campaign: international guidelines for management of sepsis and septic shock: 2016. Intensive Care Med. 2017;43(3):304–77.

71. Derkx B, Wittes J, McCloskey R, European Pediatric Meningococcal Septic Shock Trial. Randomized, placebo-controlled trial of HA-1A, a human monoclonal antibody to endotoxin, in children with meningococcal septic shock. Clin Infect Dis. 1999;28(4):770–7.

72. Levin M, Quint PA, Goldstein B, Barton P, Bradley JS, Shemie S, et al. Recombinant bactericidal/permeability-increasing protein (rBPI21) as adjunctive treatment for children with severe meningococcal sepsis: a randomised trial. Lancet. 2000;356(9234):961–7.

73. van Deuren M, Santman FW, van Dalen R, Sauerwein RW, Span LF, van der Meer JW. Plasma and whole blood exchange in meningococcal sepsis. Clin Infect Dis. 1992;15(3):424–30.

74. Garralda ME, Gledhill J, Nadel S, Neasham D, O'connor M, Shears D. Longer-term psychiatric adjustment of children and parents after meningococcal disease. Pediatr Crit Care Med. 2009;10(6):675–80.

75. Gardner P. Prevention of meningococcal disease. N Engl J Med. 2006;355(14):1466–73.

76. Tsang RS, Law DK, Deng S, Hoang L. Ciprofloxacin-resistant Neisseria meningitidis in Canada: likely imported strains. Can J Microbiol. 2017;63(3):265–8.

77. Mbaeyi SA, Bozio CH, Duffy J, Rubin LG, Hariri S, Stephens DS, et al. Meningococcal vaccination: recommendations of the Advisory Committee on Immunization Practices, United States, 2020. MMWR Recomm Rep. 2020;69(9):1–41.

78. Burman C, Serra L, Nuttens C, Presa J, Balmer P, York L. Meningococcal disease in adolescents and young adults: a review of the rationale for prevention through vaccination. Hum Vaccin Immunother. 2019;15(2):459–69.

79. Centers for Disease Control and Prevention. Meningococcal vaccine recommendations. https://www.cdc.gov/vaccines/vpd/mening/hcp/recommendations.html.

80. European Centre for Disease Prevention and Control. Recommended immunizations for meningococcal disease. http://vaccine-schedule.ecdc.europa.eu/Pages/Scheduler.aspx (accessed 2022 Nov 20).

81. MacNeil JR, Meyer SA. Meningococcal disease. In: Brunette GW, editor. CDC Yellow Book 2018. New York, United States of America: Oxford University Press; 2018.

82. World Health Organization. Health requirements and recommendations for travellers to Saudi Arabia for Hajj and Umrah. (Access Date 20 Nov 22) https://www.moh.gov.sa/en/Hajj/HealthGuidelines/HealthGuidelinesDuringHajj/Pages/HealthRequirements.aspx.

83. Organization WH. The immunological basis for immunization series: module 15: meningococcal disease. Immunological basis for immunization series, module 15. 2020.

84. Centers for Disease Control and Prevention (CDC). Exposure to patients with meningococcal disease on aircrafts—United States, 1999-2001. MMWR Morb Mortal Wkly Rep. 2001;50(23):485–9.

85. Dinleyici M, Iseri Nepesov M, Sipahi OR, Carman KB, Kilic O, Dinleyici EC. The attitudes, behaviors, and knowledge of healthcare professionals towards the diagnosis, treatment, and prevention of bacterial meningitis in Turkey. Hum Vaccin Immunother. 2019;15(1):134–40.

86. Pepe F, Akıncı E, Bodur H. What to know about travel related infections. Mediterranean J Infect Microbes Antimicrob. 2018:7.

Influenza in Travellers

19

Richard Pebody, Gavin Dabrera, and Joanna Ellis

Abstract

Influenza is a widespread respiratory infection that can have serious implications for travellers. Those going overseas can undertake a range of precautions before, during and after their visit to prevent or mitigate the impact of both seasonal and avian influenza. Health care workers in both primary and secondary care should be aware of influenza as an important infection in returning travellers and the interventions that must be promptly implemented to minimize the potential serious health consequences for the patient and those around them.

19.1 Background

Although the influenza virus was only first isolated from humans using ferrets in 1933 by Patrick Laidlow and his team at the Medical Research Council laboratories in Mill Hill [1], the history of influenza extends back much further. The annual epidemics of acute respiratory illness associated with seasonal influenza, particularly in temperate areas of the world, had been recognized for many centuries before, though the aetiological agent was unclear. Indeed, the ability of this virus to emerge and spread globally (i.e. a pandemic) was observed on several occasions, particularly during the nineteenth century and then most notably in 1918, where a pandemic of a now recognized novel A(H1N1) influenza virus was associated

R. Pebody (✉) · G. Dabrera · J. Ellis
UK Health Security Agency, London, UK
e-mail: Richard.Pebody@ukhsa.gov.uk; Gavin.dabrera@ukhsa.gov.uk; Joanna.Ellis@ukhsa.gov.uk

© The Author(s), under exclusive license to Springer Nature Switzerland AG 2024
H. Leblebicioglu et al. (eds.), *Emerging and Re-emerging Infections in Travellers*, https://doi.org/10.1007/978-3-031-49475-8_19

with over 40 million deaths, many in previously healthy, young adults at the end of the first World War. This ability of a new influenza strain to emerge and globally infect a susceptible human population has since been observed on several occasions as influenza pandemics starting in 1957, 1968, 1977 and most recently in 2009.

19.2 Aetiology

Influenza is an RNA virus of the Orthomyxovirus family. Although there are four types of influenza, only two are of clinical and public health importance to humans—influenza A and B. Two influenza A surface glycoproteins, haemagglutinin (HA) and neuraminidase (NA), are responsible for the successful attachment, replication and release of the virus in human cells, particularly in the epithelial cells of the respiratory tract. Influenza A is divided into subtypes based on the properties of the HA and NA they possess; 18 different HA and eleven different NA subtypes have been identified. The combination of these HA and NA proteins leads to the naming of the many influenza A virus subtypes e.g. A(H3N2). Influenza B viruses are not divided into subtypes but can be differentiated into lineages and strains. In addition, as an RNA virus, the influenza viral genome undergoes continuous genetic evolution. This genetic variation can result in changes in antigenicity, allowing the virus to evade the human immune system and thus successfully replicate in the host.

Three forms of influenza are described: avian influenza (where a wide range of subtypes circulate in birds and mammalian species), seasonal influenza, and pandemic influenza (when a novel influenza A virus has acquired a major change in HA and/or NA and the ability for sustained person-to-person transmission in a susceptible population).

19.3 Transmission

The virus is excreted in birds' faeces and saliva for avian influenza. Human infection can occur when the virus is in the air and a person breathes it in or gets it in their eyes, mouth and nose. Alternatively, they may touch surfaces which are contaminated with the virus.

For seasonal influenza, once a person has been infected, they usually start to shed the virus up to 24 h before the first symptoms start. Shedding can continue for 5–7 days, with children shedding more virus than adults. The virus is spread from person to person by several potential mechanisms: direct contact (e.g. a handshake); indirect (e.g. contact with an intermediate object such as a fomite); droplet spread (e.g. coughing, sneezing) and bioaerosol (which are fine, air-borne particles).

19.4 Epidemiology

19.4.1 Avian Influenza

Avian influenza is defined as a High Consequence Infectious Disease (HCID)—an acute infectious disease that can be air-borne with a high case-fatality ratio ([2] https://www.gov.uk/guidance/high-consequence-infectious-diseases-hcid).   Avian influenza viruses can circulate in a wide range of bird species—particularly aquatic birds, but can also spillover into mammals. Swine influenza is an acute respiratory illness caused by influenza A that circulates amongst pigs. Many of these viruses will circulate in birds or pigs without causing infection in humans exposed to those animals. Occasionally, the virus can spill over from animal to human, resulting in a zoonotic infection. The resulting infection can be serious, resulting in significant morbidity and sometimes death. This is particularly associated with certain influenza A subtypes. If these recently adapted viruses gain the ability to spread from human to human in a sustained fashion and population immunity is low, the virus can spread more widely and a pandemic influenza virus has potentially emerged [3].

Avian influenzas of human significance occur in a number of geographical locations. For example, A(H7N9) has circulated in poultry flocks in China, with human cases detected from 2013 onwards. More recently A(H5N1) clade 2.3.4.4b emerged in 2020 and has now spread globally leading to large numbers of deaths in wild birds and poultry around the world. The distribution of these avian influenzas, particularly H5 and H7 subtypes, is monitored by the World Organization for Animal Health (WOAH), with up-to-date information maintained at www.oie. http://www.oie.int/animal-health-in-the-world/avian-influenza-portal/. These are also listed on the UKHSA website (https://www.gov.uk/guidance/high-consequence-infectious-disease-country-specific-risk). Human cases of A(H5N1) and A(H7N9) (and indeed other avian influenzas) should be reported by member states to the World Health Organization under the International Health Regulations. Human cases invariably report recent close contact with poultry and historically have often had a severe outcome. Monitoring and follow-up of close contacts of human cases is critical to enable early detection of possible human-to-human transmission. Such onward spread has only been observed on sporadic occasions for A(H7N9) and A(H5N1), with no suggestion of sustained transmission to date.

19.4.2 Seasonal Influenza

Seasonal influenza circulates globally and continuously in humans, independent of an animal reservoir. In temperate climates, epidemic activity occurs each winter, whereas in tropical/sub-tropical climates, circulation occurs all year around.

Although a variety of influenza A subtypes can be found in animal species, only certain HA and NA subtypes have been found to infect humans. At present, two influenza A subtypes (A(H3N2) and A(H1N1)pdm09) and two influenza B lineages (B/Victoria and B/Yamagata) co-circulate in the human population, although following the disruption of seasonal influenza circulation during the COVID-19 pandemic, B/Yamagata has largely disappeared since 2022. Continuous genetic mutations in the influenza HA and NA proteins can result in antigenic drift whereby new A(H3N2) and A(H1N1)pdm09 strains emerge on a regular basis with antigenic changes in the virus such that they evade the body's immune system. This occurred, for example, during the 2014/15 influenza season in the Northern hemisphere, when a drifted A(H3N2) virus emerged.

19.5 Clinical Presentation

Influenza infection typically results in an acute self-limiting respiratory illness associated with high fever, myalgia, cough and other upper respiratory tract symptoms. A number of other respiratory viruses, such as rhinovirus and now SARS-C0V-2, can cause very similar symptoms. A significant minority of those infected with influenza will be asymptomatic or present with only mild respiratory symptoms. However, a proportion of those who are infected will develop complications, particularly lower respiratory tract signs such as pneumonia. These complications are much more common amongst groups such as older adults and those who have underlying clinical risk factors such as chronic respiratory or cardiovascular disease.

19.6 Risks for International Travellers

Travellers can be at elevated risk of avian and seasonal influenza depending upon their travel destination, timing of their journey and planned activities.

Travellers to countries with animal reservoirs for avian influenza with potential for human infection are at potential risk of infection. Certain activities will increase this risk, for example, those that might bring a visitor into close contact with infected poultry, such as visiting wet bird markets in South East Asia or long-term visitors staying with relatives in settings where they are in contact with back-yard flocks of birds.

Travellers can also be at elevated risk of seasonal influenza infection and potentially severe disease, particularly if they are in an eligible group for vaccination and not recently immunised. This risk will increase if travel occurs during annual epidemics in the winter period of temperate countries or potentially all year around in more tropical climes. Participating in mass gatherings, such as the Hajj, where transmission of acute respiratory infections is increased, will also increase the risk of seasonal influenza infection. There have been several documented accounts of seasonal influenza outbreaks on board cruise ships, highlighting the potential for transmission in what represents a closed setting containing a large number of people. In addition, there is published evidence of influenza transmission associated with commercial air travel during the 2009 pandemic.

Travellers will be at elevated risk of severe disease following infection if they are in certain vulnerable groups such as those over 65 years of age or those with long-standing underlying clinical problems, such as chronic lung or heart disease. These risk factors form the basis of the current annual seasonal influenza vaccination recommendations in the United Kingdom, delivered each autumn (Chapter 19, Green book).

19.7 Laboratory Diagnosis

Laboratory diagnosis of influenza is usually based on samples taken from the upper respiratory tract e.g. nasopharyngeal and throat swabs, ideally taken early in the illness, primarily by reverse transcription-polymerase chain reaction (RT-PCR) testing used to detect the presence of influenza viral RNA. During the influenza season, laboratory diagnosis of every case is not required, particularly in the community, as symptoms of acute influenza-like illness have a high predictive value for influenza infection.

More recently, point of care tests (POCTs) are becoming more widely used—particularly in health care settings—where they can provide more rapid diagnosis of influenza. Some of these POCTs may lack sensitivity, so care is required in their interpretation. It is important to ensure that samples from influenza cases are still sent for virus characterisation to understand which strains are circulating and how well they match the current season's influenza vaccine. This is particularly important in returning travellers, who may be infected with influenza strains during travel abroad, distinct from those circulating within the domestic population.

19.8 Prevention Advice for Travellers

There are a number of behavioural measures a traveller can employ to reduce their risk of influenza infection while overseas.

19.8.1 Respiratory and Hand Hygiene

Travellers can reduce their risk of influenza infection and other acute respiratory infections and of onward spread through careful hand and respiratory hygiene. This involves catching coughs and sneezes in a tissue, discarding it in a bin and regularly washing hands; wearing a mask in crowded places and minimizing contact with others if travellers have an acute respiratory illness. All these measures have been shown to reduce the spread of influenza.

19.8.2 Contact with Poultry (in Affected Countries)

Travellers to countries where avian influenza of potential significance to humans is circulating in animal reservoirs, such as wild birds and poultry, should be assiduous in avoiding direct/indirect contact. The latest country-specific travel health advice is summarized in the NathNac country guidance [4] and the UKHSA HCID website [2].

> **Box 19.1: Example of Avian Influenza Avoidance Advice for Travellers**
> - Wash hands regularly
> - Avoid visiting live bird and animal markets (known as wet markets in China) and poultry farms
> - Do not touch sick or dead birds
> - Avoid contact with untreated bird feathers or any animal waste
> - Avoid consuming or handling raw or undercooked egg, poultry or duck dishes
>   Source: UKHSA/NathNac

19.8.3 Vaccination

Travellers in existing influenza vaccine risk groups (such as pregnant women, immunocompromised or elderly) should ensure they take up their offer of free influenza vaccination available through the NHS each autumn [5]. This should provide protection against the seasonal strains that are most likely to circulate that winter in the United Kingdom, but also elsewhere globally for up to 12 months, though protection does wane over time. Seasonal influenza vaccine contains two influenza A and two B viruses (for quadrivalent vaccines)—an (H1N1)pdm09 and H3N2 virus and a B/Yamagata and B/Victoria lineage virus. It is an annual vaccination as the strains often require updating and protection is not long-term. It is thus important that those who are eligible get vaccinated each year.

19.8.4 Antivirals

The use of antivirals as prophylaxis is only recommended for those travellers who are in existing influenza vaccine risk groups as described and have been directly exposed to an individual who has been clinically assessed as having seasonal influenza. Antiviral prophylaxis for the duration of a whole trip is not routinely recommended and would require an individual risk assessment for the patient; in addition, this would be affected by maximum duration for prophylaxis, which vary between different antiviral medicines [6].

19.9   Management Advice for Health Care Workers

A range of pharmaceutical and non-pharmaceutical interventions can be used to prevent and mitigate the impact of traveller-associated influenza, whether seasonal or avian:

- It is important that doctors in both primary and secondary care are aware of the most common clinical presentation of influenza—acute onset of fever together with acute respiratory symptoms. This coupled with a travel history at any time of the year should raise suspicion of influenza.
- It is important to ascertain whether the patient has any underlying demographic or clinical factors that may increase their risk of developing complications of influenza, whether they have recently been vaccinated (within the previous 12 months) and whether they have undertaken any activities that may have exposed them to infection with avian influenza.
- If a patient meets the UKHSA case definition for possible or confirmed avian influenza (an example of the current UKHSA avian influenza case definition is provided in Box 19.2), then it is critical that, as an HCID, UKHSA guidelines are followed [3]. In particular, appropriate infection control measures need to be rapidly deployed to minimize the risk of onward transmission; the

---

Box 19.2: Case Definition for Possible Cases of Avian influenza
Clinical:
(a) Fever $\geq$ 38 °C
     or
(b) Acute respiratory symptoms (cough, hoarseness, nasal discharge or congestion, shortness of breath, sore throat, wheezing or sneezing)
     or
(c) Other severe or life-threatening illnesses suggestive of an infectious process

Additionally, patients must fulfil a condition in either category 1 or 2 of the exposure criteria below.
    AND

Exposure, consisting of:
(1) Close contact (within 1 m) with live, dying or dead domestic poultry or wild birds, including live bird markets, in an area of the world affected by avian influenza** or with any confirmed infected animal, in the 10 days before the onset of symptoms
    or
(2) In the 10 days before the onset of symptoms, close contact* with:
  • A confirmed human case of avian influenza

- Human case(s) of unexplained illness resulting in death from affected areas**
- Human cases of severe unexplained respiratory illness from affected areas**

*This includes handling laboratory specimens from cases without appropriate precautions or was within 1 m distance, directly providing care, touching a case or within close vicinity of an aerosol-generating procedure from 1 day prior to symptom onset and for duration of symptoms or positive virological detection.
**For H7N9, H5N1 and H5N6 see the HCID country list.
Source: UKHSA

correct biological samples need to be taken for rapid testing to enable avian influenza infection to be definitively excluded. Finally antivirals should be prescribed promptly to mitigate the impact of possible influenza infection pending the results of testing (https://www.gov.uk/government/publications/avian-influenza-guidance-and-algorithms-for-managing-human-cases)
- If a patient is diagnosed with suspected seasonal influenza with either a severe presentation or with underlying clinical risk factors for serious disease, then appropriate influenza antivirals should be prescribed as per UKHSA antiviral guidance.

19.10 Conclusions

In conclusion, influenza is a widespread respiratory infection that can have serious implications for travellers. Those going overseas can undertake a range of precautions before, during and after their visit to prevent or mitigate the impact of both seasonal, but also avian influenza. Avian influenza is one of many high-consequence infectious diseases. Health care workers in both primary and secondary care should be aware of influenza as an important infection in returning travellers and the interventions that must be promptly deployed to minimize the potential serious clinical and public health consequences.

Box 19.3: Things Commonly Forgotten
- Severe presentations of Avian Influenza may be clinically similar to other respiratory infections; therefore, travel history informs considerations of other infections causing severe acute respiratory illness and often associated with travel such as MERS and Legionnaires' disease.

Acknowledgments We would like to acknowledge the helpful comments that Dr Jake Dunning from Public Health England provided.

Declarations of Conflict of InterestNo conflicts of interest to declare.

References

1. Smith W, Andrewes C, Laidlow P. A virus obtained from influenza patients. Lancet. 1933;222:66–8. https://doi.org/10.1016/S0140-6736(00)78541-2.
2. UKHSA. High consequence infectious diseases. https://www.gov.uk/guidance/high-consequence-infectious-diseases-hcid
3. Collection. Avian influenza: guidance, data and analysis. London: Public Health England; 2019. Available from: https://www.gov.uk/government/collections/avian-influenza-guidance-data-and-analysis
4. Travel Health PR. Avian influenza (Bird Flu). London: National Travel Health Network and Centre (NaTHNaC); 2018. Available from : https://travelhealthpro.org.uk/disease/216/avian-influenza-bird-flu
5. Guidance. Chapter 19: Influenza. In: Ramsay M, editor. Immunisation against infectious disease. London: UKHSA; 2023. p. 1–29.
6. UK Health Security Agency. Guidance on use of antiviral agents for the treatment and prophylaxis of seasonal influenza. London: Public Health England; 2019. Available from: https://www.gov.uk/government/publications/influenza-treatment-and-prophylaxis-using-anti-viral-agents

Middle East Respiratory Syndrome Coronavirus (MERS-CoV) in Travellers

20

Jaffar A. Al-Tawfiq and Ziad A. Memish

Abstract

Middle East respiratory Syndrome Coronavirus (MERS-CoV) emerged in 2012 in the Kingdom of Saudi Arabia. Since then, it has been reported from 27 countries, and all cases were epidemiologically linked to the Arabian Peninsula. The transmission of MERS-CoV is thought be either through intra-familial transmission or large healthcare-associated infections, in addition to sporadic isolated cases. The clinical presentation includes asymptomatic, mild cases, and severe fatal disease. The best diagnostic test relies on molecular identification of MERS-CoV by PCR. The mainstay of therapy for patients with MERS relies on supportive care. The MIRACLE study, a randomized controlled trial, utilized lopinavir-ritonavir and interferon-β1b vs. placebo with the start of treatment within 7 days after symptom onset. The study showed a reduction in the 90-day

J. A. Al-Tawfiq
Specialty Internal Medicine, Johns Hopkins Aramco Healthcare, Dhahran, Saudi Arabia

Quality and Patient Safety Department, Johns Hopkins Aramco Healthcare, Dhahran, Saudi Arabia

Departemnt of Medicine, Indiana University School of Medicine, Indiana, IN, USA

Department of Medicine, Johns Hopkins University School of Medicine, Baltimore, MD, USA
e-mail: jaffar.tawfiq@jhah.com

Z. A. Memish (✉)
College of Medicine, Alfaisal University, Riyadh, Saudi Arabia

King Saud Medical City, Riyadh, Saudi Arabia

Hubert Department of Global Health, Rollins School of Public Health, Emory University, Atlanta, GA, USA

© The Author(s), under exclusive license to Springer Nature Switzerland AG 2024

H. Leblebicioglu et al. (eds.), *Emerging and Re-emerging Infections in Travellers*, https://doi.org/10.1007/978-3-031-49475-8_20

mortality with a relative risk of 0.19 (95% CI, 0.05–0.75). In addition, using a human polyclonal IgG antibody (SAB-301) was safe and well tolerated in phase I clinical trials.

20.1 Background

20.1.1 Brief History

The Middle East Respiratory Syndrome Coronavirus (MERS-CoV) was first described in 2012 in a 60-year-old male who was hospitalized with community-acquired pneumonia and subsequently had renal and respiratory failure. He unfortunately had progressive disease, which resulted in death [1].

20.1.2 Importance of the Disease

Since the emergence of MERS-CoV in 2012, there have been more than 2260 laboratory-confirmed cases of MERS-CoV infection in 27 countries, mainly in the Middle East and specifically in the Kingdom of Saudi Arabia [2]. In addition, MERS-CoV disease continues to be associated with a high case fatality rate of 35.6% [2]. One of the characteristics of MERS-CoV is the association with large hospital-associated outbreaks in KSA [3–14] and in the Republic of Korea in 2015 [4, 7, 15–17].

20.1.3 Why It Is Classified as Emerging and/or Reemerging

MERS-CoV was discovered in 2012 and has caused significant sporadic disease as well as multiple hospital outbreaks with a high case fatality rate. A summary of the main hospital outbreaks and associated case fatality rates are listed in Table 20.1.

Table 20.1 A summary of major reported MERS-CoV hospital outbreaks

Date of incidence	City and country	Number of involved hospitals	Number of infected cases	Percentage of infected healthcare workers	Case fatality rate	Reference
2012 April	Zarqa, Jordan	1	9	67%	22%	[26]
2013 April	Al-Hasa, KSA	4	23	9%	65%	[3]
2014 April	Jeddah, KSA	1	78	20.5%	N/A	[36]
2014 April	Riyadh, KSA	1	45	51%	29%	[9]
2014 September	Taif & Riyadh, KSA	4	38	34%	55.2%	[6]
2015 May	Seoul & others, Republic of Korea	16	186	13.4%	19.4%	[37]
2015 June	Riyadh, KSA	1	130	33%	53%	[12]

KSA Kingdom of Saudi Arabia

20.2 Aetiology

The MERS-CoV is a Coronavirus. These viruses belong to a family of viruses with adaptation to multiple species. MERS CoV is a betacoronavirus of this family [18] and is classified as clade c (lineage 3) coronavirus. The most recent common ancestor of MERS CoV was estimated at approximately 44 years ago. MERS-CoV evolved in camels, and there was an initial bat-to-camel host switching [19]. The genome of MERS-CoV has 30,119 nucleotides and has seven open reading frames (ORFs) (1a, 1b, 3, 4a, 4b, 5, 8b) and four structural genes encoding the spike (S), nucleocapsid (N), membrane (M) and envelope (E) proteins [20, 21].

20.3 Transmission

There are three patterns of transmissions [17, 22]: sporadic community cases from presumed non-human exposure [22], family clusters arising from contact with a family index case [23–25], and healthcare-acquired infections among patients and from patients to healthcare workers [3–14, 22, 26–33]. Community transmission is mainly linked to camel exposure, with possible seasonal exposure in two seasons: spring (March–May) and fall (September–November) [17]. However, other studies did not confirm seasonal variation [34]. Phylogenetic analysis of outbreaks in the community and healthcare showed multiple introductions of MERS-CoV into these outbreaks [25, 27, 28].

20.4 Epidemiology

20.4.1 Geographic Distributions

Epidemiological studies showed that MERS-CoV has limited circulation to the Arabian Peninsula. However, MERS-CoV was reported by the World Health Organization to have caused a total of 2279 laboratory-confirmed cases from 27 countries [35]. These countries include Saudi Arabia, United Arab Emirates, Qatar, Jordan, Oman, Kuwait, Egypt, Yemen, Lebanon, Iran, Turkey, Austria, the United Kingdom, Germany, France, Italy, Greece, the Netherlands, Tunisia, Algeria, Malaysia, the Philippines, and the United States [35] (Figs. 20.1 and 20.2).

20.4.2 Recent Epidemics/Outbreaks

The key characteristic of MERS-CoV is the rapid and efficient transmission in healthcare facilities, leading to large, explosive and prolonged hospital-associated outbreaks [3, 6, 9, 12, 26, 36, 37].

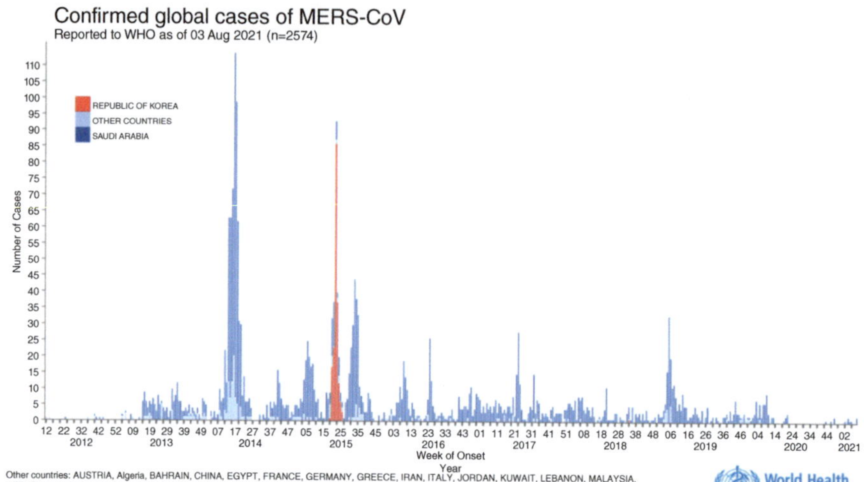

Fig. 20.1 Epicurve of MERS-CoV infections around the globe (from: https://www.who.int/images/default-source/health-topics/mers-cov/global-mers-cases-2021-08-03.jpg?sfvrsn=48d4d177_4)

20.4.3 Risk Factors

Risk factors for acquiring MERS-CoV include contacts with dromedary camels [38]. Presence of comorbidities predisposes to increased risk of MERS-CoV and correlates with increased fatality rates [39]. In addition, higher viral load [Lower cycle threshold (CT)] is associated with severe disease, risk of pneumonia and risk of death, causing significantly higher mortality [40, 41]. Increasing age is also a predictor of increased mortality, with an OR of 4.39 [29, 42].

20.4.4 Risks for International Travellers

There have been >20 travel-related MERS-CoV [43], and the disease has been reported infrequently among pilgrims performing Umrah [43, 44]. In 2012, 1.74 million foreign pilgrims performed the Hajj, and there were no reported MERS-CoV cases [45–49]. No reported cases were linked to the annual Hajj mass gathering despite systematic screening of pilgrims [48, 50–66]. There were sporadic cases of travel-associated infections, and a large outbreak in South Korea was ignited by a traveller [37, 43, 67, 68]. In addition, two reported MERS-CoV cases related to the mini-Hajj, Umrah, were reported in May 2014 [69]. Travel-related MERS cases were reviewed and summarized [43, 68, 70].

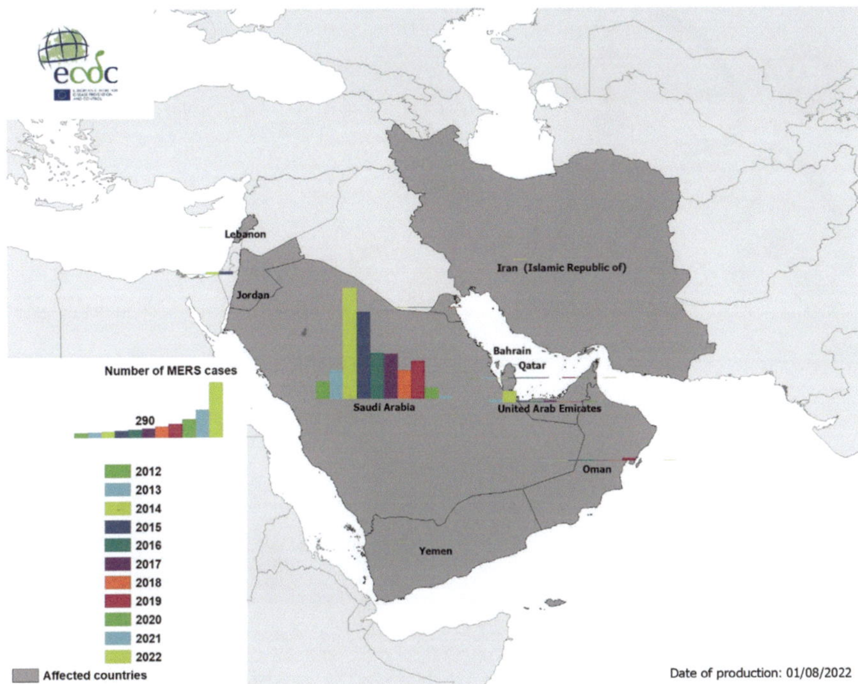

Fig. 20.2 Geographic distribution of MERS cases per country and year (from: https://www.ecdc.europa.eu/en/publications-data/geographical-distribution-confirmed-cases-mers-cov-country-infection-and-year)

20.4.5 Differing Issues for Migrants and Those "Visiting Friends and Relations" (VFR)

It is advised that people visiting countries where MERS-CoV had been reported to avoid contact with camels and eat well-coked food.

20.5 Pathogenesis

Viral entry is the first step in the cycle of MERS-CoV and is facilitated by type-I transmembrane glycoprotein, the S protein [71] or through an auxiliary pathway on the cell surface utilizing transmembrane proteases [72]. This process is followed by viral replication, cleavage, fusion and subsequent release of viral particles. The pathogenesis of MERS-CoV infection can be summarized in three phases [73]. An illustration of the MERS-CoV replication cycle and the main structures of the MERS-CoV virus is shown in Fig. 20.3. The virologic replication phase is characterized by fever and constitutional symptoms; the immunopathological phase

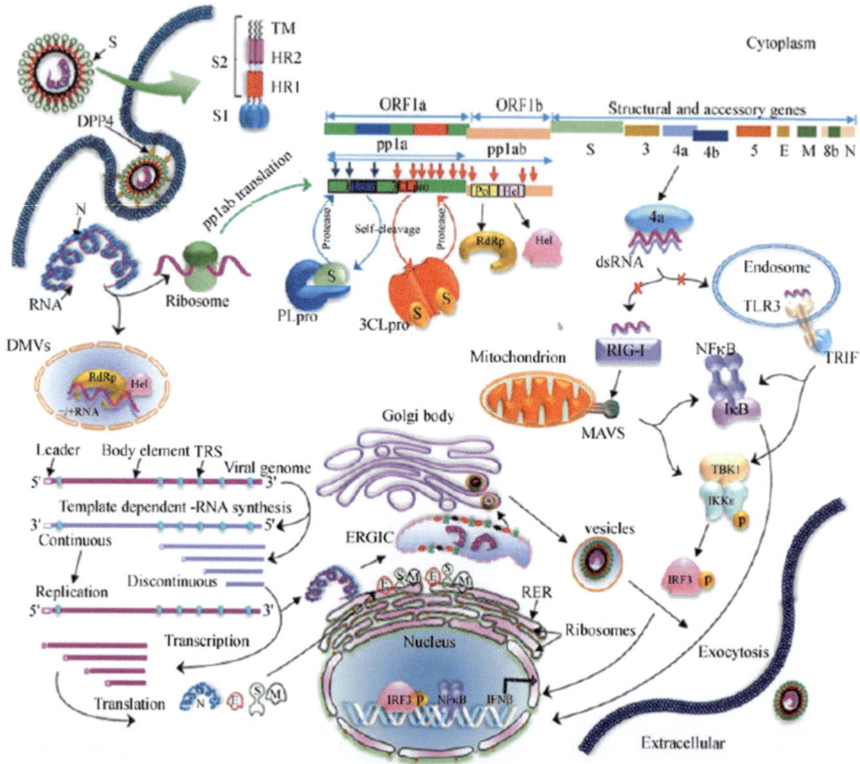

Fig. 20.3 MERS-CoV replication cycle and main structures of the virus (from: Durai et al., 2015, Middle East respiratory syndrome coronavirus: transmission, virology and therapeutic targeting to aid in outbreak control; available from: http://www.nature.com/emm/journal/v47/n8/full/emm201576a.html; licensed under a) Creative Commons Attribution 4.0 International License: https://creativecommons.org/licenses/by/4.0/legalcode

includes resolution of fever, increased oxygen desaturation, and radiological deterioration. The third phase follows with either further deterioration or resolution of symptoms [73]. Limited post-mortem studies are available. These studies showed that the virus is localized to the pulmonary and extrapulmonary tissue [74, 75]. The histopathological studies showed diffuse alveolar pulmonary damage, necrotizing pneumonia, acute kidney injury, hepatitis and myositis [74, 75]. In addition, viral particles were found in pulmonary macrophages, pneumocytes, and proximal renal tubular epithelial cells [74, 75].

20.6 Clinical Findings

The incubation period of MERS-CoV infection is 5–7 days and can reach 12 days [3, 39]. There are various clinical signs and symptoms that may be present in patients with MERS-CoV. Tachypnea was present in 27% of MERS patients compared to 60% of controls, and respiratory distress was present in 15% and 51% of cases and controls, respectively [76]. In initially described cases, 14% had leucopenia, 34% had lymphocytopenia, 11% had lymphocytosis, and 36% had thrombocytopenia [39]. Patients were also reported to have elevated lactate dehydrogenase (49%), alanine transferase (11%) and aspartate transaminase (5%) levels [39]. In addition, other studies described the elevation of urea and creatinine levels [39, 77, 78]. There is a wide range of radiological features on chest X-rays of MERS-CoV patients, and these findings include ground glass opacification, consolidation (either patchy or confluent), reticular opacities, nodular opacities and reticulo-nodular infiltrates [39]. A retrospective analysis of chest CT findings for 15 confirmed MERS-CoV patients revealed that ground glass appearance was the commonest and the earliest appearing finding, followed by a combination of consolidation and ground glass appearance, pleural effusion, and interlobular thickening [79].

20.7 Laboratory Diagnosis

Laboratory diagnosis of MERS-CoV relies on the detection of the virus by PCR. Currently, there are three PCR-based assays: real-time reverse transcriptase PCR (RT-PCR) with a sensitivity for upE gene of 3.4 copies per reaction [80–82], reverses transcription-loop-mediated isothermal amplification (RT-RTPA) which detects as few as 3.4 copies of MERS-CoV RNA [83] and reverses transcription-recombinase polymerase amplification (RT-LAMP) and this test was as sensitive as real-time RT-PCR (10 RNA molecules), rapid (3–7 min) and mobile [84]. For the PCR-based diagnosis, the detection of the regions upstream of the E gene ("up-E") is used most frequently in addition to either ORF1a or ORF1b for confirmation [80–82].

Studies showed that lower respiratory samples produce a higher yield of MERS-CoV positivity when compared to upper respiratory samples. Thus, they are the preferred samples [39, 85], and lower respiratory samples might be positive despite negative upper respiratory samples [73]. Consistent with these findings, the WHO recommends that both upper and lower respiratory tract specimens be used to diagnose MERS-CoV [86]. Moreover, repeat testing is needed in patients presenting with pneumonia to confirm or rule out MERS-CoV [85, 87].

Serology is not commonly used for the diagnosis of MERS-CoV infection. However, a screening test is an enzyme-linked immunosorbent assay (ELISA) [88]. The assay detects IgG and IgM against the S1 receptor-binding subunit of the spike protein of MERS-CoV [88]. However, additional confirmatory testing utilizing microneutralization assay is needed [89]. It is important to note that serology-based tests are for surveillance or investigational purposes, not diagnostic purposes [89].

20.8 Differential Diagnosis

The differential diagnosis of MERS-CoV infection should include any etiologic agent of upper respiratory infection and community-acquired pneumonia. In a study of the surveillance of MERS-CoV among all admitted patients, the prevalence of influenza was found to be more common than MERS-CoV [90]. MERS-CoV may coexist with influenza [91] or pulmonary tuberculosis [92], or with COVID-19, [93] which should be considered in the differential diagnosis.

20.8.1 Diagnostic Hints

Unfortunately, MERS-CoV patients have no differentiating factors compared to those who did not have MERS-CoV [76]. In addition, the use of specific visual trial scores did not aid in the diagnosis of MERS-CoV. When a visual triaging score was used, the percentage of patients with a score of ≥ 4 was 75% in MERS CoV patients compared with 85% in patients without MERS-CoV infection ($P = 0.0001$) [94]. However, in MERS-CoV non-endemic countries, any patient with community-acquired pneumonia who had visited countries or lives in countries with reported MERS-CoV should be promptly evaluated. MERS-CoV infection must be ruled out.

20.9 Management

There are no approved drugs for the treatment of human MERS-CoV infection. Several laboratory trials using cell or animal models and few human studies have been conducted to assess the efficacy of various drugs. Different interferon regimens, ribavirin and lopinavir/ritonavir, were used to manage human MERS-CoV [95–97]. A summary of the therapeutic agents used for MERS-CoV infection is listed in Table 20.2. The first study used interferon-a2b and ribavirin among five MERS-CoV-infected critically ill patients, all of whom died as a result of multiple organ failure. Of note, all patients had comorbid conditions (such as chronic renal disease) and initiation of treatment was delayed from the time of admission (median 19 days, range 10–22 days) [95]. Thus, these factors may have had a negative impact on the outcome. In another study of 44 MERS-CoV-infected patients, treatment with a combined regimen of pegylated interferon alfa-2a and ribavirin was initiated at a median of three days from diagnosis and there was no significant difference in survival rate at day 28 [97]. A retrospective study of a combination of IFN-a2a or IFN-b1a with ribavirin showed no impact on mortality [96]. There was a case report of the triplet regimen of lopinavir/ritonavir, pegylated interferon and ribavirin with reduced viral shedding [98]. South Korean authors recommended this triplet regimen for the treatment of MERS-CoV infections [99]. Interestingly, a clinical trial yet to be published is evaluating convalescent plasma (i.e. plasma containing anti-MERS-CoV antibodies drawn from individuals with prior MERS-CoV infection) for the treatment of human MERS-CoV infections [100]. The MIRACLE study, a randomized controlled trial, utilized lopinavir-ritonavir and interferon-β1b vs. placebo with the start of treatment within 7 days after symptom onset. The study showed a reduction in the 90-day mortality with a relative risk of 0.19 (95% CI, 0.05–0.75) [101]. In addition, the use of a human polyclonal IgG antibody (SAB-301) was shown to be safe and well tolerated in phase I clinical trials [102].

Table 20.2 Summary of therapeutic agents for MERS-CoV infection

Study type	Treatment	Time to initiation of therapy	Treatment group, n/N (% survival)	Control group	Reference
Case series	Ribavirin and interferon-alfa 2b	19 days post-admission	0/5 (0)	None	[95]
Retrospective cohort study	Ribavirin and interferon-alfa 2a	3 days of onset	14/20 (70 at 14 days); 6/20 (30 at 28 days)	24; survival at 14 days 29% and 17% at 28 days	[97]
Case series	Ribavirin and interferon-alfa 2a	6 days of onset	11/11 (100)	None	[125]
Case series	Ribavirin and interferon-alfa 2a	1 day following diagnosis	11/13 (85)	None	[96]
Case series	Ribavirin and interferon-b1a	1 day following diagnosis	7/11 (64)	None	[96]
Case series	Interferon beta	Not indicated	18/23 (78.3)	None	[126]
Case series	Interferon alpha	Not indicated	6/8 (75)	None	[126]
Case series	Ribavirin	Not indicated	13/19 (68.4)	None	[126]
Case series	Mycophenolate mofetil	Not indicated	8/8 (100)	None	[126]
Case report	Lopinavir/ ritonavir, ribavirin and interferon-α	Not indicated	none	4	[127]
Case report	Pegylated interferon, ribavirin and lopinavir/ritonavir	From Day 13 of illness	?	None	[98]
Case report	Ribavirin and interferon-alfa 2a	Day 1 of admission	survived	None	[128]
Case report	Ribavirin and interferon-alfa 2a	Day 12 from onset	died	None	[129]
Case series	Ribavirin and interferon-alfa 2b	1–2 days in survivals and 12–19 days in those who died	3/6 (50)	None	[130]
Randomized controlled trial	Lopinavir-ritonavir and interferon-β1b vs. placebo	Within 7 days after symptom onset	31/43 (72%)	23/52 (56%)	[101]

Public health responses evolve around the management of an individual case, such as isolation measures, laboratory safety and protocols, contact precautions, advice and management for patient contacts of healthcare and household and other close contacts.

Various studies have shown that dromedary camels harbour MERS-CoV. However, infected animals exhibit only minor clinical signs of disease, and most infections are asymptomatic [103]. In natural camel infections, MERS-CoV RNA was detected more frequently in nasal swabs than oral swabs and less frequently in rectal swabs [104–106]. In addition, MERS-CoV RNA was detected in milk samples [107, 108]. The positivity of camels by PCR extends to two weeks from initial positive results [107, 109].

For healthcare workers (HCWs), it is important to apply basic infection control measures [3], and the US CDC recommends that HCWs also apply airborne infection isolation (AII) precautions when caring for patients with suspected or proven MERS-CoV [110]. However, the World Health Organization (WHO) and the Saudi Ministry of Health recommend using AII precautions when dealing with patients requiring high-risk procedures or aerosol-generating procedures [111, 112].

20.10 Prevention and advice for travellers:

(a) **General advice pre-travel and during travel**: No specific recommendations for pilgrims are available in regard to MERS-CoV infection. However, pilgrims must practice proper hand hygiene, protective behaviours, cough etiquette, and avoid camel contact [113].

(b) **Specific advice for healthcare workers**: The WHO recommends the isolation of asymptomatic PCR-positive individuals and daily follow-up for the occurrence of symptoms. Those individuals should be tested at least weekly and HCWs should not return to work until two consecutive upper respiratory tract samples are RT-PCR negative [114]. There is a special need to rapidly identify suspected cases to quarantine them as early as possible to avoid unprotected contact with others. Limiting visitors is strongly advised.

(c) **Specific advice for special people (e.g. pregnant, immunocompromised, very young, elderly ([65] or more):** There are no specific recommendations for these people apart from the general recommendations.

20.11 Gaps in Knowledge that Need to be Addressed

A gap remains in the specific chain of events leading to and surrounding circumstances facilitating human-to-human transmission leading to multiple outbreaks [17]. Camel had been associated with primary human cases; however, there remains a number of primary cases that had no camel exposure. Thus, it is important to elucidate all factors leading to primary cases. Although asymptomatic cases have been reported [115], it is not clear what is the actual prevalence and contribution of those individuals to the overall transmission and epidemiology of the disease. It remains unclear why MERS cases are limited to the Arabian Peninsula even though camels in many countries were reported to be positive for MERS-CoV [107]. However, recent data had emerges and suggested differences in the MERS-CoV strains in different countries [116]. There is a need to have effective therapy and potentially effective vaccines. There are a number of potential MERS-CoV vaccines in the pipeline [72], and a few clinical trials were conducted [117–124]. The vaccines use either DNA platforms (GLS-5300 (INO-4700)) [117, 118] or viral vectors such as the modified vaccinia virus-based vaccine [119, 120] and adenovirus-vectored vaccine [121–124]. Phase 1 clinical trials were also conducted [117–119, 121]. In a clinical trial, a second dose showed that 9 (75%) of 12 volunteers in the low-dose group and 11 (100%) in the high-dose group developed anti-MERS-CoV S1 ELISA with no serious side effects [119]. Anti-MERS-CoV S1-ELISA was observed in 59 (86%) of 69 participants with no serious side effects [117]. The third trial showed the development of neutralizing anti-MERS-CoV antibodies in 4 (44%) of 9 participants in the high-dose group [121].

Box 20.1: Key Websites for Travellers and Healthcare Workers
(1) WHO updates with cases. http://www.who.int/csr/don/archive/disease/coronavirus_infections/en/
(2) ECDC risk assessment. http://ecdc.europa.eu/en/healthtopics/coronavirus-infections/Pages/publications.aspx
(3) WHO with links to maps: http://www.who.int/emergencies/mers-cov/en/

Box 20.2: Things Commonly Forgotten
A single negative PCR test does not exclude MERS-CoV
   Repeated and multiple PCR tests of respiratory samples are needed
   Lower respiratory samples have better yield than upper respiratory samples
   Asymptomatic persons especially healthcare workers need isolation

---

Acknowledgments None.

Declarations of Conflict of Interest None.

References

1. Zaki AM, van Boheemen S, Bestebroer TM, Osterhaus ADME, Fouchier RAM. Isolation of a novel coronavirus from a man with pneumonia in Saudi Arabia. N Engl J Med. 2012;367:1814–20. https://doi.org/10.1056/NEJMoa1211721.
2. WHO. Middle East respiratory syndrome coronavirus (MERS-CoV)—update: 2 December 2013; 2013. http://www.who.int/csr/don/2013_12_02/en/.
3. Assiri A, McGeer A, Perl TM, Price CS, Al Rabeeah AA, Cummings DAT, et al. Hospital outbreak of Middle East respiratory syndrome coronavirus. N Engl J Med. 2013;369:407–16. https://doi.org/10.1056/NEJMoa1306742.

4. Oboho IK, Tomczyk SM, Al-Asmari AM, Banjar AA, Al-Mugti H, Aloraini MS, et al. 2014 MERS-CoV outbreak in Jeddah—a link to health care facilities. N Engl J Med. 2015;372:846–54. https://doi.org/10.1056/NEJMoa1408636.

5. Nazer RI. Outbreak of Middle East respiratory syndrome-coronavirus causes high fatality after cardiac operations. Ann Thorac Surg. 2017;104:e127–9. https://doi.org/10.1016/j.athoracsur.2017.02.072.

6. Assiri A, Abedi GR, Bin Saeed AA, Abdalla MA, al-Masry M, Choudhry AJ, et al. Multifacility outbreak of Middle East respiratory syndrome in Taif, Saudi Arabia. Emerg Infect Dis. 2016;22:32–40. https://doi.org/10.3201/eid2201.151370.

7. Drosten C, Muth D, Corman VM, Hussain R, Al Masri M, HajOmar W, et al. An observational, laboratory-based study of outbreaks of Middle East respiratory syndrome coronavirus in Jeddah and Riyadh, Kingdom of Saudi Arabia, 2014. Clin Infect Dis. 2015;60:369–77. https://doi.org/10.1093/cid/ciu812.

8. Alraddadi B, Bawareth N, Omar H, Alsalmi H, Alshukairi A, Qushmaq I, et al. Patient characteristics infected with Middle East respiratory syndrome coronavirus infection in a tertiary hospital. Ann Thorac Med. 2016;11:128–31. https://doi.org/10.4103/1817-1737.180027.

9. Fagbo SF, Skakni L, Chu DKW, Garbati MA, Joseph M, Peiris M, et al. Molecular epidemiology of hospital outbreak of Middle East respiratory syndrome, Riyadh, Saudi Arabia, 2014. Emerg Infect Dis. 2015;21:1981–8. https://doi.org/10.3201/eid2111.150944.

10. Memish ZA, Al-Tawfiq JA, Alhakeem RF, Assiri A, Alharby KD, Almahallawi MS, et al. Middle East respiratory syndrome coronavirus (MERS-CoV): a cluster analysis with implications for global management of suspected cases. Travel Med Infect Dis. 2015;13:311–4. https://doi.org/10.1016/j.tmaid.2015.06.012.

11. El Bushra HE, Abdalla MN, Al Arbash H, Alshayeb Z, Al-Ali S, Latif ZA-A, et al. An outbreak of Middle East respiratory syndrome (MERS) due to coronavirus in Al-Ahssa Region, Saudi Arabia, 2015. East Mediterr Health J. 2016;22:468–75.

12. Balkhy HH, Alenazi TH, Alshamrani MM, Baffoe-Bonnie H, Al-Abdely HM, El-Saed A, et al. Notes from the field: nosocomial outbreak of Middle East respiratory syndrome in a large tertiary care hospital—Riyadh, Saudi Arabia, 2015. MMWR Morb Mortal Wkly Rep. 2016;65:163–4. https://doi.org/10.15585/mmwr.mm6506a5.

13. Balkhy HH, Alenazi TH, Alshamrani MM, Baffoe-Bonnie H, Arabi Y, Hijazi R, et al. Description of a hospital outbreak of Middle East respiratory syndrome in a large tertiary care hospital in Saudi Arabia. Infect Control Hosp Epidemiol. 2016;37:1147–55. https://doi.org/10.1017/ice.2016.132.

14. Assiri AM, Biggs HM, Abedi GR, Lu X, Bin Saeed A, Abdalla O, et al. Increase in Middle East respiratory syndrome-coronavirus cases in Saudi Arabia linked to hospital outbreak with continued circulation of recombinant virus, July 1–August 31, 2015. Open Forum Infect Dis. 2016;3:ofw165. https://doi.org/10.1093/ofid/ofw165.

15. Majumder MS, Brownstein JS, Finkelstein SN, Larson RC, Bourouiba L. Nosocomial amplification of MERS-coronavirus in South Korea, 2015. Trans R Soc Trop Med Hyg. 2017;111:261–9. https://doi.org/10.1093/trstmh/trx046.

16. Park SH, Kim Y-S, Jung Y, Choi SY, Cho N-H, Jeong HW, et al. Outbreaks of Middle East respiratory syndrome in two hospitals initiated by a single patient in Daejeon, South Korea. Infect Chemother. 2016;48:99–107. https://doi.org/10.3947/ic.2016.48.2.99.

17. Al-Tawfiq JA, Auwaerter PG. Healthcare-associated infections: the hallmark of Middle East respiratory syndrome coronavirus with review of the literature. J Hosp Infect. 2019;101:20–9. https://doi.org/10.1016/j.jhin.2018.05.021.

18. van Boheemen S, de Graaf M, Lauber C, Bestebroer TM, Raj VS, Zaki AM, et al. Genomic characterization of a newly discovered coronavirus associated with acute respiratory distress syndrome in humans. MBio. 2012;3:e00473-12. https://doi.org/10.1128/mBio.00473-12.

19. Corman VM, Ithete NL, Richards LR, Schoeman MC, Preiser W, Drosten C, et al. Rooting the phylogenetic tree of MERS-Coronavirus by characterization of a conspecific virus from an African bat. J Virol. 2014;88:11297–303. https://doi.org/10.1128/JVI.01498-14.

20. Forni D, Cagliani R, Mozzi A, Pozzoli U, Al-Daghri N, Clerici M, et al. Extensive positive selection drives the evolution of nonstructural proteins in lineage C betacoronaviruses. J Virol. 2016;90:3627–39. https://doi.org/10.1128/JVI.02988-15.

21. Mackay IM, Arden KE. MERS coronavirus: diagnostics, epidemiology and transmission. Virol J. 2015;12:222. https://doi.org/10.1186/s12985-015-0439-5.

22. Al-Tawfiq JA, Memish ZA. Drivers of MERS-CoV transmission: what do we know? Expert Rev Respir Med. 2016;10:331–8. https://doi.org/10.1586/17476348.2016.1150784.

23. Omrani AS, Matin MA, Haddad Q, Al-Nakhli D, Memish ZA, Albarrak AM. A family cluster of middle east respiratory syndrome coronavirus infections related to a likely unrecognized asymptomatic or mild case. Int J Infect Dis. 2013;17:e668–72. https://doi.org/10.1016/j.ijid.2013.07.001.

24. Memish ZA, Zumla AI, Al-Hakeem RF, Al-Rabeeah AA, Stephens GM. Family cluster of Middle East respiratory syndrome coronavirus infections. N Engl J Med. 2013;368:2487–94. https://doi.org/10.1056/NEJMoa1303729.

25. Memish ZA, Cotten M, Watson SJ, Kellam P, Zumla A, Alhakeem RF, et al. Community case clusters of Middle East respiratory syndrome coronavirus in Hafr Al-Batin, Kingdom of Saudi Arabia: a descriptive genomic study. Int J Infect Dis. 2014;23:63–8. https://doi.org/10.1016/j.ijid.2014.03.1372.

26. Al-Abdallat MM, Payne DC, Alqasrawi S, Rha B, Tohme RA, Abedi GR, et al. Hospital-associated outbreak of Middle East respiratory syndrome coronavirus: a serologic, epidemiologic, and clinical description. Clin Infect Dis. 2014;59:1225–33. https://doi.org/10.1093/cid/ciu359.

27. Hijawi B, Abdallat M, Sayaydeh A, Alqasrawi S, Haddadin A, Jaarour N, et al. Novel coronavirus infections in Jordan, April 2012: epidemiological findings from a retrospective investigation. East Mediterr Heal J. 2013;19(Suppl. 1):S12–8.

28. Almekhlafi GA, Albarrak MM, Mandourah Y, Hassan S, Alwan A, Abudayah A, et al. Presentation and outcome of Middle East respiratory syndrome in Saudi intensive care unit patients. Crit Care. 2016;20:123. https://doi.org/10.1186/s13054-016-1303-8.

29. Saad M, Omrani AS, Baig K, Bahloul A, Elzein F, Matin MA, et al. Clinical aspects and outcomes of 70 patients with Middle East respiratory syndrome coronavirus infection: a single-center experience in Saudi Arabia. Int J Infect Dis. 2014;29:301–6. https://doi.org/10.1016/j.ijid.2014.09.003.

30. Hunter JC, Nguyen D, Aden B, Al Bandar Z, Al Dhaheri W, Abu Elkheir K, et al. Transmission of Middle East respiratory syndrome coronavirus infections in healthcare settings, Abu Dhabi. Emerg Infect Dis. 2016;22:647–56. https://doi.org/10.3201/eid2204.151615.

31. Cauchemez S, Van Kerkhove MD, Riley S, Donnelly CA, Fraser C, Ferguson NM. Transmission scenarios for middle east respiratory syndrome coronavirus (MERS-CoV) and how to tell them apart. Euro Surveill. 2013;18(24) pii: 20503

32. Cauchemez S, Fraser C, Van Kerkhove MD, Donnelly CA, Riley S, Rambaut A, et al. Middle East respiratory syndrome coronavirus: quantification of the extent of the epidemic, surveillance biases, and transmissibility. Lancet Infect Dis. 2014;14:50–6. https://doi.org/10.1016/S1473-3099(13)70304-9.

33. Chowell G, Abdirizak F, Lee S, Lee J, Jung E, Nishiura H, et al. Transmission characteristics of MERS and SARS in the healthcare setting: a comparative study. BMC Med. 2015;13:210. https://doi.org/10.1186/s12916-015-0450-0.

34. Al-Tawfiq JA, Memish ZA. Lack of seasonal variation of Middle East respiratory syndrome coronavirus (MERS-CoV). Travel Med Infect Dis. 2019;27:125–6. https://doi.org/10.1016/j.tmaid.2018.09.002.

35. Harcourt JL, Rudoler N, Tamin A, Leshem E, Rasis M, Giladi M, et al. The prevalence of Middle East respiratory syndrome coronavirus (MERS-CoV) antibodies in dromedary camels in Israel. Zoonoses Public Health. 2018; https://doi.org/10.1111/zph.12482.

36. Hastings DL, Tokars JI, Abdel Aziz IZAM, Alkhaldi KZ, Bensadek AT, Alraddadi BM, et al. Outbreak of Middle East respiratory syndrome at tertiary care hospital, Jeddah, Saudi Arabia, 2014. Emerg Infect Dis. 2016;22:794–801. https://doi.org/10.3201/eid2205.151797.

37. Korea Centers for Disease Control and Prevention. Middle East respiratory syndrome coronavirus outbreak in the Republic of Korea, 2015. Osong Public Heal Res Perspect. 2015;6:269–78. https://doi.org/10.1016/j.phrp.2015.08.006.

38. Al-Tawfiq JA, Memish ZA. Middle East respiratory syndrome coronavirus in the last two years: health care workers still at risk. Am J Infect Control. 2019;47:1167–70. https://doi.org/10.1016/j.ajic.2019.04.007.

39. Assiri A, Al-Tawfiq JA, Al-Rabeeah AA, Al-Rabiah FA, Al-Hajjar S, Al-Barrak A, et al. Epidemiological, demographic, and clinical characteristics of 47 cases of Middle East respiratory syndrome coronavirus disease from Saudi Arabia: a descriptive study. Lancet Infect Dis. 2013;13:752–61. https://doi.org/10.1016/S1473-3099(13)70204-4.

40. Al-Tawfiq JA, Memish ZA. An update on Middle East respiratory syndrome: 2 years later. Expert Rev Respir Med. 2015;9:327–35. https://doi.org/10.1586/17476348.2015.1027689.

41. Feikin DR, Alraddadi B, Qutub M, Shabouni O, Curns A, Oboho IK, et al. Association of higher MERS-CoV virus load with severe disease and death, Saudi Arabia, 2014. Emerg Infect Dis. 2015;21:2029–35. https://doi.org/10.3201/eid2111.150764.

42. Alfaraj SH, Al-Tawfiq JA, Assiri AY, Alzahrani NA, Alanazi AA, Memish ZA. Clinical predictors of mortality of Middle East respiratory syndrome coronavirus (MERS-CoV) infection: a cohort study. Travel Med Infect Dis. 2019;29:48–50. https://doi.org/10.1016/j.tmaid.2019.03.004.

43. Sridhar S, Brouqui P, Parola P, Gautret P. Imported cases of Middle East respiratory syndrome: an update. Travel Med Infect Dis. 2015;13:106–9. https://doi.org/10.1016/j.tmaid.2014.11.006.

44. Al-Tawfiq JA, Zumla A, Memish ZA. Travel implications of emerging coronaviruses: SARS and MERS-CoV. Travel Med Infect Dis. 2014;12:422–8. https://doi.org/10.1016/j.tmaid.2014.06.007.

45. Khan K, Sears J, Hu VW, Brownstein JS, Hay S, Kossowsky D, et al. Potential for the international spread of middle east respiratory syndrome in association with mass gatherings in saudi arabia. PLoS Curr. 2013:5. https://doi.org/10.1371/currents.outbreaks.a7b70897ac2fa4f79b59f90d24c860b8.

46. Kandeel A, Deming M, Elkreem EA, El-Refay S, Afifi S, Abukela M, et al. Pandemic (H1N1) 2009 and Hajj Pilgrims who received predeparture vaccination, Egypt. Emerg Infect Dis. 2011;17:1266–8. https://doi.org/10.3201/eid1707.101484.

47. Rashid H, Shafi S, Haworth E, El Bashir H, Memish ZA, Sudhanva M, et al. Viral respiratory infections at the Hajj: comparison between UK and Saudi pilgrims. Clin Microbiol Infect. 2008;14:569–74. https://doi.org/10.1111/j.1469-0691.2008.01987.x.

48. Al-Tawfiq JA, Smallwood CAH, Arbuthnott KG, Malik MSK, Barbeschi M, Memish ZA. Emerging respiratory and novel coronavirus 2012 infections and mass gatherings. East Mediterr Heal J. 2013;19:48–54. https://doi.org/10.26719/2013.19.suppl.s48.

49. Memish ZA, Zumla A, Al-Tawfiq JA. How great is the risk of Middle East respiratory syndrome coronavirus to the global population? Expert Rev Anti Infect Ther. 2013;11:979–81. https://doi.org/10.1586/14787210.2013.836965.

50. Barasheed O, Rashid H, Alfelali M, Tashani M, Azeem M, Bokhary H, et al. Viral respiratory infections among Hajj pilgrims in 2013. Virol Sin. 2014;29:364–71. https://doi.org/10.1007/s12250-014-3507-x.

51. Griffiths K, Charrel R, Lagier J-C, Nougairede A, Simon F, Parola P, et al. Infections in symptomatic travelers returning from the Arabian peninsula to France: a retrospective cross-sectional study. Travel Med Infect Dis. 2016;14:414–6. https://doi.org/10.1016/j.tmaid.2016.05.002.

52. Memish ZA, Assiri A, Turkestani A, Yezli S, Al Masri M, Charrel R, et al. Mass gathering and globalization of respiratory pathogens during the 2013 Hajj. Clin Microbiol Infect. 2015;21(571):e1–8. https://doi.org/10.1016/j.cmi.2015.02.008.

53. Benkouiten S, Charrel R, Belhouchat K, Drali T, Nougairede A, Salez N, et al. Respiratory viruses and bacteria among pilgrims during the 2013 Hajj. Emerg Infect Dis. 2014;20:1821–7. https://doi.org/10.3201/eid2011.140600.

54. Ma X, Liu F, Liu L, Zhang L, Lu M, Abudukadeer A, et al. No MERS-CoV but positive influenza viruses in returning Hajj pilgrims, China, 2013–2015. BMC Infect Dis. 2017;17:715. https://doi.org/10.1186/s12879-017-2791-0.

55. Al-Abdallat MM, Rha B, Alqasrawi S, Payne DC, Iblan I, Binder AM, et al. Acute respiratory infections among returning Hajj pilgrims—Jordan, 2014. J Clin Virol. 2017;89:34–7. https://doi.org/10.1016/j.jcv.2017.01.010.

56. Koul PA, Mir H, Saha S, Chadha MS, Potdar V, Widdowson M-A, et al. Influenza not MERS CoV among returning Hajj and Umrah pilgrims with respiratory illness, Kashmir, north India, 2014–15. Travel Med Infect Dis. 2017;15:45–7. https://doi.org/10.1016/j.tmaid.2016.12.002.

57. Gautret P, Charrel R, Benkouiten S, Belhouchat K, Nougairede A, Drali T, et al. Lack of MERS coronavirus but prevalence of influenza virus in French pilgrims after 2013 Hajj. Emerg Infect Dis. 2014;20:728–30. https://doi.org/10.3201/eid2004.131708.

58. Memish ZA, Almasri M, Turkestani A, Al-Shangiti AM, Yezli S. Etiology of severe community-acquired pneumonia during the 2013 Hajj-part of the MERS-CoV surveillance program. Int J Infect Dis. 2014;25:186–90. https://doi.org/10.1016/j.ijid.2014.06.003.

59. Gautret P, Charrel R, Belhouchat K, Drali T, Benkouiten S, Nougairede A, et al. Lack of nasal carriage of novel corona virus (HCoV-EMC) in French Hajj pilgrims returning from the Hajj 2012, despite a high rate of respiratory symptoms. Clin Microbiol Infect. 2013;19:E315–7. https://doi.org/10.1111/1469-0691.12174.

60. Baharoon S, Al-Jahdali H, Al Hashmi J, Memish ZA, Ahmed QA. Severe sepsis and septic shock at the Hajj: etiologies and outcomes. Travel Med Infect Dis. 2009;7:247–52. https://doi.org/10.1016/j.tmaid.2008.09.002.

61. Memish ZA, Assiri A, Almasri M, Alhakeem RF, Turkestani A, Al Rabeeah AA, et al. Prevalence of MERS-CoV nasal carriage and compliance with the Saudi health recommendations among pilgrims attending the 2013 Hajj. J Infect Dis. 2014;210:1067–72. https://doi.org/10.1093/infdis/jiu150.

62. Annan A, Owusu M, Marfo KS, Larbi R, Sarpong FN, Adu-Sarkodie Y, et al. High prevalence of common respiratory viruses and no evidence of Middle East respiratory syndrome coronavirus in Hajj pilgrims returning to Ghana, 2013. Trop Med Int Heal. 2015;20:807–12. https://doi.org/10.1111/tmi.12482.

63. Refaey S, Amin MM, Roguski K, Azziz-Baumgartner E, Uyeki TM, Labib M, et al. Cross-sectional survey and surveillance for influenza viruses and MERS-CoV among Egyptian pilgrims returning from Hajj during 2012–2015. Influenza Other Respi Viruses. 2017;11:57–60. https://doi.org/10.1111/irv.12429.

64. Atabani SF, Wilson S, Overton-Lewis C, Workman J, Kidd IM, Petersen E, et al. Active screening and surveillance in the United Kingdom for Middle East respiratory syndrome coronavirus in returning travellers and pilgrims from the Middle East: a prospective descriptive study for the period 2013–2015. Int J Infect Dis. 2016;47:10–4. https://doi.org/10.1016/j.ijid.2016.04.016.

65. ProMed. Novel coronavirus—Eastern Mediterranean (03): Saudi comment, 12 February 2013 2013. http://promedmail.org/post/20130326.1603038.

66. Aberle JH, Popow-Kraupp T, Kreidl P, Laferl H, Heinz FX, Aberle SW. Influenza A and B viruses but not MERS-CoV in Hajj Pilgrims, Austria, 2014. Emerg Infect Dis. 2015;21:726–7. https://doi.org/10.3201/eid2104.141745.

67. Kim Y, Lee S, Chu C, Choe S, Hong S, Shin Y. The characteristics of Middle Eastern respiratory syndrome coronavirus transmission dynamics in South Korea. Osong Public Heal Res Perspect. 2016;7:49–55. https://doi.org/10.1016/j.phrp.2016.01.001.

68. Pavli A, Tsiodras S, Maltezou HC. Middle East respiratory syndrome coronavirus (MERS-CoV): prevention in travelers. Travel Med Infect Dis. 2014;12:602–8. https://doi.org/10.1016/j.tmaid.2014.10.006.

69. Kraaij-Dirkzwager M, Timen A, Dirksen K, Gelinck L, Leyten E, Groeneveld P, et al. Middle East respiratory syndrome coronavirus (MERS-CoV) infections in two returning travellers in the Netherlands, May 2014. Euro Surveill. 2014;19. pii: 20817

70. Carias C, O'Hagan JJ, Jewett A, Gambhir M, Cohen NJ, Haber Y, et al. Exportations of symptomatic cases of MERS-CoV infection to countries outside the Middle East. Emerg Infect Dis. 2016;22:723–5.

71. Xia S, Liu Q, Wang Q, Sun Z, Su S, Du L, et al. Middle East respiratory syndrome coronavirus (MERS-CoV) entry inhibitors targeting spike protein. Virus Res. 2014;194:200–10. https://doi.org/10.1016/j.virusres.2014.10.007.

72. Skariyachan S, Challapilli SB, Packirisamy S, Kumargowda ST, Sridhar VS. Recent aspects on the pathogenesis mechanism, animal models and novel therapeutic interventions for middle east respiratory syndrome coronavirus infections. Front Microbiol. 2019;10:569. https://doi.org/10.3389/fmicb.2019.00569.

73. Al-Tawfiq JA, Hinedi K. The calm before the storm: clinical observations of Middle East respiratory syndrome (MERS) patients. J Chemother. 2018;30:179–82. https://doi.org/1 0.1080/1120009X.2018.1429236.

74. Alsaad KO, Hajeer AH, Al Balwi M, Al Moaiqel M, Al Oudah N, Al Ajlan A, et al. Histopathology of Middle East respiratory syndrome coronovirus (MERS-CoV) infection— clinicopathological and ultrastructural study. Histopathology. 2018;72:516–24. https://doi.org/10.1111/his.13379.

75. Ng DL, Al Hosani F, Keating MK, Gerber SI, Jones TL, Metcalfe MG, et al. Clinicopathologic, immunohistochemical, and ultrastructural findings of a fatal case of Middle East respiratory syndrome coronavirus infection in the United Arab Emirates, April 2014. Am J Pathol. 2016;186:652–8. https://doi.org/10.1016/j.ajpath.2015.10.024.

76. Al-Tawfiq JA, Hinedi K, Ghandour J, Khairalla H, Musleh S, Ujayli A, et al. Middle east respiratory syndrome coronavirus: a case-control study of hospitalized patients. Clin Infect Dis. 2014;59:160–5. https://doi.org/10.1093/cid/ciu226.

77. Choi WS, Kang C-I, Kim Y, Choi J-P, Joh JS, Shin H-S, et al. Clinical presentation and outcomes of Middle East respiratory syndrome in the Republic of Korea. Infect Chemother. 2016;48:118–26. https://doi.org/10.3947/ic.2016.48.2.118.

78. Arabi YM, Arifi AA, Balkhy HH, Najm H, Aldawood AS, Ghabashi A, et al. Clinical course and outcomes of critically ill patients with Middle East respiratory syndrome coronavirus infection. Ann Intern Med. 2014;160:389–97. https://doi.org/10.7326/M13-2486.

79. Das KM, Lee EY, Enani MA, AlJawder SE, Singh R, Bashir S, et al. CT correlation with outcomes in 15 patients with acute Middle East respiratory syndrome coronavirus. AJR Am J Roentgenol. 2015;204:736–42. https://doi.org/10.2214/AJR.14.13671.

80. Corman VM, Eckerle I, Bleicker T, Zaki A, Landt O, Eschbach-Bludau M, et al. Detection of a novel human coronavirus by real-time reverse-transcription polymerase chain reaction. Eurosurveillance. 2012;17. https://doi.org/10.2807/ese.17.39.20285-en.

81. Corman VM, Ölschläger S, Wendtner C-M, Drexler JF, Hess M, Drosten C. Performance and clinical validation of the RealStar MERS-CoV Kit for detection of Middle East respiratory syndrome coronavirus RNA. J Clin Virol. 2014;60:168–71. https://doi.org/10.1016/j. jcv.2014.03.012.

82. Corman VM, Müller MA, Costabel U, Timm J, Binger T, Meyer B, et al. Assays for laboratory confirmation of novel human coronavirus (hCoV-EMC) infections. Euro Surveill. 2012;17:49.

83. Shirato K, Yano T, Senba S, Akachi S, Kobayashi T, Nishinaka T, et al. Detection of Middle East respiratory syndrome coronavirus using reverse transcription loop-mediated isothermal amplification (RT-LAMP). Virol J. 2014;11:139. https://doi.org/10.1186/1743-422X-11-139.

84. El Wahed AA, Patel P, Heidenreich D, Hufert FT, Weidmann M. Reverse transcription recombinase polymerase amplification assay for the detection of middle east respiratory syndrome coronavirus. PLoS Curr. 2013;5. https://doi.org/10.1371/currents.outbreaks.62df1c7c75ffc9 6cd59034531e2e8364.

85. Memish ZA, Al-Tawfiq JA, Makhdoom HQ, Assiri A, Alhakeem RF, Albarrak A, et al. Respiratory tract samples, viral load, and genome fraction yield in patients with middle east respiratory syndrome. J Infect Dis. 2014;210:1590–4. https://doi.org/10.1093/infdis/jiu292.

86. World Health Organization. Laboratory testing for Middle Easr respiratory syndrome coronavirus (MERS CoV): interim guidance; 2015. p. 6. http://apps.who.int/iris/bitstream/10665/176982/1/WHO_MERS_LAB_15.1_eng.pdf?ua=1 (accessed December 20, 2016)

87. Alfaraj SH, Al-Tawfiq JA, Memish ZA. Middle East respiratory syndrome coronavirus intermittent positive cases: implications for infection control. Am J Infect Control. 2019;47:290–3. https://doi.org/10.1016/j.ajic.2018.08.020.

88. Reusken C, Mou H, Godeke GJ, van der Hoek L, Meyer B, Müller MA, et al. Specific serology for emerging human coronaviruses by protein microarray. Euro Surveill. 2013;18:20441.

89. CDC. MERS-CoV | Laboratory Testing for MERS-CoV | CDC n.d. https://www.cdc.gov/coronavirus/mers/lab/lab-testing.html (accessed May 10, 2019).

90. Al-Tawfiq JA, Rabaan AA, Hinedi K. Influenza is more common than Middle East respiratory syndrome coronavirus (MERS-CoV) among hospitalized adult Saudi patients. Travel Med Infect Dis. 2017;20:56–60. https://doi.org/10.1016/j.tmaid.2017.10.004.

91. Alfaraj SH, Al-Tawfiq JA, Alzahrani NA, Altwaijri TA, Memish ZA. The impact of co-infection of influenza A virus on the severity of Middle East respiratory syndrome coronavirus. J Infect. 2017;74:521–3. https://doi.org/10.1016/j.jinf.2017.02.001.

92. Alfaraj SH, Al-Tawfiq JA, Altuwaijri TA, Memish ZA. Middle East respiratory syndrome coronavirus and pulmonary tuberculosis coinfection: implications for infection control. Intervirology. 2017;60:53–5. https://doi.org/10.1159/000477908.

93. Elhazmi A, Al-Tawfiq JA, Sallam H, Al-Omari A, Alhumaid S, Mady A, Al Mutair A. Severe acute respiratory syndrome coronavirus 2 (SARSCoV-2) and Middle East Respiratory Syndrome Coronavirus (MERS-CoV) coinfection: A unique case series. Travel Med Infect Dis. 2021;41:102026. https://doi.org/10.1016/j.tmaid.2021.102026.

94. Alfaraj SH, Al-Tawfiq JA, Gautret P, Alenazi MG, Asiri AY, Memish ZA. Evaluation of visual triage for screening of Middle East respiratory syndrome coronavirus patients. New Microbes New Infect. 2018;26:49–52. https://doi.org/10.1016/j.nmni.2018.08.008.

95. Al-Tawfiq JA, Momattin H, Dib J, Memish ZA. Ribavirin and interferon therapy in patients infected with the Middle East respiratory syndrome coronavirus: an observational study. Int J Infect Dis. 2014;20:42–6. https://doi.org/10.1016/j.ijid.2013.12.003.

96. Shalhoub S, Farahat F, Al-Jiffri A, Simhairi R, Shamma O, Siddiqi N, et al. IFN-α2a or IFN-β1a in combination with ribavirin to treat Middle East respiratory syndrome coronavirus pneumonia: a retrospective study. J Antimicrob Chemother. 2015;70:2129–32. https://doi.org/10.1093/jac/dkv085.

97. Omrani AS, Saad MM, Baig K, Bahloul A, Abdul-Matin M, Alaidaroos AY, et al. Ribavirin and interferon alfa-2a for severe Middle East respiratory syndrome coronavirus infection: a retrospective cohort study. Lancet Infect Dis. 2014;14:1090–5. https://doi.org/10.1016/S1473-3099(14)70920-X.

98. Spanakis N, Tsiodras S, Haagmans BL, Raj VS, Pontikis K, Koutsoukou A, et al. Virological and serological analysis of a recent Middle East respiratory syndrome coronavirus infection case on a triple combination antiviral regimen. Int J Antimicrob Agents. 2014;44:528–32. https://doi.org/10.1016/j.ijantimicag.2014.07.026.

99. Chong YP, Song JY, Bin SY, Choi J-P, Shin H-S, Rapid Response Team. Antiviral treatment guidelines for Middle East respiratory syndrome. Infect Chemother. 2015;47:212–22. https://doi.org/10.3947/ic.2015.47.3.212.

100. Arabi Y, Balkhy H, Hajeer AH, Bouchama A, Hayden FG, Al-Omari A, et al. Feasibility, safety, clinical, and laboratory effects of convalescent plasma therapy for patients with Middle East respiratory syndrome coronavirus infection: a study protocol. Springerplus. 2015;4:709. https://doi.org/10.1186/s40064-015-1490-9.

101. Arabi YM, Asiri AY, Assiri AM, Balkhy HH, Al Bshabshe A, Al Jeraisy M, et al. Interferon Beta-1b and Lopinavir–Ritonavir for Middle East respiratory syndrome. N Engl J Med. 2020;383:1645–56. https://doi.org/10.1056/nejmoa2015294.

102. Beigel JH, Voell J, Kumar P, Raviprakash K, Wu H, Jiao JA, et al. Safety and tolerability of a novel, polyclonal human anti-MERS coronavirus antibody produced from transchromosomic

cattle: a phase 1 randomised, double-blind, single-dose-escalation study. Lancet Infect Dis. 2018;18:410–8. https://doi.org/10.1016/S1473-3099(18)30002-1.

103. Chu DKW, Poon LLM, Gomaa MM, Shehata MM, Perera RAPM, Zeid DA, et al. MERS coronaviruses in dromedary camels. Egypt. Emerg Infect Dis. 2014;20:1049–53. https://doi.org/10.3201/eid2006.140299.

104. Sabir JSM, Lam TT, Mohamed MM, Li L, Shen Y, Abo-aba SEM, et al. Co-circulation of three camel coronavirus species and recombination of MERS-CoVs in Saudi Arabia. Science. 2015;351:1–6. https://doi.org/10.1126/science.aac8606.

105. Van Doremalen N, Hijazeen ZSK, Holloway P, Al Omari B, Mcdowell C, Adney D, et al. High prevalence of middle east respiratory coronavirus in young dromedary camels in Jordan. Vector-Borne Zoonotic Dis. 2017;17:155–9. https://doi.org/10.1089/vbz.2016.2062.

106. Hemida MG, Alnaeem A, Chu DK, Perera RA, Chan SM, Almathen F, et al. Longitudinal study of Middle East Respiratory Syndrome coronavirus infection in dromedary camel herds in Saudi Arabia, 2014–2015. Emerg Microbes Infect. 2017;6:e56. https://doi.org/10.1038/emi.2017.44.

107. Ali MA, Shehata MM, Gomaa MR, Kandeil A, El-Shesheny R, Kayed AS, et al. Systematic, active surveillance for Middle East respiratory syndrome coronavirus in camels in Egypt. Emerg Microbes Infect. 2017;6:e1. https://doi.org/10.1038/emi.2016.130.

108. Reusken CB, Farag EA, Jonges M, Godeke GJ, El-Sayed AM, Pas SD, et al. Middle east respiratory syndrome coronavirus (MERS-CoV) RNA and neutralising antibodies in milk collected according to local customs from dromedary camels, Qatar, April 2014. Eurosurveillance. 2014;19 https://doi.org/10.2807/1560-7917.ES2014.19.23.20829.

109. Muhairi SA, Hosani FA, Eltahir YM, Mulla MA, Yusof MF, Serhan WS, Hashem FM, Elsayed EA, Marzoug BA, Abdelazim AS. Epidemiological investigation of Middle East respiratory syndrome coronavirus in dromedary camel farms linked with human infection in Abu Dhabi Emirate, United Arab Emirates. Virus Genes. 2016;52:848–54. https://doi.org/10.1007/s11262-016-1367-1.

110. CDC. Interim Infection Prevention and Control Recommendations for Hospitalized Patients with Middle East Respiratory Syndrome Coronavirus (MERS-CoV); 2015. https://www.cdc.gov/coronavirus/mers/infection-prevention-control.html (accessed March 9, 2017).

111. World Health Organization. Infection prevention and control during health care for probable or confirmed cases of Middle East respiratory syndrome coronavirus (MERS-CoV) infection; 2015.

112. Saudi Ministry of Health. Middle East Respiratory Syndrome Coronavirus 2018 Guidelines for Healthcare Professionals; 2018. https://www.moh.gov.sa/CCC/healthp/regulations/Documents/MERS-CoV Guidelines for Healthcare Professionals—May 2018—v5.1%281%29.pdf (accessed May 23, 2019).

113. Al-Tawfiq JA, Memish ZA. The Hajj: updated health hazards and current recommendations for 2012. Euro Surveill. 2012;17:20295.

114. WHO. Management of asymptomatic persons who are RT- PCR positive for Middle East respiratory syndrome coronavirus (MERS-CoV); 2018, pp. 1–3. http://apps.who.int/iris/bitstream/handle/10665/180973/WHO_MERS_IPC_15.2_eng.pdf;jsessionid=F362DEB01D8550505DDF4C962CD62479?sequence=1 (accessed July 22, 2018).

115. Al-Tawfiq JA, Gautret P. Asymptomatic Middle East respiratory syndrome coronavirus (MERS-CoV) infection: extent and implications for infection control: a systematic review. Travel Med Infect Dis. 2019;27:27–32. https://doi.org/10.1016/j.tmaid.2018.12.003.

116. Shirato K, Melaku SK, Kawachi K, Nao N, Iwata-Yoshikawa N, Kawase M, Kamitani W, Matsuyama S, Tessema TS, Sentsui H. Middle East respiratory syndrome coronavirus in dromedaries in Ethiopia is antigenically different from the Middle East isolate EMC. Front Microbiol. 2019;10:1326.

117. Modjarrad K, Roberts CC, Mills KT, Castellano AR, Paolino K, Muthumani K, et al. Safety and immunogenicity of an anti-Middle East respiratory syndrome coronavirus DNA vaccine: a phase 1, open-label, single-arm, dose-escalation trial. Lancet Infect Dis. 2019;19:1013–22. https://doi.org/10.1016/S1473-3099(19)30266-X.

118. Evaluate the Safety, Tolerability and Immunogenicity Study of GLS-5300 in healthy volunteers—full text view—ClinicalTrials.gov n.d. https://clinicaltrials.gov/ct2/show/NCT03721718 (accessed March 26, 2021).

119. Koch T, Dahlke C, Fathi A, Kupke A, Krähling V, Okba NMA, et al. Safety and immunogenicity of a modified vaccinia virus Ankara vector vaccine candidate for Middle East respiratory syndrome: an open-label, phase 1 trial. Lancet Infect Dis. 2020;20:827–38. https://doi.org/10.1016/S1473-3099(20)30248-6.

120. Safety and Immunogenicity of the Candidate Vaccine MVA-MERS-S_DF-1 against MERS—full text view—ClinicalTrials.gov n.d. https://clinicaltrials.gov/ct2/show/NCT04119440 (accessed March 26, 2021).

121. Folegatti PM, Bittaye M, Flaxman A, Lopez FR, Bellamy D, Kupke A, et al. Safety and immunogenicity of a candidate Middle East respiratory syndrome coronavirus viral-vectored vaccine: a dose-escalation, open-label, non-randomised, uncontrolled, phase 1 trial. Lancet Infect Dis. 2020;20:816–26. https://doi.org/10.1016/S1473-3099(20)30160-2.

122. A clinical trial to determine the safety and immunogenicity of healthy candidate MERS-CoV vaccine (MERS002)—full text view—ClinicalTrials.gov n.d. https://clinicaltrials.gov/ct2/show/NCT04170829 (accessed March 26, 2021).

123. Gamaleya Research Institute of Epidemiology and Microbiology HM of the RF. Study of Safety and Immunogenicity of BVRS-GamVac-Combi—full text view—ClinicalTrials.gov. Clin Trials 2019. https://clinicaltrials.gov/ct2/show/NCT04128059 (accessed March 26, 2021).

124. Study of Safety and Immunogenicity of BVRS-GamVac—full text view—ClinicalTrials.gov n.d. https://clinicaltrials.gov/ct2/show/NCT04130594 (accessed March 26, 2021).

125. Khalid I, Alraddadi BM, Dairi Y, Khalid TJ, Kadri M, Alshukairi AN, et al. Acute management and long-term survival among subjects with severe middle east respiratory syndrome coronavirus pneumonia and ARDS. Respir Care. 2016;61:340–8. https://doi.org/10.4187/respcare.04325.

126. Al Ghamdi M, Alghamdi KM, Ghandoora Y, Alzahrani A, Salah F, Alsulami A, et al. Treatment outcomes for patients with Middle Eastern respiratory syndrome coronavirus (MERS CoV) infection at a coronavirus referral center in the Kingdom of Saudi Arabia. BMC Infect Dis. 2016;16:174. https://doi.org/10.1186/s12879-016-1492-4.

127. Kim UJ, Won E-J, Kee S-J, Jung S-I, Jang H-C. Combination therapy with lopinavir/ritonavir, ribavirin and interferon-alpha for Middle East respiratory syndrome: a case report. Antivir Ther. 2015; https://doi.org/10.3851/IMP3002.

128. Khalid M, Al Rabiah F, Khan B, Al Mobeireek A, Butt TS, Al ME. Ribavirin and interferon-α2b as primary and preventive treatment for Middle East respiratory syndrome coronavirus: a preliminary report of two cases. Antivir Ther. 2015;20:87–91. https://doi.org/10.3851/IMP2792.

129. Malik A, El Masry KM, Ravi M, Sayed F. Middle east respiratory syndrome coronavirus during pregnancy, Abu Dhabi, United Arab Emirates, 2013. Emerg Infect Dis. 2016;22:515–7. https://doi.org/10.3201/eid2203.151049.

130. Khalid M, Khan B, Al Rabiah F, Alismaili R, Saleemi S, Rehan-Khaliq AM, et al. Middle Eastern respiratory syndrome corona virus (MERS CoV): case reports from a tertiary care hospital in Saudi Arabia. Ann Saudi Med. 2014;34:396–400. https://doi.org/10.5144/0256-4947.2014.396.

Multi-drug Resistant Tuberculosis in Travellers

21

Geraint Rhys Davies

Abstract

Tuberculosis remains a major global public health crisis, and multidrug-resistant tuberculosis (MDR-TB) has become a threat to disease control in many countries. More than 20% of humanity is latently infected with TB, and an estimated 450,000 people develop MDR-TB disease annually. While the risk to casual travellers is low, even during long-haul air travel, healthcare and humanitarian workers, migrants and refugees from high-burden countries and the immunocompromised may be at substantial risk. BCG vaccination may offer modest protection, and screening strategies for latent infection can identify who may be at risk of future disease after exposure, but the best approach to management of latent MDR-TB infection remains unclear. MDR-TB disease should be suspected in those with relevant symptoms and signs after possible exposure. Rapid molecular testing and susceptibility prediction can speed up diagnosis, while novel all-oral treatment regimens have significantly shortened and simplified the treatment of MDR-TB in recent years.

21.1 Background

Tuberculosis (TB) is among humans' most ancient and co-evolved pathogens, likely emerging as early as the Neolithic period [1]. The ongoing worldwide pandemic of TB dates from the period of rapid global urbanization and expansion

G. R. Davies (✉)
Department of Clinical Infection, Microbiology and Immunology, University of Liverpool, Liverpool, UK
e-mail: gerrydavies@doctors.org.uk

© The Author(s), under exclusive license to Springer Nature Switzerland AG 2024
H. Leblebicioglu et al. (eds.), *Emerging and Re-emerging Infections in Travellers*, https://doi.org/10.1007/978-3-031-49475-8_21

331

of trade over the last three hundred years. While TB is not a new pathogen, in the decade preceding the COVID-19 pandemic, it remained the single biggest cause of mortality from an infectious agent with a disproportionate impact on younger adults. Though effective treatment for the disease has been available for more than 70 years, efforts to control TB on a global scale have not resulted in a reduction in the burden of the disease until 2012, and the decline in incidence since then has been slow [2]. Furthermore, the advent and expansion of strains of *M. tuberculosis* (MTB) resistant to both of the key anti-tuberculosis drugs rifampicin (RIF) and isoniazid (INH) (multi-drug resistant or MDR-TB) since the 1990s and the more recent emergence of fluoroquinolone-resistant MDR-TB poses an important threat to this recent and fragile public health progress in many parts of the world [3].

21.2 Aetiology

TB is caused by members of the MTB species complex, which, while relatively genetically homogenous, is currently subdivided into nine lineages whose distribution varies geographically [4]. While *M. tuberculosis sensu stricto* and *M africanum* are strictly human pathogens, infection may also be caused by other sub-species typically restricted to other mammals such as *M.bovis* and *M. microti*. Emerging evidence suggests that lineage characteristics may have biological and clinical significance. The ancestral Lineage 1 (Indo-Oceanic) has been linked with an extra-pulmonary pattern of disease [5], while Lineages 5 and 6 (West African) may be associated with slower progression to and of disease [6]. Lineage 2 (East Asian) produces an abundant phenolic glycolipid postulated to be an important virulence factor, appears more transmissible and may be more commonly associated with drug resistance [7].

Resistance in MTB is invariably due to single nucleotide polymorphisms (SNPs) in key target genes rather than the mobile genetic elements frequently found in other bacteria [8]. Resistance to INH is most commonly due to loss-of-function SNPs in the *katG* locus, which codes for the catalase enzyme responsible for activating the drug within the mycobacterial cell. Less commonly, mutations occur in the *inhA* locus, which codes for an enoyl-acyl carrier protein that facilitates the synthesis of mycolic acids in the mycobacterial cell wall, which is the ultimate target of INH. Resistance to RIF is due to SNPs in the small "hotspot" area of the MTB *rpoB* gene coding for the bacterial RNA polymerase enzyme, which prevents the drug's binding to its target, allowing protein synthesis to continue. Resistance to fluoroquinolones is typically caused by a small number of mutations in the resistance-determining region (RDR) of the *gyrA* gene coding for the key mycobacterial gyrase/topoisomerase enzyme responsible for DNA super-coiling [9].

21.3 Transmission

MTB is transmitted by small airborne droplets typically produced by people with sputum smear-positive pulmonary TB. Risk of transmission has traditionally been linked to close and prolonged contact, though recent aerobiology studies have demonstrated differences in the efficiency of droplet production between index cases, which may be biologically significant. While guidance typically defines people with positive sputum smears as infectious for public health and screening purposes, there is also reliable evidence that transmission may occur in some circumstances from people with pulmonary disease who do not meet this criterion [10]. While major outbreaks of MDR-TB are well-described [11], there is little evidence that MDR-TB strains are inherently more transmissible than drug-susceptible strains of MTB, since though they may, in theory, enjoy a selective advantage in their ability to survive the effects of first-line drugs, in vitro experiments show that there is likely a fitness cost to acquisition of drug resistance, particularly the loss of catalase activity with *katG* mutations, reducing resilience to oxidative stress [12].

21.4 Epidemiology

TB is distributed worldwide, though the incidence varies geographically. A simple epidemiological model helps frame clinical and public health decision-making (see Fig. 21.1). It is estimated from tuberculin skin test surveys and mathematical modelling of notification data that slightly more than 20% of the global population is latently infected with MTB [13]. Replenishment of this reservoir of infection is driven by contact with infectious individuals in affected communities while the annual risk of subsequently developing disease varies according to key host factors, including HIV co-infection, diabetes mellitus, cigarette smoking, undernutrition and poverty [2]. While immaturity and senescence of the immune system are similarly thought to explain the typical age distribution of disease, specific forms of

Fig. 21.1 Simplified model of TB epidemiology. R_o = average number of secondary cases resulting from each case

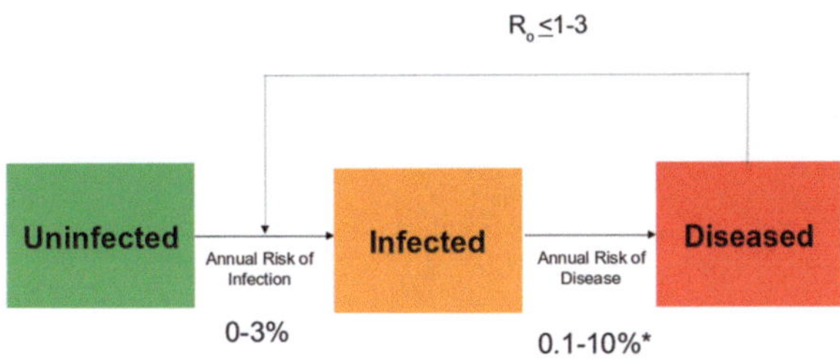

immunosuppression have also been closely associated with TB, including TNF-alpha blockade and hypovitaminosis D as well as rare defects in the IFN-gamma and IL-12 signalling pathways. With an average lifetime risk of developing disease estimated at 2.5–5%, 10.6 million cases of TB disease are notified each year, resulting in 1.6 million deaths annually [2]. Almost 90% occur in 30 high-burden countries (see Fig. 21.2).

Due to incomplete coverage of susceptibility testing in many countries, data on MDR-TB is less certain, but the best estimate suggests that 450,000 people were living with the disease worldwide in 2021, approximately 3.6% of people presenting with TB for the first time. This figure disguises significant regional variations, however, ranging from 1.5% (Philippines) to 38% (Russian Federation) among the seven countries with the highest burden of TB (Fig. 21.3). Currently only a third of people suffering from MDR-TB are enrolled in treatment programmes [2].

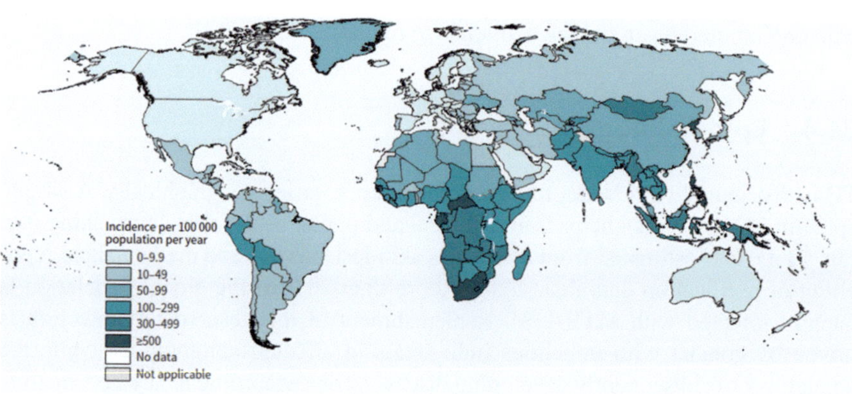

Fig. 21.2 Incidence rate of TB by country. (Source WHO Global TB Report 2022)

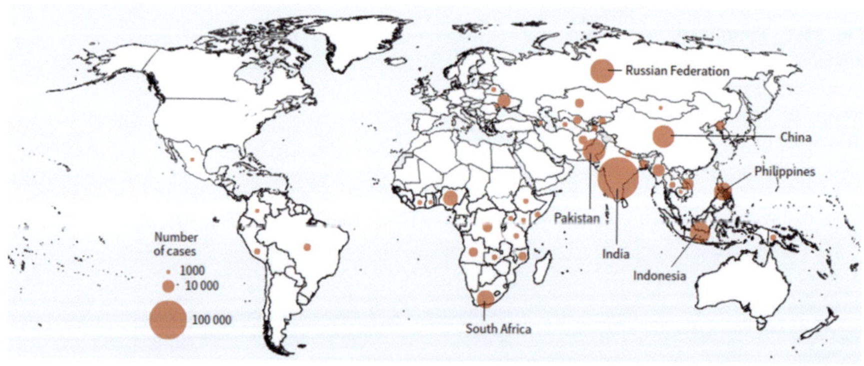

Fig. 21.3 Incidence of MDR-TB by country. The seven named countries contribute two-thirds of the burden of MDR-TB. (Source WHO Global TB Report 2022)

The risk to travellers from MDR-TB is linked to the geographical distribution of disease and the personal risks related to their activities and health status. Among those at highest risk are healthcare workers who may encounter people with infectious MDR-TB in affected communities or health facilities in high-burden countries. There is reliable evidence that the risk of TB infection is increased in healthcare workers in such countries, even in general or emergency care settings [14, 15].

People originating from a high MDR-TB burden country or who travel often or for prolonged periods to visit relatives or friends are also an important risk group. In many low-incidence countries, the majority of the burden of TB is in people born outside their current country of residence, and measures for pre-immigration, port-of-entry or early screening are usual. Despite these measures, a global observational cohort study conducted from 2008 to 2020 found that 97.5% of imported cases of MDR-TB were in migrants from high-burden countries. However, in almost half it was not possible to exclude the possibility of transmission due to crowded accommodation, transport and incarceration en route [16].

The risks associated with routine recreational travel are low, with an estimated risk of TB infection and active disease of 1.6% and 0.3%, respectively, in people travelling or volunteering abroad for up to 6 months [15]. While there have been incidents of possible transmission of MDR-TB to passengers on long-haul international flights [17], international guidance suggests that these are rare and that the zone of infectivity of index cases is likely confined to immediately adjoining seats and adjacent rows in the cabin [18].

21.5 Pathogenesis

The outcome of primary infection with MTB is determined by the state of immunity of the host and the ability of their alveolar and intra-pulmonary macrophages to contain replication and spread of the organisms. MTB has numerous adaptations that enable it to resist phagolysosomal fusion within phagocytes, and containment typically relies on the formation of granulomas after the onset of cell-mediated immunity and macrophage activation provoked by antigen presentation in regional lymph nodes. In 95% of instances, primary infection results in a state of latent infection with a reduced load of MTB organisms contained within functional granulomas that persist while immunity remains effective. Only when immune control wanes with time or never develops does disease in the lungs and other body sites or disseminated infection result [19].

21.6 Clinical Findings

TB most commonly affects the lungs with the cardinal symptoms of chronic cough lasting more than 2–3 weeks, fever, night sweats and weight loss. Advanced pulmonary disease may present characteristic imaging appearances such as cavitation and lymphadenopathy (Fig. 21.4) and suitable respiratory specimens can usually

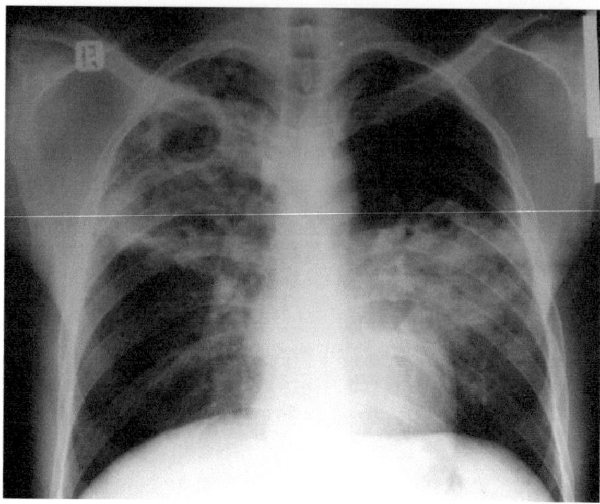

Fig. 21.4 Plain chest radiograph with characteristic appearances of advanced pulmonary TB

be readily obtained to confirm the diagnosis. However, any body system may be affected by TB, and extrapulmonary disease may pose diagnostic challenges, particularly in those with associated immunosuppression, such as HIV co-infection. Commoner presentations may include cervical and/or mediastinal lymphadenopathy, pleural and pericardial effusions, abdominal lymphadenopathy, ascites and spinal disease. Though less common, disseminated disease and tuberculous meningitis are associated with the highest mortality. Reaching a confirmed diagnosis of extrapulmonary TB relies on the use of appropriate imaging modalities and more invasive means of obtaining tissue or fluid suitable for mycobacterial culture or rapid molecular testing. However, TB treatment often needs to be initiated in some clinical situations prior to microbiological confirmation, which may never be obtained in about half of people with extrapulmonary TB due to lower rates of culture positivity.

21.7 Laboratory Diagnosis

Latent infection with TB/MDR-TB may be diagnosed using the traditional tuberculin skin test and/or the more modern interferon-gamma release assays. The latter are more specific and have a higher positive predictive value for disease within 2 years, though in both cases this is low, and neither has real clinical value in the diagnosis of active TB [20]. Confirming active TB depends on the site of infection. In most cases, this will be pulmonary and spontaneous respiratory specimens may readily confirm the diagnosis by direct visualization by microscopy using the traditional Ziehl-Neelson or Auramine stains, solid or liquid mycobacterial culture or increasingly nucleic acid amplification testing (NAAT) such as the GeneXpert MTB-RIF test [21]. In extrapulmonary TB, a variety of specimens may be used to confirm the diagnosis on histology or culture. NAATs are also clinically useful on some of these specimens (including lymph nodes, pleural and cerebrospinal fluid). NAATs are also the means of rapidly evaluating whether RIF resistance is present. Line probe (HAIN) and real-time PCR (Xpert) assays are available for this purpose and prevent the delay of more than 6 weeks which is typically required for mycobacterial culture and phenotypic testing to be completed. Susceptibility testing for second-line drugs still relies on culture in most high-burden countries but rapid molecular methods for some drugs are now available and resistance prediction from whole genome sequencing is rapidly becoming a reality in some higher-income countries [22].

21.8 Differential Diagnosis

TB should be suspected in anyone with a chronic cough lasting more than 2–3 weeks especially when associated with constitutional symptoms and weight loss, where there was no previous pulmonary disease and initial treatment with antibiotics has been ineffective. Pulmonary imaging appearances are very variable and not specific, mimicking many causes of lower respiratory tract infection. The cavitating lesions associated with advanced severe disease may be confused with anaerobic bacterial or fungal infection, but these will often be much less likely in the clinical context. Extrapulmonary manifestations of TB are manifold and may be confused with many different conditions, particularly other chronic bacterial infections, haematological malignancies and auto-immune disorders. The possibility of MDR-TB should always be considered in people with a history of contact with MDR-TB, a previous history of TB treatment, travel to or origin in a high-burden MDR-TB country or who do not respond to treatment as expected.

21.9 Management

Treatment of MDR-TB is more prolonged, clinically complex and costly than first-line treatment, and until recently, outcomes were sub-optimal. Traditional, longer (18–24 months) regimens comprising four to six drugs remained the norm until 2017, but the advent of newer and more effective second-line drugs, in particular the identification of a critical set of Group A drugs (Bedaquiline, Linezolid, and Fluoroquinolones), has led to rapid changes in WHO and national guidelines [23]. Shorter (9–12 months) all-oral regimens comprising seven drugs have now been used successfully in many countries and will be supplanted in the near future by a novel four-drug, 6-month regimen composed of bedaquiline, pretomanid, linezolid and moxifloxacin, recommended by WHO in 2022 [24]. Despite these advances, tolerability and toxicity of second-line drugs, particularly linezolid, remains an issue, and considerable clinical experience and support is still needed to ensure good clinical outcomes.

Anyone diagnosed with TB in a health facility requires precautionary isolation to prevent onward transmission to unexposed individuals, and close contacts in the community should be screened using skin or interferon-gamma release testing and/or chest radiography if symptomatic. In drug-sensitive TB, contacts testing positive are typically offered treatment of their latent TB infection with 6 months of isoniazid or 3 months of rifampicin and isoniazid (though 1-month rifapentine-isoniazid regimens are increasingly available in some countries). Once 2 weeks of treatment have elapsed and respiratory symptoms have subsided, most people are considered non-infectious and can be released from isolation, whether in hospital or at home. In MDR-TB the consequences of transmission and a lack of evidence on appropriate treatment for latent infection mandate a more cautious approach. Isolation is more prolonged with a higher level of personal respiratory protection for carers, and documented stable sputum smear (and ideally culture) conversion is recommended for release from isolation. People with MDR-TB should not be permitted to travel by air until two negative cultures have been obtained [16]. The use of moxifloxacin for the treatment of latently infected contacts is often suggested. Still, little randomized evidence is yet available to support this practice, and its clinical usefulness depends on the index strain's susceptibility pattern [25].

21.10 Prevention and Advice for Travellers

Given the geographical and occupational variability in the risk of TB exposure, travel advice should be tailored to the individual. Those at higher risk may include health or social care workers, people visiting relatives in high-burden countries and longer-term travellers. Reassurance can be provided on the very low risks of TB transmission during air travel, and generic advice to limit contact with those exhibiting signs of respiratory infection, particularly in higher-risk areas such as homeless hostels, healthcare facilities or prisons, may be appropriate. Though BCG is a part of the global primary immunization schedule and may modestly reduce the risk of TB in adults [26], it is not generally recommended for travellers for whom significant exposure is unlikely unless they are under 16 years of age and have not received primary vaccination. Healthcare workers likely to be in prolonged contact with TB sufferers, especially in countries with a high burden of MDR-TB, should be offered advice about the appropriate use of personal protective equipment and tuberculin skin or interferon-gamma release assay testing prior to departure and, if negative, BCG vaccination. Post-travel follow-up for repeat testing and, if necessary, consideration of chemoprophylaxis will usually be required when returning to employment in their home country [27]. This approach may also be considered in some other high-risk groups based on risk assessment. Travellers with a higher risk of progression to TB disease should they become infected may also be offered pre-travel screening for TB infection, if not already determined, and repeat testing after the return. While the effectiveness of this practice is well-evidenced in those with HIV infection [28], recommendations are less consistent in people with transplants or therapeutic immunosuppression for other reasons and careful clinical consideration and interpretation of testing may be required.

21.11 Knowledge Gaps That Need to Be Addressed

Novel tests that determine not just an individual's infection status but also their risk of progression to disease in the near term would be valuable in decision-making around latent TB infection. The recent development of tests based on transcriptomic signatures may have a modestly increased positive predictive value over the traditional methods but are currently only available for research.

The best strategies for the treatment of latent infection in MDR-TB contacts are currently very unclear. While observational evidence suggests that fluoroquinolone monotherapy may be effective, the results of clinical trials are awaited, and the use of newer drugs with lower rates of pre-existing resistance has yet to be evaluated.

Box 21.1: Key Websites for Travellers and Healthcare Workers
CDC Yellow Book Travel Advice on Tuberculosis https://wwwnc.cdc.gov/travel/yellowbook/2024/infections-diseases/tuberculosis

World Health Organization. Tuberculosis and air travel: guidelines for prevention and control, 3rd edition. 2008. Available from: www.who.int/publications/i/item/9789241547505

World Health Organisation, Tuberculosis topic page https://www.who.int/health-topics/tuberculosis#tab=tab_1

TB Drug Monographs Available at : http://www.tbdrugmonographs.co.uk/

Box 21.2: Things Commonly Forgotten
MDR-TB strains do not appear to be more transmissible than drug-sensitive strains

More than 95% of individuals with latent TB infection never develop TB disease

BCG vaccination confers limited protection against adult disease but may still be indicated in healthcare workers at the highest risk of contact with MDR-TB

Interferon-gamma release assays are not a test for TB disease and have low positive predictive value

Evidence is lacking on the best regimens for treatment of latent MDR-TB infection and the susceptibility pattern of the index case will often be unknown

---

Box 21.3: Information Resources for Patients
TB Alert The truth about TB: Your essential guide to TB. Available at : https://www.thetruthabouttb.org/

CDC patient and general public materials. Available at : https://www.cdc.gov/tb/education/patient_edmaterials.htm

Acknowledgments None.

Declarations of Conflict of Interest None.

References

1. Donoghue H. Paleomicrobiology of human tuberculosis. Microbiol Spectr. 2016;4(4) https://doi.org/10.1128/microbiolspec.PoH-0003-2014.
2. World Health Organisation 2022 Global tuberculosis report. https://www.who.int/teams/global-tuberculosis-programme/tb-reports/global-tuberculosis-report-2022
3. Dean AS, Tosas Auguet O, Glaziou P, Zignol M, Ismail N, Kasaeva T, Floyd K. 25 years of surveillance of drug-resistant tuberculosis: achievements, challenges, and way forward. Lancet Infect Dis. 2022;22:e191–6.
4. Coscolla M, Gagneux S, Menardo F, Loiseau C, Ruiz-Rodriguez P, Borrell S, Otchere I, Asante-Poku A, Asare P, Sanchez-Buso L, Gehre F, Sanoussi N, Antonio M, Affolabi D, Fyfe J, Beckert P, Niemann S, Alabi AS, Grobusch M, Kobbe R, Parkhill J, Beisel C, Fenner L, Bottger EC, Meehan CJ, Harris RS, de Jong B, Yeboah-Manu D, Brites D. Phylogenomics of *Mycobacterium africanum* reveals a new lineage and a complex evolutionary history. Microb Genom. 2021;7:000477. https://doi.org/10.1099/mgen.0.000477.
5. Du DH, Geskus RB, Zhao Y, Codecasa LR, Cirillo DM, van Crevel R, Pascupurnama DN, Chaidir L, Niemann S, Diel R, Omar SV, Grandjean L, Rokadiya S, Ortitz RT, Lan NH, Ha D, Smith EG, Robinson E, Dedicoat M, Nhat L, Thwaites G, Van L, Thuong N, Walker T. The effect of M. tuberculosis lineage on clinical phenotype. PLOS Global Public Health. medRxiv. Preprint. 2023; https://doi.org/10.1101/2023.03.14.23287284.
6. de Jong BC, Antonio M, Gagneux S. Mycobacterium africanum—review of an important cause of human tuberculosis in West Africa. PLoS Negl Trop Dis. 2010;4:e744. https://doi.org/10.1371/journal.pntd.0000744.
7. Karmakar M, Trauer JM, Ascher DB, Denholm JT. Hyper transmission of Beijing lineage Mycobacterium tuberculosis: systematic review and meta-analysis. J Infect. 2019;79:572–81. https://doi.org/10.1016/j.jinf.2019.09.016.
8. Dookie N, Rambaran S, Padayatchi N, Mahomed S, Naidoo K. Evolution of drug resistance in Mycobacterium tuberculosis: a review on the molecular determinants of resistance and implications for personalized care. J Antimicrob Chemother. 2018;73:1138–51. https://doi.org/10.1093/jac/dkx506.
9. Walker TM, Miotto P, Koser C, Fowler P, Knaggs J, Iqbal Z, Hunt M, Chindelevich L, Farhat M, Cirillo DM, Comas I, Posey J, Omar SV, Peto T, Suresh A, Uplekar S, Laurent S, Colman RE, Nathanson C, Zignol M, Walker SA, CryPTIC Consortium, Seq&Treat consortium, Crook DW, Ismail N, Rodwell T. The 2021 WHO catalogue of Mycobacterium tuberculosis complex mutations associated with drug resistance: a genotypic analysis. Lancet Microbe. 2022;3:e265–73.
10. Williams CM, Abdulwhhab M, Birring SS, De Kock E, Garton NJ, Townsend E, Pareek M, Al-Taie A, Pan J, Ganatra R, Stoltz AC, Haldar P, Barer MR. Exhaled Mycobacterium tuberculosis output and detection of subclinical disease by face-mask sampling: prospective observational studies. Lancet Infect Dis. 2020;20:607–17. https://doi.org/10.1016/S1473-3099(19)30707-8.
11. Cohen KA, Abeel T, Manson McGuire A, Desjardins CA, Munsamy V, Shea TP, Walker BJ, Bantubani N, Almeida DV, Alvarado L, Chapman SB, Mvelase NR, Duffy EY, Fitzgerald MG, Govender P, Gujja S, Hamilton S, Howarth C, Larimer JD, Maharaj K, Pearson MD, Priest ME, Zeng Q, Padayatchi N, Grosset J, Young SK, Wortman J, Mlisana KP, O'Donnell MR, Birren BW, Bishai WR, Pym AS, Earl AM. Evolution of extensively drug-resistant tuberculosis over four decades: whole genome sequencing and dating analysis of Mycobacterium tuberculosis isolates from KwaZulu-Natal. PLoS Med. 2015;12:e1001880. https://doi.org/10.1371/journal.pmed.1001880.

12. Alame Emane AK, Guo X, Takiff HE, Liu S. Drug resistance, fitness and compensatory mutations in Mycobacterium tuberculosis. Tuberculosis (Edinb). 2021;129:102091. https://doi.org/10.1016/j.tube.2021.102091.

13. Houben RM, Dodd PJ. The global burden of latent tuberculosis infection: a re-estimation using mathematical modelling. PLoS Med. 2016;13:e1002152. https://doi.org/10.1371/journal.pmed.1002152.

14. Joshi R, Reingold AL, Menzies D, Pai M. Tuberculosis among healthcare workers in low- and middle-income countries: a systematic review. PLoS Med. 2006;3:e494. https://doi.org/10.1371/journal.pmed.0030494.

15. Diefenbach-Elstob TR, Alabdulkarim B, Deb-Rinker P, Pernica JM, Schwarzer G, Menzies D, Shrier I, Schwartzman K, Greenaway C. Risk of latent and active tuberculosis infection in travellers: a systematic review and meta-analysis. J Travel Med. 2021;28:taaa214. https://doi.org/10.1093/jtm/taaa214.

16. Eimer J, Patimeteeporn C, Jensenius M, Gkrania-Klotsas E, Duvignaud A, Barnett ED, Hochberg NS, Chen LH, Trigo-Esteban E, Gertler M, Greenaway C, Grobusch MP, Angelo KM, Hamer DH, Caumes E, Asgeirsson H. Multidrug-resistant tuberculosis imported into low-incidence countries-a GeoSentinel analysis, 2008–2020. J Travel Med. 2021;28:taab069. https://doi.org/10.1093/jtm/taab069.

17. Kenyon TA, Valway SE, Ihle WW, Onorato IM, Castro KG. Transmission of multidrug-resistant Mycobacterium tuberculosis during a long airplane flight. N Engl J Med. 1996;334:933–8. https://doi.org/10.1056/NEJM199604113341501.

18. Abubakar I. Tuberculosis and air travel: a systematic review and analysis of policy. Lancet Infect Dis. 2010;10:176–83. https://doi.org/10.1016/S1473-3099(10)70028-1.

19. Pai M, Behr MA, Dowdy D, Dheda K, Divangahi M, Boehme CC, Ginsberg A, Swaminathan S, Spigelman M, Getahun H, Menzies D, Raviglione M. Tuberculosis. Nat Rev Dis Primers. 2016;2:16076. https://doi.org/10.1038/nrdp.2016.76.

20. Zhou G, Luo Q, Luo S, Teng Z, Ji Z, Yang J, Wang F, Wen S, Ding Z, Li L, Chen T, Abi ME, Jian M, Luo L, Liu A, Bao F. Interferon-γ release assays or tuberculin skin test for detection and management of latent tuberculosis infection: a systematic review and meta-analysis. Lancet Infect Dis. 2020;20:1457–69. https://doi.org/10.1016/S1473-3099(20)30276-0.

21. Horne DJ, Kohli M, Zifodya JS, Schiller I, Dendukuri N, Tollefson D, Schumacher SG, Ochodo EA, Pai M, Steingart KR. Xpert MTB/RIF and Xpert MTB/RIF Ultra for pulmonary tuberculosis and rifampicin resistance in adults. Cochrane Database Syst Rev. 2019;6:CD009593. https://doi.org/10.1002/14651858.CD009593.pub4.

22. CRyPTIC Consortium and the 100,000 Genomes Project, Allix-Béguec C, Arandjelovic I, Bi L, Beckert P, Bonnet M, Bradley P, Cabibbe AM, Cancino-Muñoz I, Caulfield MJ, Chaiprasert A, Cirillo DM, Clifton DA, Comas I, Crook DW, De Filippo MR, de Neeling H, Diel R, Drobniewski FA, Faksri K, Farhat MR, Fleming J, Fowler P, Fowler TA, Gao Q, Gardy J, Gascoyne-Binzi D, Gibertoni-Cruz AL, Gil-Brusola A, Golubchik T, Gonzalo X, Grandjean L, He G, Guthrie JL, Hoosdally S, Hunt M, Iqbal Z, Ismail N, Johnston J, Khanzada FM, Khor CC, Kohl TA, Kong C, Lipworth S, Liu Q, Maphalala G, Martinez E, Mathys V, Merker M, Miotto P, Mistry N, Moore DAJ, Murray M, Niemann S, Omar SV, Ong RT, Peto TEA, Posey JE, Prammananan T, Pym A, Rodrigues C, Rodrigues M, Rodwell T, Rossolini GM, Sánchez Padilla E, Schito M, Shen X, Shendure J, Sintchenko V, Sloutsky A, Smith EG, Snyder M, Soetaert K, Starks AM, Supply P, Suriyapol P, Tahseen S, Tang P, Teo YY, Thuong TNT, Thwaites G, Tortoli E, van Soolingen D, Walker AS, Walker TM, Wilcox M, Wilson DJ, Wyllie D, Yang Y, Zhang H, Zhao Y, Zhu B. Prediction of susceptibility to first-line tuberculosis drugs by DNA sequencing. N Engl J Med. 2018;379:1403–15. https://doi.org/10.1056/NEJMoa1800474.

23. World Health Organisation. WHO consolidated guidelines on tuberculosis. Module 4: treatment—drug-resistant tuberculosis treatment, 2022 update. Available at : https://www.who.int/publications/i/item/9789240063129.

24. Nyang'wa BT, Berry C, Kazounis E, Motta I, Parpieva N, Tigay Z, Solodovnikova V, Liverko I, Moodliar R, Dodd M, Ngubane N, Rassool M, McHugh TD, Spigelman M, Moore DAJ, Ritmeijer K, du Cros P, Fielding K, TB-PRACTECAL Study Collaborators. A 24-week, all-

oral regimen for Rifampicin-resistant tuberculosis. N Engl J Med. 2022;387:2331–43. https://doi.org/10.1056/NEJMoa2117166.

25. Kherabi Y, Tunesi S, Kay A, Guglielmetti L. Preventive therapy for contacts of drug-resistant tuberculosis. Pathogens. 2022;11:1189.
26. Mangtani P, Abubakar I, Ariti C, Beynon R, Pimpin L, Fine PE, Rodrigues LC, Smith PG, Lipman M, Whiting PF, Sterne JA. Protection by BCG vaccine against tuberculosis: a systematic review of randomized controlled trials. Clin Infect Dis. 2014;58:470–80. https://doi.org/10.1093/cid/cit790.
27. Seaworth BJ, Armitige LY, Aronson NE, Hoft D, Fleenor M, Gardner AF, Harris DA, Stricof RL, Nardell EA. Multidrug-resistant tuberculosis. Recommendations for reducing risk during travel for healthcare and humanitarian work. Ann Am Thorac Soc. 2014;11:286–95. https://doi.org/10.1513/AnnalsATS.201309-312PS.
28. British HIV Association. BHIVA guidelines for the management of tuberculosis in adults living with HIV 2018 (2023 interim update). Available at: https://www.bhiva.org/TB-guidelines

Malaria in Travellers

22

Eskild Petersen and Martin P. Grobusch

Abstract

Travellers visiting areas where transmission of malaria occurs are at risk of infection. Detailed knowledge of malaria endemicity is therefore needed to be able to provide travellers with guidance on the prevention of malaria. In returning travellers, the key symptom of malaria infection is fever, and any patients presenting to the health care system should be asked, "Have you been travelling?" Diagnostics are reviewed. Imported malaria is a rare diagnosis, and expertise in microscopy may be difficult to maintain. Rapid diagnostic tests and molecular methods are replacing microscopy for initial diagnosis.

Treatment options are discussed, and especially in patients with severe malaria, the hospital taking care of the patient must have artesunate available. Treatment is special risk groups such as pregnant women and children are discussed.

E. Petersen (✉)
Institute for Clinical Medicine, Faculty of Health Science, University of Aarhus, Aarhus, Denmark

ESCMID Emerging Infections Task Force, Basel, Switzerland

M. P. Grobusch
Center of Tropical Medicine and Travel Medicine, Department of Infectious Diseases, Amsterdam University Medical Centers, University of Amsterdam, Amsterdam, The Netherlands
e-mail: m.p.grobusch@amsterdamumc.nl

© The Author(s), under exclusive license to Springer Nature Switzerland AG 2024
H. Leblebicioglu et al. (eds.), *Emerging and Re-emerging Infections in Travellers*, https://doi.org/10.1007/978-3-031-49475-8_22

22.1   Introduction

Diagnosing and managing malaria as an infrequently encountered infectious disease are challenging for many physicians in non-endemic areas. Malaria symptoms are non-specific and cannot easily be distinguished from other febrile conditions on clinical grounds alone [1, 2]. Thus, a high degree of suspicion is needed, and a travel history is mandatory for any febrile patient presenting with non-specific, often flu-like signs and symptoms.

22.2   Epidemiology of Imported Malaria

The pattern of imported malaria is defined by traffic between endemic and non-endemic areas. Between 2005 and 2015, the West Africa region accounted for 56% (13,947/24941) of all imported cases to non-endemic countries. France and the United Kingdom received the highest number of cases, with an average of over 4000 reported cases per year [3]. Malaria in migrants and travellers visiting friends and relatives (VFRs) in malaria-endemic areas continues to increase and is as important as malaria in returning travellers [4, 5].

Countries strongly linked by movements of imported cases are grouped by historical, language, and travel ties; and there is strong spatial clustering of Plasmodium species according to country of infection. The WHO recently introduced the 'Global Technical Strategy for Malaria 2016–2030,' aiming to reduce malaria morbidity and mortality by 90% by 2030 [6]. A new component in the fight against malaria is the use of the RTS,S vaccine [6]. However, the vaccine will not currently be offered to travellers where chemoprophylaxis has higher protective efficacy. Still, successor vaccines are on the horizon [7], of which some are of potential interest for further development as traveller vaccines, as well as people living in areas of highly seasonal endemicity. However, we will not cover malaria vaccines at the time of writing in this chapter.

It is estimated that 25–30 million individuals travel annually from Europe to areas with malaria transmission. Malaria imported to Europe is seen in travellers returning from endemic areas and migrants living in Europe returning from visiting friends and relatives (VFR) [3, 5]. VFR children are particularly at risk. In 2019, the ECDC reported 8641 malaria cases in the EU/EEA [8]. The majority of imported cases remains uncomplicated [1, 5], and the mortality of imported *Plasmodium falciparum* malaria cases varies from 0.4% in a large cohort from France up to 5% in a cluster of cases imported from The Gambia [9, 10].

One study found that the crude malaria risk for travellers (all species) varied from 1 per 100,000 travellers to Central America and the Caribbean to 357 per 100,000 in Central Africa [11].

In a 20-year (1998–2018) EuroTravNet cohort of almost 120,000 patients with imported infectious diseases to Europe, malaria was the number-two diagnosis for patients seen during and after travel, amounting to 7195 or 6.9% of all cases. Most (6370; 88.5%) were from sub-Saharan Africa, of which 5082 (79.8%) were falciparum malaria. Of all cases, 3407/7195 (47.3%) were in VRFs. Among 11,239 migrants, 337 (3.0%) had falciparum malaria, and 204 (1.8%) had vivax malaria [5]. In this largest cohort of travellers described to date, the overall proportion of deaths was below 0.05%); however, malaria patients had a 2,5:1 risk ratio of dying as compared to all patients with other diagnoses [5].

More than 5 million African migrants may currently be living in Europe, one-third of them originating from sub-Saharan Africa. VFRs travelling to sub-Saharan Africa have more than eight times the risk of being diagnosed with malaria compared to tourists and more than twice the odds of being diagnosed with malaria after travel to Asia [12]. VFR children are particularly at risk [13]. Malaria chemoprophylaxis is effective, but when and where to use it in addition to repellents and long-lasting impregnated bednets, especially in low-risk areas, is not generally agreed upon [14].

22.2.1 Rare Modes of Transmission

Rare modes of transmission mean that patients with fever and without a travel history to endemic areas might need to be tested for malaria. These include so-called 'airport malaria', or 'Odyssean malaria' [15], where *Anopheles* mosquitoes carrying malaria parasites are transported by aeroplane to a non-endemic area and take a blood meal from someone living close to the destination airport [16]. Malaria parasites can also be transmitted in blood as a consequence of intravenous drug use and blood transfusion [17, 18] or even nosocomially transmitted in hospitals with no apparent mode of transmission [19]. Organ transplants are also a risk [20].

22.3 Clinical Symptoms

22.3.1 Clinical Symptoms in Non-immune Individuals (Persons Not Born and Raised in Endemic Areas)

It is important to distinguish between complicated and uncomplicated malaria (Table 22.1).

Management of complicated malaria needs a multi-speciality team and often requires admission to an intensive care unit, ICU, for ventilator treatment, pressor support and dialysis. The management of complicated malaria is outside the scope of this chapter.

The WHO has published detailed guidelines, but the key is that in non-immune subjects, a parasitaemia below 2% is regarded as uncomplicated except for symptoms like hypotension, kidney failure, or acidosis [21]. However, unlike in other species, the vast majority of the parasite biomass is sequestered in falciparum malaria; thus, parasitaemia is an unreliable proxy for severity. With regard to management, early suspicion and subsequent swift diagnosis and treatment are key to management, which also needs to account for pathophysiological peculiarities such

Table 22.1 Laboratory indicators of a poor clinical prognosis in severe malaria

Hyperparasitaemia	>250.000/µl or > 2% of infected erythrocytes in non-immunes and > 5% in semi-immune individuals
	Schizonts of *P. Falciparum* in peripheral blood
Haemoglobin	< 5 g/dl or packed cell volume (haematocrit) < 0.15
Coagulation disturbances	Platelets (thrombocytes) < 50.000/µl
	Prothrombin time prolonged > 3 s
	Prolonged partial thromboplastin time
	Fibrinogen < 200 mg/dl
	Low antithrombin III levels
Hypoglycaemia	<2.2 mmol/l (<40 mg/dl)
Acidosis	Venous HCO_3 < 15 mmol/l and/or arterial pH < 7.3
	Lactate > 5 mmol/l
Renal function	Serum creatinine > 3.0 mg/dl (>265 mmol/l)
	Estimated creatinin clearance
	Blood urea nitrogen > 60 mg/dl
	Haemoglobinuria
Liver function	More than threefold elevation of aminotransferases (AST, ALT)

as restrictive fluid management to avoid iatrogenic aggravation of the disease course [22].

Most infections due to *P. falciparum* in non-immunes become symptomatic mostly shortly after a minimum incubation period of 10 days until about 42 days after return from a malaria-endemic area, but longer incubation periods are seen with the other species and in persons with semi-immunity from previous exposures [21].

A study from Portugal including 284 patients (46% non-immunes and 54% semi-immunes) found that the diagnosis was made between the day of return from the malarious area and up to 47 days later; a single non-immune patient was first diagnosed on the 120th day after leaving Angola [23].

Prodromal symptoms, which may precede fever for up to 2 days, are fatigue, loss of appetite, headache and body pains. In non-immune patients, malaria usually starts suddenly with a severe feeling of sickness and fever, often reaching 39 °C or higher [1, 2]. Not all patients show fever paroxysms, and the absence of fever should not alleviate the suspicion of malaria in an ill patient until proven otherwise. A regular fever pattern is not always present. Especially in *P. falciparum* malaria, the fever is usually not regular, at least not during the first few days, which is essential in establishing a timely diagnosis before progression to severe disease is imminent. If present, the frequency of the febrile episodes depends on the parasite species, occurring every 48 h (tertian) for *P. vivax* and *P. ovale*, every 72 h (quartan) for *P. malariae* and 24 h (quotidian) for *P. knowlesi*.

Very common symptoms are headache and myalgia. Other signs and symptoms may include nausea, vomiting, dry cough, confusion and respiratory distress. Compromised circulation leads to low blood pressure, renal failure and impaired tissue perfusion, resulting in acidosis. Gastrointestinal complaints unrelated to treatment, including vomiting and diarrhoea are less frequent. Patients with significant fever paroxysms may initially have a normal temperature between the fevers and feel relatively well.

Clinical examination is non-specific or even completely unremarkable. It often takes some days before anaemia develops. Splenomegaly is seen regularly very early due to the sequestering of parasitized erys, and usually resolves promptly after successful treatment. Coryza, swelling of lymph nodes and eosinophilia are not seen in malaria [21].

22.3.2 Clinical Symptoms in Persons Migrating from Malaria-Endemic Areas

Malaria in adult migrants from malaria-endemic areas usually exhibit some degree of natural immunity. This immunity is not sterile and malaria parasites can still be found either in asymptomatic infections or in the clinical disease characterized by a milder clinical presentation, lower levels of parasitaemia, shorter parasite clearance time after treatment and shorter fever duration compared to malaria in travellers due to previously acquired semi-immunity [2, 21, 24, 25]. Children born in Europe to migrant parents are not immune.

A high proportion of migrants have few symptoms and are present long after arrival in the host country [26], with periods of months up to more than 14 years recorded [27]. If semi-immunity is lost, migrants who travel to their country of origin would have a risk of clinical malaria approaching that of travellers born in non-endemic countries. However, a degree of clinical immunity against severe malaria may be retained. A high prevalence (from 7.1% to 31.8%) of *P. falciparum* infection (detected by PCR) has been found among asymptomatic sub-Saharan African migrants after their migration to Europe [28].

22.4 Indications for Malaria Diagnostics

Diagnostic tests for malaria should be performed in any ill patient who has a history of travel to a malaria endemic area, whether or not they are febrile at presentation and whether or not malaria chemoprophylaxis has been used. Testing should be extended to persons with fever with no obvious course, as rare modes of transmission is possible.

22.4.1 Non-specific Laboratory Results

The most consistent finding is thrombocytopaenia, and a study from the United Kingdom found that children with malaria and a platelet count of <50,000 per ml had an odds ratio of 8.3 for admission to intensive care units [29]. However, it should be noted that thrombocytes retain their full functionality and that malaria patients 'do not bleed' on the grounds of thrombocytopaenia only unless there are complicating factors such as translocation of non-typhoidal salmonellae into the bloodstream, with resulting disseminated intravascular coagulation as a complication.

With the white blood cell count remaining unafflicted in uncomplicated malaria, an elevated neutrophil count suggests bacteria co-infection and potential progression towards sepsis. The C-reactive protein, procalcitonin, fibrinogen may be raised during a malaria attack. Thrombocytopaenia with decreased concentration of fibrinogen and elevated fibrin degradation products strongly suggest disseminated intravascular coagulation (DIC). Bicarbonate concentration is reduced and lactate may be elevated in metabolic acidosis.

Serum creatinine and urea, total and conjugated bilirubin and liver transaminases may be raised. Hypoglycaemia may occur and is related to high parasitaemia and severe lactic acidosis [30]. Signs and symptoms indicating severe and complicated malaria are shown in Table 22.1.

Blood cultures should be obtained on admission as malaria infection can be complicated by septicaemia [31]; in any case if a patient does not defervescence (becomes afebrile) within an appropriate timeframe after therapy initiation, and if the white blood cell count deviates from normal. All patients with malaria should have the following obtained at the time of diagnosis: haemoglobin, MCV, MCHC, differential white blood cell (WBC) count, platelets, blood urea nitrogen or creatinine, alanine transferase, basic phosphatase and LDH. In complicated malaria, this should be supplemented with tests for DIC and arterial blood for pH, lactate (arterial), blood gases and blood cultures. Additional potentially useful parameters include chest x-ray, urine culture, ECG, potassium, urea, ALT,

haptoglobin, fibrinogen.

22.4.2 Malaria-Specific Diagnostics

The gold standard for malaria diagnosis is light microscopy of Giemsa-stained thin and thick blood films, which requires a high level of expertise [32].

This is not always available around the clock outside specialized centres and rapid diagnostic tests (RDTs) are increasingly used. Unless expert microscopy is warranted, they follow WHO guidelines mandatorily preceding treatment initiation in resource-poor settings. However, RDTs come with limitations, and once a malaria diagnosis has been made, the infecting species present must be determined [33].

Parasitaemia (expressed as the number of parasites per microlitre of blood or as a percentage of red cells infected) is an essential parameter for determining whether the patient has complicated malaria or not and to monitor treatment efficacy.

Early diagnosis is important to prevent uncomplicated malaria from progressing into a complicated disease. Patients with malaria should be managed in centres with the ability to quantify the parasitaemia. Expert malaria microscopy has a threshold of around five parasites per microliter of blood [34].

After the start of treatment, there is a lag phase before the parasite density begins to decline [35], and there may even be an increase in the first 24 h after starting treatment.

For *P.falciparum* malaria, many RDTs yield a close-to-100% parasite detection score down to a parasite density level of 200 per microlitre, equivalent to a parasitaemia of approximately 0.004% [33]. Polymerase chain reaction (PCR) can detect parasites down to a density of 0.01 parasites per microlitre after a lysis procedure and one parasite per microlitre without lysis [36] but are impractical for routine ad-hoc emergency diagnosis [37]. RDTs are increasingly used in medical centres with limited access to experienced microscopists; however, a rapid test (even if a 'pan-specific' aldolase or pLDH is used as antigen, with the latter being advantageous if non-falciparum species are suspected based on epidemiological reasoning) cannot determine the parasite density and may miss infections with *P.ovale, P.vivax, P.malariae* and *P.knowlesi*. Mutations in the HRP2 gene may also result in false negative tests [38].

Microscopy and rapid diagnostic tests (RDTs) are the primary choices for diagnosing malaria in the field. Still, neither method is capable of detecting low-density malaria infections, which are common in both low- and high-transmission settings. Nucleic acid amplification tests (NAATs) enable sensitive detection of low-density malaria infections (below one parasite/μL). The use of NAATs can be broadly divided into four roles: qualitative or quantitative parasite detection, determination of the multiplicity of infection, genotyping to distinguish recrudescence from reinfection and detection of drug resistance mutations [39].

Clinicians using rapid tests should be instructed that no RDT test so far is 100% reliable and that they should be used in parallel to and not instead of blood film examination. To reduce the risk of missing malaria, testing with blood films and RDTs should be performed on three blood samples taken at daily intervals for patients with high suspicion of malaria. If the suspicion of malaria remains after three negative samples, expert advice should be obtained from a tropical or infectious diseases specialist. Once the diagnosis has been made, the patient should have daily blood films until they are negative for asexual parasites (i.e. rings, trophozoites, schizonts). Gametocytes do not multiply or cause clinical illness and may remain after clearance of the asexual parasitaemia.

It is important that centres managing malaria patients are able to count the parasite density, i.e. know the parasitaemia [40]. RDTs and NAAT do not provide validated parasite density assessment, so microscopy is needed.

22.5 Treatment of Uncomplicated *P. Falciparum* Malaria

Treatment should provide rapid clinical and parasitological cure within 3 days. Oral artemisinin combination therapy, ACT, is the standard treatment of uncomplicated malaria as recommended by WHO, see Table 22.2 [41]. Currently, artemether/lumefantrine and dihydroartemisinin/piperaquine, another ACT formulation marketed in many countries, are the drug combinations of choice. Artemether/lumefantrine is

Table 22.2 Treatment of uncomplicated falciparum malaria in adults (WHO 2022)

Artemether/lumefantrine (Riamet™; 20/120 mg)	
Dosage	Twice daily for 3 days >35 kg: 4 tablets each 20 mg/120 mg for 6 doses (0–8–24–36–48–60 h)
	Take with fatty food
Dihydroartemisinin/piperaquine (Eurartesim™)	
Dosage	Once daily for 3 days 36 < 75 kg: 3 tablets each 320 mg/40 mg, 75–100 kg: 4 tablets each 320 mg/40 mg, daily for 3 days
	Fasting, at least 3 h after last meal
Atovaquone/proguanil (Malarone™)	
Dosage	Once daily for 3 days >40 kg: 4 tablets each 250/100 mg
	Take with fatty food
Mefloquine (Lariam™)	Total dose divided into 2–3 doses 6–8 h apart
	45–60 kg: 5 tablets (3 + 2 tablets) >60 kg: 6 tablets (3 + 2 + 1 tablets)

Other drug combinations that is recommended by the WHO is: artesunate + amodiaquine; artesunate + mefloquine; artesunate + sulfadoxine–pyrimethamine (SP) (WHO 2022 pp. 82, 5.2.1)

well tolerated and highly effective in all endemic regions except for *P. falciparum* infections acquired in Cambodia and the border regions of Thailand with Myanmar, where multidrug-resistant *P. falciparum* strains are highly prevalent.

Artemether/lumefantrine has to be administered with fatty food to obtain optimal plasma drug concentrations, see Table 22.2 [42].

Atovaquone/proguanil can be used as first-line treatment for uncomplicated malaria and needs to be administered with fatty food to increase bioavailability. However, parasite clearance times are slower than ACTs, so ACTs should be preferred before atovaquone-proguanil is used.

Second-line anti-malarial treatments include mefloquine monotherapy but a high prevalence of mefloquine resistance is common in Thailand, Myanmar and Cambodia. Quinine drug combinations have excellent efficacy, but tolerability is generally poor due to prolonged treatment courses and the occurrence of characteristic adverse effects [43].

The use of chloroquine is not recommended for the treatment of *P. falciparum* malaria because of widespread resistance. In the case of failed anti-malarial chemoprophylaxis, an anti-malarial drug different from the chemoprophylactic drug taken should be used for treatment. Finally, it is important to note that even though oral anti-malarials are recommended for the treatment of uncomplicated malaria, it is sometimes necessary for the responsible physician to use intravenous treatment with artesunate as recommended for treating severe malaria. This decision may be made based on evidence of important co-morbidities, intractable vomiting, or clinical concerns of the physician. The clinical criteria for severe malaria are shown in Table 22.1. The WHO defined a parasitaemia of 2% or more as severe malaria in non-immunes and 5% or more in patients from endemic areas [21].

Patients suffering from *P. falciparum* malaria should, in general, be admitted to a hospital since monitoring of prognostic parameters, including parasitaemia, treatment adherence, and, if needed, transfer to intensive care units, should be instantly available. Repeated blood pressure monitoring, urinary output and oxygen saturation may be indicated. However, management as outpatients may be considered in uncomplicated cases in some healthcare systems where daily follow-up until clearance of parasitaemia and fever and monitoring of treatment adherence can be undertaken. Persons migrating from malaria-endemic regions may fall into this category.

In low-transmission areas, a single dose of 0.25 mg/kg primaquine with ACT is given to patients with *P. falciparum* malaria (except pregnant women, infants aged <6 months and women breastfeeding infants aged <6 months) to reduce transmission. G6PD testing is not required [21].

The management of malaria in non-endemic areas may vary between centres. For example, in a prospective study of over 500 patients from five European countries treated between 2003 and 2009, 18 different combination regimens were used [44]. To standardize management based on current evidence, this paper reviews malaria management for non-specialists and advocates how it should be practised in Europe.

22.5.1 Treatment of Complicated Falciparum Malaria

The clinical criteria for severe malaria are shown in Table 22.1. Severe malaria may also be caused by species other than *P. falciparum*, especially *P. knowlesi* and *P. vivax*.

22.5.2 Intravenous Artesunate (IVA)

IVA is superior to intravenous quinine (IVQ) in overall survival and safer and simpler to administer [45, 46]. IVA is administered as 2.4 mg per kilogram of body weight every 12 h on day 1 and then once daily up to 12 mg per kilogram in five doses over 3 days [21]. IVA should be the drug of choice for the treatment of severe malaria. IVA should be completed with an entire course of ACT, atovaquone/proguanil or mefloquine.

A recent study reported haemolytic anaemia in six out of 25 patients treated with IVA for severe imported malaria diagnosed 14–31 days after the first dose of IVA. IVA treatment may be complicated with haemolytic anaemia, and patients should be monitored twice weekly for 4 weeks following IVA for haemolysis and leukopaenia [47, 48]. Therefore, patients receiving IVA should be followed with twice weekly haemoglobin tests for 4 weeks after treatment.

There is no single supportive therapy regimen which has proven effective, and in times of artesunate therapy, exchange transfusions are obsolete. Of importance, fluid management ought to be restrictive [49].

22.6 Paediatric Malaria

Paediatric dosages are shown in Table 22.3. For imported cases, the risk of developing severe malaria is very high in VFR children without acquired semi-immunity and who are often more exposed to malaria [50]. Migrants' children are less likely

Table 22.3 Treatment of uncomplicated falciparum malaria in children (WHO 2022)

Artemether/lumefantrine (Riamet™; 20/120 mg)	
Dosage	5–14 kg: 1 tablet per dose 15–24 kg: 2 tablets per dose
	25–34 kg: 3 tablets per dose
	>35 kg: 4 tablets per dose
	Dosing: 0–8–24–36–48–60 h
Dihydroartemisinin/piperaquine (Eurartesim™)	
Dosage	5–<7 kg: 1/2 tablet 160 mg/20 mg
	7–<13 kg 1 tablet 160 mg/20 mg
	13–<24 kg: 1 tablet 320 mg/40 mg
	24–<36 kg: 2 tablets 320 mg/20 mg
	36–< 75 kg: 3 tablets 320 mg/40 mg
	75–100 kg: 4 tablets 320 mg/40 mg once daily for 3 days
Atovaquone/proguanil (Malarone Paediatric™)	
	5–8 kg: 2 tablets Malarone Paediatric 9–10 kg: 3 tablets Malarone Paediatric 11–20 kg: 1 tablet Malarone
	21–30 kg: 2 tablets Malarone
	31–40 kg: 3 tablets Malarone
	>40 kg: 4 tablets Malaroneonce daily for 3 days
Mefloquine (Lariam™)	5–10 kg: 1/2–1 tablet 10–20 kg: 1–2 tablets
	20–30 kg: 2–3 tablets (2 + 1) 30–45 kg: 3–4 tablets (2 + 2) 45–60 kg: 5 tablets (3 + 2)
	>60 kg 6 tablets (3 + 2 + 1)
	20–25 mg/kg total dose divided into 1–3 doses 6 h apart

to complain of chills, arthralgia/ myalgia or headaches. Treatment of children is comparable to treatment of adult patients and relies on the classification of uncomplicated and severe falciparum malaria (Table 22.1). Clinical assessment of the inability to walk, stand, sit, or feed is a useful clinical indicator for severe disease in endemic regions, and it may be a particularly useful clinical indicator for very young children. A study of 0.5 mg/kg/day of primaquine in children where G6PD deficiency was excluded found good tolerability [51]. Anti-malarial treatment in infants younger than 12 months of age is complex due to the lack of clinical trial data [49].

22.7 Pregnant Women

Pregnant women are at increased risk for malaria-related morbidity and mortality. This increased risk extends to the post-partum period [52]. Pregnant women visiting endemic areas or arriving from areas of malaria transmission are at greater risk of clinical malaria during pregnancy [26] than non-pregnant women. Malaria parasites cross the placenta and consequently the disease can occur in newborns from asymptomatic mothers [53].

Table 22.4 Treatment of uncomplicated malaria in pregnancy

P. falciparum	
1st trimester (1)	Quinine/clindamycin quinine monotherapy
2nd and third trimester	Artemether/lumefantrine
P. Ovale, P. Malariae and *P. Vivax* (2)	
All trimesters	Oral chloroquine
2nd and third trimester	Artemether/lumefantrine or dihydroartemisinin/piperaquine

1. Artemether/lumefantrine is not the first drug of choice due to a lack of data on lumefantrine in pregnancy but it should be used if quinine is not available
2. Primaquine should not be used because of the risk of foetal haemolytic anaemia

Suggested treatment for uncomplicated malaria in pregnant women is shown in Table 22.4. In complicated malaria, effective treatment with artesunate should be used to save the life of the mother, even if there are safety concerns regarding the drug used. Quinine, chloroquine, clindamycin and proguanil are considered safe in the first trimester but are outside the scope of this chapter, and WHO guidelines should be consulted [21]. An analysis of women exposed to mefloquine around the time of conception and in the first trimester showed no increased risk of malformations in the offspring [54].

Pregnant women presenting with malaria in the first trimester should be treated with quinine and clindamycin for 7 days. Alternatives to artemether/lumefantrine in the second and third trimesters are quinine plus clindamycin or artesunate plus clindamycin [55] for 7 days in each case or mefloquine monotherapy for regions without multidrug-resistant parasites. Primaquine and tetracyclines should not be used in pregnancy. Atovaquone/proguanil is not recommended in pregnancy due to lack of data but can be used in situations where no other drugs are available.

22.7.1 Treatment of *P. Vivax, P. Ovale, P. Malariae* and *P. Knowlesi*

Plasmodium ovale and *P. malariae* generally remain sensitive to chloroquine in all endemic areas, despite reports of delayed parasite clearance time [56]. *Plasmodium vivax* sensitivity to chloroquine has declined steadily in Indonesia, Peru and Oceania, and ACT is the drug of choice here. The use of artemether/lumefantrine has been suggested as a pragmatic choice in areas with chloroquine-resistant P. vivax [57], and it may also be used in mixed infections of *P. falciparum* with this parasite or with *P. ovale* or *P. malariae* [58]. Monotherapy with artemisinins alone should not be used except for intravenous artesunate therapy in the initial stages of treatment for severe infection.

Chloroquine is still effective for the treatment of non-falciparum malaria and still recommended as first-line therapy in some countries; however, treatment modalities for non-falciparum malaria currently undergo a paradigm change with a widely observed switch to ACT treatment for those, too, given the high efficacy and the favourable parasite and fever clearance time.

P. knowlesi may cause severe cases, with fatality rates as high as 27%, especially in older or female patients. Uncomplicated *P. knowlesi* cases can be treated with ACT, chloroquine, quinine, or atovaquone/proguanil [59]. Mefloquine may not be recommended in light of case reports of treatment failure. There is no clear evidence of latent liver stages in *P. knowlesi,* which have not been described in animal models [60]. A recent study showed that ACT cleared parasites faster than other anti-malarials. In severe *P. knowlesi* cases, the use of IVA was associated with a lower case-fatality rate (17% vs. 31%) and lower median parasite clearance time (2 days vs. 4 days) than IVQ [61].

22.7.2 Primaquine Treatment to Prevent Relapse in *P. Vivax* and *P. Ovale* Infections

P. vivax and *P. ovale* infections, but not *P. malariae* and *P. knowlesi* require treatment with primaquine (PQ) for 14 days to eradicate liver hypnozoites and thus prevent relapses. *P. vivax* strains with reduced susceptibility to primaquine are found in southern regions of Oceania and Southeast Asia. A 7 mg/kg dose was found to have no severe side effects [62]. G6PD testing is required when considering primaquine (soon possibly tafenoquine) for hypnozoite eradication following vivax and ovale malaria therapy [63, 64].

Primaquine is contraindicated in patients with the enzyme glucose-6-phosphate dehydrogenase deficiency [65]. In patients with mild G6PD deficiency, the WHO suggests using an intermittent primaquine regimen of 0.75 mg base/kg once a week for 8 weeks [65].

Conflicts of Interest The authors declare no conflicts of interest.

References

1. Grobusch MP, Kremsner PG. Uncomplicated malaria. Curr Top Microbiol Immunol. 2005;295:83–104.
2. Angelo KM, Libman M, Caumes E, Hamer DH, Kain KC, Leder K, for the GeoSentinel Network, et al. Malaria after international travel: a GeoSentinel analysis, 2003–2016. Malar J. 2017;16(1):293. https://doi.org/10.1186/s12936-017-1936-3.
3. Tatem AJ, Jia P, Ordanovich D, Falkner M, Huang Z, Howes R, Hay SI, et al. The geography of imported malaria to non-endemic countries: a meta-analysis of nationally reported statistics. Lancet Infect Dis. 2017;17(1):98–107. https://doi.org/10.1016/S1473-3099(16)30326-7.
4. Mischlinger J, Rönnberg C, Álvarez-Martínez MJ, Bühler S, Paul M, Schlagenhauf P, et al. Imported malaria in countries where malaria is not endemic: a comparison of semi-immune and non-immune travelers. Clin Microbiol Rev. 2020;33:e00104–19. https://doi.org/10.1128/CMR.00104-19.
5. Grobusch MP, Weld L, Goorhuis A, Hamer DH, Schunk M, Jordan S, et al. Travel-related infections presenting in Europe: a 20-year analysis of EuroTravNet surveillance data. Lancet Reg Health Eur. 2021;1:100001. https://doi.org/10.1016/j.lanepe.2020.100001.

6. World Health Organization. World malaria report 2023. Geneva: WHO; 2023. (http://www. who.int/malaria/world_malaria_report_2023/en/. Accesses 27th December 2022)

7. Nadeem AY, Shehzad A, Islam SU, Al-Suhaimi EA, Lee YS. Mosquirix™ RTS, S/AS01 vaccine development, immunogenicity, and efficacy. Vaccines (Basel). 2022;10:713. https://doi.org/10.3390/vaccines10050713.

8. European Center for Disease Control (ECDC). Malaria. Annual epidemiological report for 2019. https://www.ecdc.europa.eu/sites/default/files/documents/AER-malaria-2019.pdf (Accessed 24 November 2022).

9. Jelinek T, Larsen CS, Siikamäki H, Myrvang B, Chiodini P, Gascon J. European cluster of imported falciparum malaria from Gambia. Euro Surveill 2008;13:pii:19077.

10. Seringe E, Thellier M, Fontanet A, Legros F, Bouchaud O, Ancelle T, Kendjo E, Houze S, Le Bras J, Danis M, Durand R. French National Reference Center for imported malaria study group: severe imported plasmodium falciparum malaria, France, 1996–2003. Emerg Infect Dis. 2011;17:807–13.

11. Askling HH, Nilsson J, Tegnell A, Janzon R, Ekdahl K. Malaria risk in travelers. Emerg Infect Dis. 2005;11:436–41.

12. Leder K, Tong S, Weld L, Kain KC, Wilder-Smith A, von Sonnenburg F, Black J, Brown GV, Torresi J. GeoSentinel surveillance Network: illness in travelers visiting friends and relatives: a review of the GeoSentinel surveillance Network. Clin Infect Dis. 2006;43:1185–93.

13. Stäger K, Legros F, Krause G, Low N, Bradley D, Desai M, et al. Imported malaria in children in industrialized countries, 1992–2002. Emerg Infect Dis. 2009;15:185–91.

14. Schlagenhauf P, Petersen E. Malaria chemoprophylaxis: strategies for risk groups. Clin Microbiol Rev. 2008;21(3):466–72. https://doi.org/10.1128/CMR.00059-07.

15. Dlamini SK. Diagnosis and treatment of imported and odyssean malaria. S Afr Med J. 2014;104:344. https://doi.org/10.7196/samj.8306.

16. Van Bortel W, Van den Poel B, Hermans G, Vanden Driessche M, Molzahn H, Deblauwe I, et al. Two fatal autochthonous cases of airport malaria, Belgium, 2020. Euro Surveill. 2022;27:2100724. https://doi.org/10.2807/1560-7917.ES.2022.27.16.2100724.

17. Chau TT, Mai NT, Phu NH, Luxemburger C, Chuong LV, Loc PP, et al. Malaria in injection drug abusers in Vietnam. Clin Infect Dis. 2002;34:1317–22.

18. Noubouossie D, Tagny CT, Same-Ekobo A, Mbanya D. Asymptomatic carriage of malaria parasites in blood donors in Yaoundé. Transfus Med. 2012;22:63–7.

19. Verona Mesia B, López-Ruiz N, Duran-Pla E. Epidemiological investigation of a case of malaria in a non-endemic area, campo de Gibraltar, Cadiz, Spain, January 2022. Euro Surveill. 2022;27(46):2200786. https://doi.org/10.2807/1560-7917.ES.2022.27.46.2200786.

20. Clemente WT, Pierrotti LC, Abdala E, Morris MI, Azevedo LS, López-Vélez R, et al. Recommendations for management of endemic diseases and travel medicine in solid-organ transplant recipients and donors: Latin America. Transplantation. 2018;102:193–208. https://doi.org/10.1097/TP.0000000000002027.

21. World Health Organization. WHO Guidelines for malaria, 22 November 2022. Geneva: WHO; 2022. https://www.who.int/publications/i/item/guidelines-for-malaria (Accessed 2 December 2022)

22. Kalkman LC, Hänscheid T, Krishna S, Grobusch MP. Fluid therapy for severe malaria. Lancet Infect Dis. 2022;22:e160–70. https://doi.org/10.1016/j.nmni.2022.101035.

23. Santos LC, Abreu CF, Xerinda SM, Tavares M, Lucas R, Sarmento AC. Severe imported malaria in an intensive care unit: a review of 59 cases. Malar J. 2012;11:96.

24. Mascarello M, Allegranzi B, Angheben A, Anselmi M, Concia E, Laganà S, et al. Imported malaria in adults and children: epidemiological and clinical characteristics of 380 consecutive cases observed in Verona, Italy. J Travel Med. 2008;15:229–36.

25. Wertheimer ER, Brundage JF, Fukuda MM. High rates of malaria among US military members born in malaria-endemic countries, 2002–2010. Emerg Infect Dis. 2011;17:1701–3.

26. D'Ortenzio E, Godineau N, Fontanet A, Houze S, Bouchaud O, Matheron S, LeBras J. Prolonged *plasmodium falciparum* infection in immigrants. Paris Emerg Infect Dis. 2008;14:323–6.

27. Bouchaud O, Cot M, Kony S, Durand R, Schiemann R, Ralaimazava P. Do African immigrants living in France have long-term malarial immunity? Am J Trop Med Hyg. 2005;72:21–5.
28. Monge-Maillo B, Jiménez BC, Pérez-Molina JA, Norman F, Navarro M, Pérez-Ayala A, Herrero JM, Zamarrón P, López-Vélez R. Imported infectious diseases in mobile populations. Spain Emerg Infect Dis. 2009;15:1745–52.
29. Ladhani S, Garbash M, Whitty CJ, Chiodini PL, Aibara RJ, Riordan FA, Shingadia D. Prospective, national clinical and epidemiologic study on imported childhood malaria in the United Kingdom and the Republic of Ireland. Pediatr Infect Dis J. 2010;29:434–8.
30. Yeo TW, Lampah DA, Gitawati R, Tjitra E, Kenangalem E, McNeil YR, et al. Recovery of endothelial function in severe falciparum malaria: relationship with improvement in plasma L-arginine and blood lactate concentrations. J Infect Dis. 2008;198:602–8.
31. Reddy EA, Shaw AV, Crump JA. Community-acquired bloodstream infections in Africa: a systematic review and meta-analysis. Lancet Infect Dis. 2010;10:417–32.
32. World Health Organization. Malaria microscopy. Quality assurance manual—version 2.0. Geneva: WHO; 2017. https://www.who.int/teams/global-malaria-programme/casemanagement/diagnosis/microscopy; (Accessed 4 December 2022)
33. Cunningham J, Jones S, Gatton ML, Barnwell JW, Cheng Q, Chiodini PL, et al. A review of the WHO malaria rapid diagnostic test product testing programme (2008–2018): performance, procurement and policy. Malar J. 2019;18:387. https://doi.org/10.1186/s12936-019-3028-z.
34. Petersen E, Marbiah NT, New L, Gottschau A. Comparison of two methods for enumerating malaria parasites in thick blood films. Am J Trop Med Hyg. 1996;55:485–9. https://doi.org/10.4269/ajtmh.1996.55.485.
35. Flegg JA, Guerin PJ, White NJ, Stepniewska K. Standardizing the measurement of parasite clearance in falciparum malaria: the parasite clearance estimator. Malar J. 2011;10:339.
36. Imwong M, Hanchana S, Malleret B, Rénia L, Day NP, Dondorp A, et al. High-throughput ultrasensitive molecular techniques for quantifying low-density malaria parasitemias. J Clin Microbiol. 2014;52:3303–9. https://doi.org/10.1128/JCM.01057-14.
37. Hänscheid T, Grobusch MP. How useful is PCR in the diagnosis of malaria? Trends Parasitol. 2002;18:395–8. https://doi.org/10.1016/s1471-4922(02)02348-6.
38. Koita OA, Doumbo OK, Ouattara A, Tall LK, Konaré A, Diakité M, et al. False-negative rapid diagnostic tests for malaria and deletion of the histidine-rich repeat region of the HRP2 gene. Am J Trop Med Hyg. 2012;86:194–8. https://doi.org/10.4269/ajtmh.2012.10-0665.
39. World Health Organization. WHO external quality assurance scheme for malaria nucleic acid amplification testing. Geneva: Operational Manual WHO; 2017. (Accessed 4 December 2022)
40. Askling HH, Bruneel F, Burchard G, Castelli F, Chiodini PL, Grobusch MP, et al. Management of imported malaria in Europe. Malar J. 2012;11:328. https://doi.org/10.1186/1475-2875-11-328.
41. World Health Organization. Global technical strategy for malaria 2016–2030, 2021 update. 19 July 2021. https://www.who.int/publications/i/item/9789240031357 (Accessed 4 December 2022).
42. Wernsdorfer WH. Coartemether (artemether and lumefantrine): an oral antimalarial drug. Expert Rev Anti-Infect Ther. 2004;2:181–96.
43. Adegnika AA, Breitling LP, Agnandji ST, Chai SK, Schütte D, Oyakhirome S, et al. Effectiveness of quinine monotherapy for the treatment of plasmodium falciparum infection in pregnant women in Lambaréné. Gabon Am J Trop Med Hyg. 2005;73:263–6.
44. Bouchaud O, Mühlberger N, Parola P, Calleri G, Matteelli A, Peyerl-Hoffmann G, et al. Therapy of uncomplicated falciparum malaria in Europe—a prospective observational multicentre study. Malar J. 2012;11:212. https://doi.org/10.1186/1475-2875-11-212.
45. Dondorp A, Nosten F, Stepniewska K, Day N, White N. Artesunate versus quinine for treatment of severe falciparum malaria: a randomised trial. Lancet. 2005;366:717–25.
46. Dondorp AM, Fanello CI, Hendriksen IC, Gomes E, Seni A, Chhaganlal KD, et al. Artesunate versus quinine in the treatment of severe falciparum malaria in African children (AQUAMAT): an open-label, randomised trial. Lancet. 2010;376:1647–57. https://doi.org/10.1016/S0140-6736(10)61924-1.

47. Roussel C, Caumes E, Thellier M, Ndour PA, Buffet PA, Jauréguiberry S. Artesunate to treat severe malaria in travellers: review of efficacy and safety and practical implications. J Travel Med. 2017;24:taw093. https://doi.org/10.1093/jtm/taw093.

48. Foster A. Post-artesunate delayed hemolysis after treatment of malaria with intravenous artesunate: a case study. IDCases. 2022;27:e01418. https://doi.org/10.1016/j.idcr.2022.e01418.

49. Kalkman LC, Hanscheid T, Krishna S, Kremsner PG, Grobusch MP. Anti-malarial treatment in infants. Expert Opin Pharmacother. 2022;23:1711–26. https://doi.org/10.1080/1465656 6.2022.2130687.

50. Ladhani S, Aibara RJ, Riordan FA, Shingadia D. Imported malaria in children: a review of clinical studies. Lancet Infect Dis. 2007;7:349–57.

51. Betuela I, Bassat Q, Kiniboro B, Robinson LJ, Rosanas-Urgell A, Stanisic D, Siba PM, Alonso PL, Mueller I. Tolerability and safety of primaquine in Papua New Guinean children 1 to 10 years of age. Antimicrob Agents Chemother. 2012;56:2146–9.

52. Ramharter M, Grobusch MP, Kiessling G, Adegnika AA, Möller U, et al. Clinical and parasitological characteristics of puerperal malaria. J Infect Dis. 2005;191:1005–9.

53. Hagmann S, Khanna K, Niazi M, Purswani M, Robins EB. Congenital malaria, an important differential diagnosis to consider when evaluating febrile infants of immigrant mothers. Pediatr Emerg Care. 2007;23:326–9.

54. Schlagenhauf P, Blumentals WA, Suter P, Regep L, Vital-Durand G, Schaerer MT, et al. Pregnancy and fetal outcomes after exposure to mefloquine in the pre- and periconception period and during pregnancy. Clin Infect Dis. 2012;54:124–31.

55. Ramharter M, Oyakhirome S, Klein Klouwenberg P, Adégnika AA, Agnandji ST, Missinou MA, et al. Artesunate-clindamycin versus quinine-clindamycin in the treatment of *plasmodium falciparum* malaria: a randomized controlled trial. Clin Infect Dis. 2005;40:1777–84.

56. Siswantoro H, Russell B, Ratcliff A, Prasetyorini B, Chalfein F, Marfurt J, et al. In vivo and in vitro efficacy of chloroquine against *plasmodium malariae* and *P. Ovale* in Papua, Indonesia. Antimicrob Agent Chemother. 2011;55:197–202.

57. Bassat Q. The use of artemether-lumefantrine for the treatment of uncomplicated *plasmodium vivax* malaria. PLoS Negl Trop Dis. 2011;5:e1325.

58. Mombo-Ngoma G, Kleine C, Basra A, Würbel H, Diop DA, Capan M, et al. Prospective evaluation of artemether-lumefantrine for the treatment of non-falciparum and mixed-species malaria in Gabon. Malar J. 2012;11:120.

59. Singh B, Daneshvar C. *Plasmodium knowlesi* malaria in Malaysia. Med J Malaysia. 2010;65:224–30.

60. Anderios F, Noorrain A, Vythilingam I. In vivo study of human plasmodium knowlesi in Macaca fascicularis. Exp Parasitol. 2010;124:181–9.

61. William T, Menon J, Rajaram G, Chan L, Ma G, Donaldsnon S, et al. Severe *Plasmodium knowlesi* malaria in a tertiary care hospital, Sabah, Malaysia. Emerg Infect Dis. 2011;17:1248–55.

62. Chamma-Siqueira NN, Negreiros SC, Ballard SB, Farias S, Silva SP, Chenet SM, et al. Higher-dose Primaquine to prevent relapse of *plasmodium vivax* malaria. N Engl J Med. 2022;386:1244–53. https://doi.org/10.1056/NEJMoa2104226.

63. Grobusch MP, Schlagenhauf P. Primaquine and the power of adherence in radical cure. Lancet Infect Dis. 2022;22:304–5. https://doi.org/10.1016/S1473-3099(21)00389-3.

64. Fernando D, Rodrigo C, Rajapakse S. Primaquine in vivax malaria: an update and review on management issues. Malar J. 2011;10:351.

65. Leslie T, Mayan I, Mohammed N, Erasmus P, Kolaczinski J, Whitty CJ, Rowland M. A randomised trial of an eight-week, once weekly primaquine regimen to prevent relapse of plasmodium vivax in northwest Frontier Province, Pakistan. PLoS One. 2008;3:e2861.